# LASERS IN
# AESTHETIC SURGERY

Springer Science+Business Media, LLC

# LASERS IN
# AESTHETIC SURGERY

Michael I. Kulick, M.D., D.D.S.
Editor

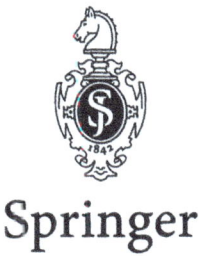

Springer

Michael I. Kulick, M.D., D.D.S.
Faculty
St. Francis Plastic Surgery Program
San Francisco, California 94109
USA

Library of Congress Cataloging-in-Publication Data
Kulick, Michael I.
    Lasers in aesthetic surgery / by Michael I. Kulick.
        p. cm.
    Includes bibliographical references and index.
    ISBN 978-0-387-94891-1    ISBN 978-1-4612-1620-9 (eBook)
    DOI 10.1007/978-1-4612-1620-9
    I. Title.
    [DNLM: 1. Surgery, Plastic—methods.  2. Laser Surgery. WO
600K955L   1997]
    RD119.K84   1997
    617.9'5—dc21                                    96-53897
Printed on acid-free paper.

Production managed by University Graphics and supervised by Lesley Poliner; manufacturing supervised by Rhea Talbert.
Typeset by University Graphics, York, PA.

9 8 7 6 5 4 3 2 1

ISBN 978-0-387-94891-1

# Preface

A compilation of more than 50 years of combined clinical experience with lasers, this book serves as a manual for physicians embarking on the utilization of lasers for aesthetic applications. The contributing authors provide a step-by-step outline of how they treat patients in their practice. The two chapters dealing with the management of cutaneous lesions convey protocol and optimal wavelengths for specific vascular and pigmented conditions. The chapters on skin resurfacing and surgical procedures provide a detailed explanation on the use of two laser systems. Clinical "pearls" with photographic support should help the reader understand educational points and avoid complications. Because of the laser options available to physicians, the chapters are designed to cover similar topics, but from the viewpoint of different experts demonstrating the options available.

One of the criticisms of lasers centers on the inability to have "one" laser perform with great efficacy and safety on all potential clinical applications. However, it is the specific properties of laser energy, the distinct wavelength that attracts one's laser energy to water or to the color of hemoglobin, that allows this surgical tool the advantage over other therapeutic modalities. Thus, the construction that makes lasers unique is what limits universal application. It is hoped that the reader will canvass this book with an open mind and understand that this technology is now emerging into the field of aesthetic surgery.

San Francisco, California                          Michael I. Kulick, M.D., D.D.S.

# Contents

# Contributors

**David B. Apfelberg, M.D.**

A graduate of the plastic surgery training program at the University of Kansas Medical Center, he serves as an assistant clinical professor at Stanford University. A founding member of the American Society for Laser Medicine and Surgery, he served as its president in 1990. He has published over 100 scientific articles and is well known for his research in the clinical application of lasers in medicine.

**Julene E. Cray, R.N., B.S.N.**

Has lectured extensively on the topic of lasers in aesthetic surgery and has focused her recent efforts as a consultant to various laser companies helping them with their educational programs and safety policies.

**Glenn D. Goldstein, M.D.**

A graduate in dermatology from the Kansas University Center he is certified by the American Board of Dermatology and American College of Mohs Micrographic Surgery and Cutaneous Oncology. He is currently the director of the Skin and Mohs Surgery Center at the Baptist Medical Center in Kansas City, Missouri.

**Donald Groot, M.D., F.R.C.P.(C), F.A.C.P.**

Holds fellowships in dermatology in both Canada and the United States. An associate clinical professor at the University of Alberta Department of Medicine, he has published numerous scientific papers and served as the editor-in-chief for the Journal of Contemporary Dermatology. In addition, he is presently the president of the Alberta Society of Dermatologists. He is best known for his expertise in dermatologic and laser surgery.

**Patricia Johnston, B.Sc., M.Cl.Sc., M.B.A.**

Patricia Johnston holds advanced degrees in clinical science and business administration. Over the past fourteen years she has assisted in the development, implementation, and publication of medical research specializing in the field of dermatology and laser surgery. Ms. Johnston is also a regular columnist for a local women's magazine and has co-authored a book entitled *Young as You Look* with Dr. Donald Groot.

As a lecturer, she teaches physicians effective business management strategies, and as a consultant, she assists physicians creating practices that meet the needs of their patients.

**Michael I. Kulick, M.D., D.D.S.**

A graduate from the Stanford University Plastic Surgery Program, he is one of the early pioneers in plastic surgery advocating the efficacy of lasers for aesthetic procedures. He has lectured both nationally and internationally and written articles centered around safety as well as integrating lasers for surgical procedures.

**Wendy Pica-Furey, R.N., M.S.N., M.B.A.**

Ms. Pica-Furey received her masters degree in nursing and master of business administration from the University of San Francisco. Her professional areas of focus include research in the area of ambulatory surgery and patient satisfaction and she is also experienced in regulatory and clinical research in the biotechnology industry.

**Contributors**

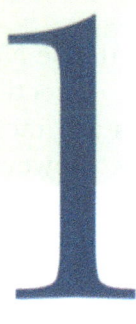

# Laser Safety for Aesthetic Procedures: Surgical and Nonsurgical

Julene E. Cray, *R.N., B.S.N.*

Wendy Pica-Furey, *R.N., M.S.N., M.B.A.*

Michael I. Kulick, *M.D., D.D.S.*

## Lasers for Aesthetic Surgical Procedures: *General Overview*

The most recent breakthrough in cosmetic laser technology has centered on carbon dioxide ($CO_2$) laser delivery methods. Historically, the $CO_2$ laser has been the "workhorse" for laser surgery since the 1960s. The $CO_2$ laser produces invisible light of 10,600 nm and is strongly absorbed by water in tissues [1]. Therefore, the energy penetrates skin very superficially compared to other lasers. This "what you see is what you get" principle has made the $CO_2$ laser a favorite among many physicians for superficial, non-vascular cutaneous lesions.

Advances in $CO_2$ laser technology for surgical procedures such as rhytidectomy, endoscopic forehead, neck lifts, and blepharoplasty have been achieved through high energy and fiber (wave guide) delivery devices. These high output, pulsed $CO_2$ lasers, more commonly referred to by the trade names of Surgipulse (Sharplan Laser, Inc.) and the UltraPulse (Coherent Medical), allow for char-free cutting and excellent coagulation. Combining this new type of technology with a very thin, flexible waveguide (fiber) inserted into the operating channel of the endoscope with the Sharplan system allows the surgeon to deliver accurate laser energy into spaces with a confined surgical field [1]. Previously, the $CO_2$ laser could only be delivered through an articulating arm with larger rigid waveguides, which made it impossible for the cosmetic surgeon to reach target tissues accessed by endoscopic techniques.

The continuous wave Nd:YAG (1,064 nm) and the KTP (potassium titanyl phosphate) (532 nm) lasers are also used for aesthetic surgical procedures. The continuous wave Nd:YAG energy is transmitted through fiberoptic channels to a handpiece fitted with either sharpened quartz fibers or contact sapphire tips. The Nd:YAG wavelength can produce thermal tissue damage up to 6 mm and is an excellent coagulator of blood vessels. This laser, unlike the $CO_2$ laser, readily penetrates through water and is absorbed by hemoglobin and other pigmented tissues. The contact probes, which come in various shapes and sizes, are used to harness this intense Nd:YAG energy primarily in the form of heat to permit tissue dissection. Advantages of the contact Nd:YAG versus the $CO_2$ lasers are tactile feedback, less bleeding, and laser plume during surgery. However, this laser generally causes greater thermal damage to the surrounding tissues. This can be a great disadvantage, especially for the cosmetic surgeon who is working on delicate tissue in the face.

The KTP laser is a doubled frequency YAG laser (1,064 nm/2-532 nm) which is also delivered through a fiberoptic cable and produces a bright green visible light. The properties of the KTP wavelength are similar to argon in that it is strongly absorbed by hemoglobin and melanin and transmitted through clear fluids. The laser energy emitted can penetrate tissue 2 to 3 mm in depth and is capable of vaporizing, cutting, and coagulating simultaneously. The delivery system provides the surgeon with tactile feedback. Thus, it is an excellent tool for aesthetic surgery.

## Lasers for Nonsurgical Aesthetic Procedures: *General Overview*

The most popular technique used by cosmetic surgeons today is $CO_2$ laser skin resurfacing of facial rhytids and superfical pigmented lesions in the perioral, periorbital, and full face areas. Laser resurfacing of the face is also effective for actinic keratosis, precancerous conditions, and other superficial dermatological imperfections.

A wide variety of other lasers are used for nonsurgical and noninvasive procedures and include the continuous wave Nd:YAG Q-switched Nd:YAG, KTP, argon, flash lamp pulsed dye (FLPD), alexandrite, and ruby lasers. These lasers are used for the treatment of dermatologic conditions such as vascular and pigmented lesions, tattoos, acne scarring, immature traumatic scars, keloids, and verruca. The laser of choice is dependent on the patient's specific condition and the surgeon's skill, and is frequently the only instrument needed for the procedure. However, to obtain an optimal result, multiple laser treatments may be necessary at various intervals for certain cutaneous conditions, e.g., port wine stain. Many of these laser treatments can be performed in the physician's office. A topical anesthetic agent (EMLA) or injected local anesthesia (nerve block) may be used to alleviate discomfort. General anesthesia is rarely necessary and is usually reserved for children requiring treatment or when large surface areas are involved.

When selecting a laser, vascular lesions such as telangectasias, port wine stains, and capillary hemangiomas may be treated using the KTP, argon, copper vapor, and FLPD lasers. Each wavelength and delivery system has its own purported advantages and, for the most part, furnishes good results when treating lesions above the heart. Deep cavernous hemangiomas have been successfully treated with the Nd:YAG laser due to the deeper penetration of the 1064 nm wavelength.

Pigmented lesions of the skin due to sun or aging ("liver" or age spots, solar lentigos, café au lait lesions) can be treated with the Q-switched Nd:YAG, ruby, or KTP lasers. Wavelengths selected for treatment depend on morphology, the surgeon's experience, and available equipment.

Tattoos can be removed with the Q-switched Nd:YAG, Q-switched ruby, and/or alexandrite lasers depending on the color of the dye in the tattoo. The Nd:YAG is best used for black, red, brown, and orange dyes, the ruby is most effective for violet and purple dyes, and the alexandrite laser has been more successful in treating green and blue dyes [2].

## Standards and Guidelines for Laser Safety

Currently, many aesthetic surgeons utilize one or more lasers in their practice for both surgical and nonsurgical procedures. Although each laser system is unique with regard to wavelength, set-up, operation, instrumentation, and accessories, the general principles of safety apply: the need for eye safety, evacuation of plume, and special filtration. Due to the rapid advancement of laser technology, the surgeon and personnel must be acutely aware of the specific safety aspects associated with each laser system. Strict adherence to laser safety is vital to the success of the physician's practice, from both a medical/legal standpoint as well as providing comfort and confidence for patients questioning the risks and hazards of laser treatment.

The United States, Australia, Great Britain, Canada, and Japan have adopted standards for laser safety. In the United States, the American National Standard for the Safe Use of Lasers in Health Care Facilities, also known as ANSI Z-136.3, is the only nationally accepted, nonregulatory guideline for laser safety [3].

Currently, there are no national certification or licensing agencies for laser surgeons, nurses, or technicians. Each institution must establish its own criteria. However, the Occupational Safety and Health Administration (OSHA) follows ANSI Z-136.3, which is the industry standard when evaluating laser safety programs in the workplace [4]. It is imperative that facilities using lasers have a copy of ANSI guidelines. Refer to Table 1-1 for an address for obtaining a copy.

Eleven of the fifty states follow statewide regulations, which in some respects are more stringent than those outlined by ANSI. Physicians practicing in Alaska, Arizona, Arkansas, Florida, Georgia, Illinois, Massachusetts, Montana, New York, Texas, or Washington must refer to their state's radiation department for the appropriate guidelines. For additional information about the overall safe use of medical lasers, refer to the available source list in Table 1-1.

## Overall Safety Precautions for Laser Use

### Posted Warning Signs

Warning signs that are clearly marked with the danger of laser radiation, including the international symbol for laser radiation, should be placed on the outside of each door leading into the area where the laser will be used. The wavelength to be used, the maximum

**Table 1-1.**
Laser Safety References

| |
|---|
| American National Standards Institute (ANSI) <br> 11 West 42nd Street <br> New York, NY 10036 <br> 212-642-4900 |
| American Society for Laser Medicine and Surgery, Inc. (ASLMS) <br> 2404 Stewart Square <br> Wausau, WI 54401 <br> 715-845-9283 |
| Association of Operating Room Nurses (AORN) <br> 2170 South Parker Road, #300 <br> Denver, CO 80231 <br> 800-755-2676 |
| Conference of Radiation Control Program Directors (CRCPD) <br> (provides information regarding individual state requirements) <br> 205 Capitol Avenue <br> Frankfort, KY 40601 <br> 502-227-4543 |
| Laser Institute of America <br> (Secretariat for the ANSI Z136.3 Standards) <br> 12424 Research Parkway <br> Orlando, FL 32826 <br> 800-345-2737 <br> 407-380-1553 |
| Occupational Safety and Health Administration (OSHA) <br> Bureau of National Affairs <br> 1231 25th Street, NW <br> Washington, DC 20037 <br> 202-452-4200 |

wattage, and the appropriate eye wear required should be indicated on the sign. In addition, protective goggles for the corresponding wavelength that will be in use should be placed next to the sign for those entering the room.

### Eye Protection: $CO_2$, Nd:YAG, and KTP Lasers

The eye is very sensitive to laser radiation. It is recommended that protective goggles, glasses, and lens covers have the appropriate filtering capabilities and optical density written on the eye wear. Whether using goggles or glasses, side guards are recommended. The patient's eyes can be covered with saline-soaked gauze secured by tape for protection when treating lesions not in close proximity to the eyelids. However, whenever laser energy is used near the eye, such as in the case of blepharoplasty or resurfacing the eyelids, metal eye shields covering the cornea and sclera are recommended. Before placement of the shields, ophthalmic tetracaine is instilled in each eye, followed by a non–water-soluble ocular lubricant.

The $CO_2$ laser can cause a corneal burn if the eyes are not protected. If the operating suite has glass windows, they do not need to be covered when the $CO_2$ laser is in use. The clear glass will protect the eyes of those looking into the room. For those in the room, however, contact lenses or prescription glasses (unless they have side shields) are not adequate protection from a stray beam. Safety glasses are clear and lightweight. Protective eye wear for those in the treatment room should be checked for scratches or other defects. A scratched surface can transmit a laser beam that could damage the wearer's eyes.

When using the Nd:YAG or KTP lasers, glasses are tinted for protective filtering of the specific wavelength used. The optical density is printed on the side of the goggles or glasses. An optical density of 4.5 is frequently used for lasers with these wavelengths in a clinical facility. Unlike the $CO_2$ laser, when using these wavelengths, all glass windows must be covered to prevent people from looking into the operating room while the laser is in use. When using an endoscope, an appropriate protective lens filter can be placed between the scope and camera. To protect the opposite eye, the surgeon may wear a specific, one-lens-only pair of glasses or close the eye during laser operation. It should be noted that ocular damage is preventable 100% of the time by wearing the appropriate protective eye wear.

## Standby Mode

It is imperative that the laser be put in the standby mode whenever there is an extended pause in usage or when the laser is not attended. Most of the accidents occurring with lasers are from misdirected laser beams [5].

Ms. Cray was teaching the staff of an operating room on laser safety as the facility had just purchased their first $CO_2$ laser The instructor repeatedly emphasized the importance of standby control. However, one week later, an accident occurred. The nurse had left the operating room, "circulating." The surgeon put the laser handpiece in the plastic electrocautery pouch to hold it on the sterile field. He then proceeded to pick up the electrosurgical handpiece and instead of stepping on the cautery foot pedal, he inadvertently stepped on the laser foot pedal. Since the laser was not in standby, the laser beam was activated, igniting the plastic pouch which ignited the paper drapes on the patient within seconds. Unfortunately, the patient received second-degree burns. When it comes to laser safety, we as health care personnel can never be too careful [6].

## Smoke Evacuation: $CO_2$, Nd:YAG, and KTP Lasers

During a $CO_2$ laser procedure on the skin surface, the smoke evacuator should be positioned so that the assistant can hold the suction-wand or tubing within 1 cm of the laser energy contact with skin. Some handpieces have integral suction parts attached to them obviating the need of the assistant to hold the suction tube. When using an endoscope, the proper $\frac{3}{16}$-inch suction tubing must be connected to the smoke evacuator's larger tubing to ensure adequate plume evacuation.

The filters in the smoke evacuator need to be changed according to the manufacturer's instructions. It should be noted that the laser plume is a potentially harmful substance capable of transferring live viral particles [7]. Wall suction is not sufficient to evacuate this smoke unless properly adapted and if used, the carbon particles within the plume may clog the entire wall evacuation system. When using lasers for treatment of vascular and pigmented lesions and tattoo removal, tissue is not vaporized. Thus, no plume is created, eliminating the need for smoke evacuation.

Two suction systems should be used when performing incisional procedures with the $CO_2$, Nd:YAG, and KTP lasers. The standard wall suction is used to evacuate blood and irrigation fluids. The high evacuation system eliminates the laser plume. The specific contents of the laser plume depend on the wavelength of the laser used. Laser generated airborne contaminants continue to be the subject of various research studies and a topic of debate. Current studies have revealed harmful effects associated with laser plume [8]. Therefore, we must acknowledge the potential danger of laser plume and take the necessary precautions with regard to high flow smoke evacuation, special masks, filters, tubing, and biohazard waste.

### Fire Hazard

To minimize the possibility of a fire hazard propagating, a basin of water should be placed on the back table readily available for emergency use. The location of the nearest industry standard fire extinguisher should be noted. A halon fire extinguisher is recommended because it does not produce residue and has low toxicity. Flammable solutions, such as alcohol or Hibiclens, should not be used on or around the laser or to clean the patient's skin. Prior to lasing along the hairline, all hair spray or hair gels, which may contain alcohol, should be removed and hairline should be thoroughly moistened.

### Endoscopic Considerations

Specific precautions must be adhered to when using the endoscope with any laser. Eye safety precautions are particularly important when using the fiberoptic Nd:YAG and KTP lasers because of their affinity for hemoglobin. The endoscope should never be placed on the dry drapes with the xenon light source activated as this can cause a fire unrelated to the laser. The endoscope may become damaged if the laser fiber is not positioned at least 1 cm past the distal end of the scope. The surgeon should be able to visualize the fiber tip before activating the laser. When inserting a sharpened fiber into the handpiece, extreme care must be taken so that the end of the fiber is not broken or the protective coating on the fiber is not fractured. Disruption of this protective coating surrounding the fiber during insertion could cause damage to the lumen of the scope if the laser is activated and energy "leaks" out during laser activation due to a discontinuity of this protective coating.

## Oxygen Considerations

External oxygen administration should be limited to minimize the chance of a fire hazard. In cases of short duration, and when sedation does not impair full patient cooperation, it is safe to insert nasal prongs into a patient's mouth and ask the patient to seal their lips to increase delivery of oxygen and prevent oxygen "leak." Alternatively, a small pediatric feeding tube can be inserted through the nose into the posterior nasopharynx to increase oxygen delivery. It should be secured well so that it does not slip out. When using supplemental oxygen, caution must be exercised to prevent laser energy from striking and penetrating the delivery tubing. This can be facilitated by covering the tubing with foil or using specially designed tubing.

## Maintenance

The laser equipment and accessories should be properly cleaned, sterilized, and stored according to the manufacturer's instructions for future use. Laser lens and safety glasses/goggles should be inspected and cleansed before each case. Disposable laser fibers should be considered "sharps" when disposed. The smoke evacuator tubing and filters should be discarded into a biohazard bag. The deployment and storage of the articulated arm of the $CO_2$ lasers should be performed carefully to avoid malalignment of the delicate mirrors within the arm that provide for accurate beam transmission. A comprehensive preventive maintenance program and documentation log book is extremely important to the success of ongoing laser usage. Laser maintenance can be provided by the specific laser manufacturer or third-party service companies. However, if a third party is used for maintenance and repairs, the manufacturer's warranty may become invalid. Safety inspections should be conducted on a regular basis, preferably quarterly if the laser is being used frequently [9].

When using a fiber, it should be checked regularly during the procedure for char build-up at the tip, which should be removed. The fiber tip should also be inspected for evidence of degradation. If present, the tip/handpiece should be replaced. The integrity of the protective coating covering the entire length of the fiber should periodically be inspected by the nurse. Repeated fiber bending may cause a fracture in the protective "cladding" or coating which keeps the laser energy contained within the fiber.

If a flash lamp pulsed dye laser is used, dye changes may be required on a regular basis which pose a potential danger. Therefore, dye kits should be handled and disposed of according to the manufacturer's instructions. Gloves, masks, and protective glasses should be worn when changing the dye kits.

## Pre-procedure Consultation and Teaching

One or more consultations may be required to educate the patient about the planned procedure, and photographs are invaluable to enhance the patient's understanding. Informed consent and post-procedure instructions are signed, acknowledging receipt and understanding of what is to transpire. It is often helpful for the office nurse to reinforce the details of the planned procedure in addition to the time the patient spends with the physician. This would include the importance of pre- and postoperative skin treatments. Often, the nurse coordinates the patient's skin care with an esthetician. During the preoperative counseling the nurse should discuss the safety aspects of the procedure and explain the eye protection protocol to allay patient fears. It is also helpful to explain the "Danger" sign which can be seen by the non-sedated patient when entering the operating room suite.

## Phases of the Laser Procedure and the Nurse's Role in Safety

The laser safety checklist is an excellent guide for the preparation of all laser procedures [Table 1-2]. It is essential to set up all equipment in a manner that is conducive to facilitate the ease and safety of the operation. The nurse gathers the necessary supplies and equipment for the procedure, including disposable goods (gauze, cotton tip applicators, local anesthetic, gloves, sterile saline, post-treatment dressing or ointments, etc.), sterile fibers, protective eye wear, and the correct laser and handpieces specific to each case. The key to the laser must be retrieved from its appropriate secure location. The laser and associated equipment should be turned on and tested before the patient is premedicated. In the case of the $CO_2$ laser, the beam is evaluated for alignment and function (tested on a wet tongue blade).

When using the $CO_2$ laser, the articulating arm should be positioned over the dominant shoulder of the surgeon for ease of maneuverability. This also prevents the arm from crossing over the sterile field and making it awkward for the surgical technician to retract and assist. The articulating arm of the laser can be covered with a sterile drape for incisional procedures. For the YAG and KTP lasers, the fibers come in prepackaged sterile containers.

The patient is moved into the procedure room and placed in a supine position. Normal saline can be used to remove EMLA cream if administered topically prior to the cutaneous procedure. For inci-

**Table 1-2.**
Laser Safety Checklist Sample

| | | |
|---|---|---|
| Laser sign on all doors | yes | no |
| All windows covered if necessary | yes | no |
| Appropriate safety glasses/protective eye cover | | |
|    patient | yes | no |
|    staff | yes | no |
| Flammable substances | | |
|    near patient | yes | no |
|    used as prep solution | yes | no |
| Electrical precautions noted | yes | no |
| Fire precautions | | |
|    water in room | yes | no |
|    fire extinguisher location known | yes | no |
| High suction smoke evacuation available | yes | no |
| Laser consent signed | yes | no |

Patient name _____ Date _____

Type of laser (wavelength & model) _____

Laser equipment setup performed by _____

Procedure performed by _____

Laser setting(s):      Anatomic site      Settings

                 _____     _____

                 _____     _____

                 _____     _____

                 _____     _____

Laser Safety Checklist performed by _____

sional procedures, skin cleansing should be performed with a solution void of alcohol content.

The circulating nurse, in addition to his or her other responsibilities, assumes the role of the laser safety advocate. Once the procedure begins, the laser operation is the nurse's number one responsibility, in addition to patient monitoring during conscious (intravenous) sedation cases. Laser operation responsibilities include confirmation that the laser checklist is complete and that the laser is in the appropriate position and its foot pedal is in front of the surgeon and isolated from all of the other foot pedals. The date, laser system used, type of treatment (skin resurfacing, vascular ablation, etc.), and area to be treated are documented on the laser treatment record in addition to a completed laser safety checklist. The nurse must be attentive to the surgeon's laser setting preferences. The laser settings used, i.e., wattage, energy (joules/cm), pulse width, and mode of delivery where applicable, are documented. This is important for legal purposes as well as serving as a guide for future treatments and assessing clinical response.

Following the operative procedure, the laser equipment is cleaned, sterilized where appropriate, and stored in a secure location. Disposable fibers are discarded as "sharps" in biohazard containers. All laser signs, glasses, and accessories are kept with the corresponding laser. Laser safety and performance documentation is completed and placed in the patient's chart. The key to the laser is kept in a secured location.

## Post-procedure Care and Discharge Teaching

Once the procedure is completed, the eye protection is removed from the patient. If scleral shields have been used, an eye wash solution is administered to help remove the ocular lubricant. Following a $CO_2$ laser skin resurfacing, a thin layer of ointment or an occlusive dressing may be applied depending on the surgeon's preference. After the treatment of localized vascular and pigmented lesions, a topical ointment is often applied with or without the prescription of systemic antibiotics depending on the extent of the lesion treated. Treated tattoos are often covered with an ointment and sterile nonadhesive dressing (Telfa) which can be changed daily.

Topical application of a cool ice pack for the first twelve hours after treatment and mild analgesics such as nonsteriodal anti-inflammatory agents or acetaminophen are usually all that is needed for the discomfort following the laser treatment of vascular and pigmented lesions. Slight localized edema is expected and superficial crusting is common. A shower can be taken the next day, however, patients are instructed not to scrub or abrade the treatment site with a towel or washcloth. Make-up can usually be applied after any superficial crusting falls off, usually four to seven days post treatment. Patients are also instructed to refrain from any activity that may traumatize the treated area for one to two weeks. Most importantly, the patient must avoid unprotected exposure to sunlight for one to four months, depending on the procedure. Treatment of vascular lesions requires approximately four weeks of sun protection, while skin resurfacing requires three to six months of cover. In addition to sunscreens, large wrap-around sunglasses and broad-brimmed hats are helpful. Patients may be more compliant if they understand that failure to wear protective sunscreen will cause sun damage that can result in new pigmented and/or vascular lesions. It is helpful to call the patient on the night of the procedure and for the next few days to reassure and monitor the patient for any adverse effects.

The surgeon and his or her staff have an enormous responsibility with regard to the safe use of each laser system used in practice today. Education, teamwork, and communication are vital to the success of a laser program. As technology provides advances in laser systems for the office setting and outpatient arenas, we as health care providers will continue to be challenged with regard to keeping laser safety a priority.

## Medical Device Reporting

Physicians, nurses, and other health care personnel may be unaware that it is now mandatory that they report device-related adverse events to the manufacturer and to the Food and Drug Administration (FDA) [Table 1-3]. Since 1984, manufacturers have been required to report product problems to the FDA. However, reporting by user facilities was voluntary until recently due to the Safe Medical Devices Act of 1990 [10]. Underreporting on the part of health care professionals has occurred not only due to lack of awareness, but because of the time and paperwork involved, concerns about confidentiality, and legal issues. Due to the advent of mandatory reporting, medical device reports have more than tripled. The FDA received 95,437 reports of device failures in 1992 compared to 29,935 for the previous year [11].

## Who Should Report

The FDA published a tentative final rule on November 26, 1991 which added provisions for the regulation of medical devices with regard to the reporting of incidences by user facilities and distributors. The Safe Medical Devices Act (SMDA) was signed into law November 28, 1990 and amended on June 16, 1992. As a result of this ruling, user facilities and distributors, including importers, are required to submit reports of death, serious illnesses, or injuries related to medical devices to the FDA and to the manufacturer [10, 12, 13]. User facilities are defined as hospitals, ambulatory surgery centers, nursing homes, and outpatient treatment centers, that are not physicians' offices [14].

## What Constitutes a Medical Device Report

Manufactures, importers, distributors, and user facilities are required to report a device-related adverse event to the FDA when they become aware of information that "reasonably suggests" that a marketed device: (1) may have caused or contributed to death or serious injury, or (2) has malfunctioned and if the malfunction were to recur, it would likely cause or contribute to a death or serious injury [10]. (see Table 1-3) A serious illness or injury is considered one that is (1) life threatening, (2) results in permanent impairment of body function or permanent impairment to body structure, (3) necessitates medical or surgical intervention by a health care professional to preclude permanent impairment of body function or permanent damage to body structure [10]. These reports must include incidences of malfunction and user error. Under [21 CFR 803.24(d) (1)] of the *Federal Register*, a medical device report is required if the device was used "beyond its labeled useful life" or "the event is due to user error" [12].

Device-related reports should include information concerning events that are (1) serious and unlabeled and (2) serious and labeled that require medical or surgical intervention or occur with more frequency or severity than labeled [12]. An event is labeled when it is

**Table 1-3.**

MEDWatch 3500 A: Mandatory Reporting Form for the Reporting of Device-related Events Involving Death, Serious Injury, or Malfunction.

# MEDWATCH
### THE FDA MEDICAL PRODUCTS REPORTING PROGRAM

For use by user-facilities, distributors and manufacturers for **MANDATORY** reporting

Page ____ of ____

| Mfr report # |
| UF/Dist report # |
| FDA Use Only |

## A. Patient information

1. Patient identifier | 2. Age at time of event:

   or _____

   Date of birth:

   *In confidence*

3. Sex
   ☐ female
   ☐ male

4. Weight
   _____ lbs
   or
   _____ kgs

## B. Adverse event or product problem

1. ☐ Adverse event   and/or   ☐ Product problem (e.g., defects/malfunctions)

2. Outcomes attributed to adverse event (check all that apply)
   ☐ death _____ (mo/day/yr)
   ☐ life-threatening
   ☐ hospitalization – initial or prolonged
   ☐ disability
   ☐ congenital anomaly
   ☐ required intervention to prevent permanent impairment/damage
   ☐ other: _____

3. Date of event (mo/day/yr)

4. Date of this report (mo/day/yr)

5. Describe event or problem

6. Relevant tests/laboratory data, including dates

7. Other relevant history, including preexisting medical conditions (e.g., allergies, race, pregnancy, smoking and alcohol use, hepatic/renal dysfunction, etc.)

## C. Suspect medication(s)

1. Name (give labeled strength & mfr/labeler, if known)
   #1
   #2

2. Dose, frequency & route used
   #1
   #2

3. Therapy dates (if unknown, give duration) from/to (or best estimate)
   #1
   #2

4. Diagnosis for use (indication)
   #1
   #2

5. Event abated after use stopped or dose reduced
   #1 ☐ yes ☐ no ☐ doesn't apply
   #2 ☐ yes ☐ no ☐ doesn't apply

6. Lot # (if known)
   #1
   #2

7. Exp. date (if known)
   #1
   #2

8. Event reappeared after reintroduction
   #1 ☐ yes ☐ no ☐ doesn't apply
   #2 ☐ yes ☐ no ☐ doesn't apply

9. NDC # – for product problems only (if known)
   __ – __

10. Concomitant medical products and therapy dates (exclude treatment of event)

## D. Suspect medical device

1. Brand name

2. Type of device

3. Manufacturer name & address

4. Operator of device
   ☐ health professional
   ☐ lay user/patient
   ☐ other: _____

6.
   model # _____
   catalog # _____
   serial # _____
   lot # _____
   other # _____

5. Expiration date (mo/day/yr)

7. If implanted, give date (mo/day/yr)

8. If explanted, give date (mo/day/yr)

9. Device available for evaluation? (Do not send to FDA)
   ☐ yes   ☐ no   ☐ returned to manufacturer on _____ (mo/day/yr)

10. Concomitant medical products and therapy dates (exclude treatment of event)

## E. Initial reporter

1. Name, address & phone #

2. Health professional?
   ☐ yes ☐ no

3. Occupation

4. Initial reporter also sent report to FDA
   ☐ yes ☐ no ☐ unk

FDA

FDA Form 3500A (6/93)

Submission of a report does not constitute an admission that medical personnel, user facility, distributor, manufacturer or product caused or contributed to the event.

# Medication and Device Experience Report
(continued)

Refer to guidelines for specific instructions

Submission of a report does not constitute an admission that medical personnel, user facility, distributor, manufacturer or product caused or contributed to the event.

Page ____ of ____

U.S. DEPARTMENT OF HEALTH AND HUMAN SERVICES
Public Health Service • Food and Drug Administration

FDA Use Only

## F. For use by user facility/distributor–devices only

**1. Check one**
☐ user facility  ☐ distributor

**2. UF/Dist report number**

**3. User facility or distributor name/address**

**4. Contact person**

**5. Phone Number**

**6. Date user facility or distributor became aware of event** (mo/day/yr)

**7. Type of report**
☐ initial
☐ follow-up # ____

**8. Date of this report** (mo/day/yr)

**9. Approximate age of device**

**10. Event problem codes** (refer to coding manual)
patient code  ☐☐☐ – ☐☐☐ – ☐☐☐
device code  ☐☐☐ – ☐☐☐ – ☐☐☐

**11. Report sent to FDA?**
☐ yes ____ (mo/day/yr)
☐ no

**12. Location where event occurred**
☐ hospital      ☐ outpatient diagnostic facility
☐ home          ☐ ambulatory surgical facility
☐ nursing home
☐ outpatient treatment facility
☐ other: ____
specify

**13. Report sent to manufacturer?**
☐ yes ____ (mo/day/yr)
☐ no

**14. Manufacturer name/address**

## G. All manufacturers

**1. Contact office – name/address (& mfring site for devices)**

**2. Phone number**

**3. Report source** (check all that apply)
☐ foreign
☐ study
☐ literature
☐ consumer
☐ health professional
☐ user facility
☐ company representative
☐ distributor
☐ other: ____

**4. Date received by manufacturer** (mo/day/yr)

**5.**
(A)NDA # ____
IND # ____
PLA # ____
pre-1938  ☐ yes
OTC product  ☐ yes

**6. If IND, protocol #**

**7. Type of report** (check all that apply)
☐ 5-day     ☐ 15-day
☐ 10-day    ☐ periodic
☐ initial   ☐ follow-up # ____

**8. Adverse event term(s)**

**9. Mfr. report number**

## H. Device manufacturers only

**1. Type of reportable event**
☐ death
☐ serious injury
☐ malfunction (see guidelines)
☐ other: ____

**2. If follow-up, what type?**
☐ correction
☐ additional information
☐ response to FDA request
☐ device evaluation

**3. Device evaluated by mfr?**
☐ not returned to mfr.
☐ yes  ☐ evaluation summary attached
☐ no (attach page to explain why not) or provide code: ____

**4. Device manufacture date** (mo/yr)

**5. Labeled for single use?**
☐ yes  ☐ no

**6. Evaluation codes** (refer to coding manual)
method  ☐☐☐ – ☐☐☐ – ☐☐☐ – ☐☐☐
results  ☐☐☐ – ☐☐☐ – ☐☐☐ – ☐☐☐
conclusions  ☐☐☐ – ☐☐☐ – ☐☐☐ – ☐☐☐

**7. If remedial action initiated, check type**
☐ recall       ☐ notification
☐ repair       ☐ inspection
☐ replace      ☐ patient monitoring
☐ relabeling   ☐ modification/adjustment
☐ other: ____

**8. Usage of device**
☐ initial use of device
☐ reuse
☐ unknown

**9. If action reported to FDA under 21 USC 360i(f), list correction/removal reporting number:**

**10.** ☐ Additional manufacturer narrative  and/or  **11.** ☐ Corrected data

The public reporting burden for this collection of information has been estimated to average one-hour per response, including the time for reviewing instructions, searching existing data sources, gathering and maintaining the data needed, and completing and reviewing the collection of information. Send your comments regarding this burden estimate or any other aspect of this collection of information, including suggestions for reducing this burden to:

Reports Clearance Officer, PHS
Hubert H. Humphrey Building, Room 721-B
200 Independence Avenue, S.W.
Washington, DC 20201
ATTN: PRA

and to:
Office of Management and Budget
Paperwork Reduction Project (0910-0291)
Washington, DC 20503

Please do NOT return this form to either of these addresses

FDA Form 3500A - back

identified in nature, severity, and frequency in the current manufacturer's device manuals or brochures [12].

### User Facility Reporting Guidelines

Medical device reports must be submitted by user facilities no later than ten working days after the initial receipt of information that suggests that there is a reasonable probability that the device caused or contributed to death, serious illness, or injury [10, 12 ,13]. The SMDA requires that user facilities report device-related deaths directly to the FDA and to the manufacturer. However, reports of serious illness or injury may be reported only to the manufacturer. If the manufacturer is not known, then reports must be sent to the FDA. User facilities should attempt to identify the manufacturer whose device is involved in a reportable event [12, 13].

User facilities are also required to submit semi-annual summaries of all reports submitted to the FDA and to the manufacturer [12, 13]. Semi-annual summaries must include information concerning the identification of the device, user facility, manufacturer, and a brief description of the event. User facilities are required to maintain a file for each event that may be device-related and must retain these records for two years [14].

### Reporting by Phone, Fax, or Computer Modem

One may also report medical device-related events by calling 1-800-FDA-1088 or 301-427-7500 [13, 14]. The FDA is capable of answering multiple calls and encourages that reports be made between 8:00 and 4:30 p.m. EST. Calls received before 8:00 a.m. and after 4:30 p.m. Monday through Friday and on the weekends and holidays will be answered by a telephone recording machine. The recorder will prompt the caller for his or her name, the name of the firm or facility, telephone number, and type of event such as death, serious illness, injury, or malfunction [12].

For approval of computer-generated facsimiles, contact MED-Watch: The FDA Medical Products Reporting Program, Food and Drug Administration, 5600 Fishers Lane, Rockville, MD 20857 [15]. The fax number is 1-800-FDA-0178. One may also report by computer modem by calling 1-800-FDA-7737 [16].

### Recommendations for User Facilities

A centralized hospital reporting system that collects internal reports and transmits them to the outside should also be developed for appropriate data collection, device tracking, and trend analysis. In addition, a system for retrieving device-related information, including labels and packaging, is necessary to identify the product problem associated with the device and determine if labeling was deficient [17].

It is further advised that a procedure and policy for preserving a medical device and impounding equipment, supplies, and accessories be formulated. However, legal advice with regard to the development of these policies is warranted [17]. Following a device-related incident, the issue of whether the device belongs to the hospital or to the manufacturer may arise. Devices involved in a reportable event should never be relinquished to the manufacturer without legal consultation. Most manufacturers cooperate with hospitals in the investigation of device-related events. However, there have been some cases in which destruction and loss of evidence which would have benefited the hospital has occurred [17]. When a device-related incident occurs, the user facility may begin its own investigation. However, while this investigation is being conducted, the facility must make sure that any device-related incidences be reported within the appropriate time frame. The submission of device-related reports should not be detained because the facility is conducting an investigation.

### References

1. Keller G, Cray J. Laser-assisted surgery of the aging face. *Facial Plast Surg Clin North Am* 1995;3:319–341.

2. Zelickson B, Mehregan D, Zarrin A, et al. Clinical, histological and ultrastructural evaluation of tattoos treated with three laser systems. *Lasers Surg Med* 1994;15:364–372.

3. Smalley PJ. Laser technology: A nursing perspective. *Derm Nursing* 1991;3:241–245.

4. Anonymous. Simple measures can ensure compliance . . . surprise OSHA inspections are rare, but be prepared. *Clin Laser Monthly* 1994;12:128–130.

5. Anonymous. Laser use and safety. *Health Devices* 1992;21:306–310.

6. Ball K. *Lasers—The Perioperative Challenge, 1st edition.* St. Louis. CV Mosby Company, 1990.

7. Garden JM, Bakus AD. Health safety issues of laser generated plume. Presented at American Society for Laser Medicine and Surgery 13th annual meeting, New Orleans, LA. April 18–20, 1993.

8. Baggish M. Laser plume danger? Questions remain, caution advised. *Clin Laser Monthly* 1988; 111–112.

9. Lanzafame R. Laser safety programs in general surgery. *J Laser Applications* 1994;6:111–114.

10. *Federal Register*, Wednesday September 1, 1993 Part V. Department of Health and Human Services, Food and Drug Administration (21 CFR Parts 804 and 807) Medical Devices; Medical Device Distributor Reporting; Final Rules.

11. Gardner E. Device failure reports triple modern healthcare 1993;23:57.

12. U.S. Department of Health and Human Services, Public Health and Service, Food and Drug Administration, Center for Devices and Radiologic Health, Rockville, Maryland 20857. *Medical Device Reporting Questions and Answers* 1998;1–44.

13. U.S. Department of Health and Human Services, Food and Drug Administration, Center for Devices and Radiologic Health Service/Food and Drug Administration Center for Devices and Radiologic Health. *The Safe Medical Devices Act of 1990 and the Medical Device Amendments of 1992*;1–14.

14. *Federal Register*, Tuesday November 26, 1991 Part VI. Department of Health and Human Services, Food and Drug Administration (21 CFR Parts 803 and 807) Medical Devices; Medical Device User Facility, Distributor, and Manufacturer Reporting, Certification, and Registration; Proposed Rule.

15. Merriman J. New federal program encourages health professionals to report drug, device problems. *AORN* 1993;58:594–597.

16. *Medical Device Reporting Participant's Guide.* September 27, 1994. Food and Drug Administration and the Food and Drug Law Institute. Video Teleconference. Part I MedWatch.

17. Kock A, Solomon R. The Safe Medical Devices Act: What nurses know about user reporting, implant tracking. *AORN* 1993;55:537, 540–548.

# Laser Treatment of Cutaneous Vascular Lesions

Glenn D. Goldstein, *M.D.*

Currently, there is no one laser that can treat all cutaneous lesions with excellent results. One must have a clear understanding of the laser to skin tissue interaction before treating a patient to minimize any undesirable outcomes. The morphology, configuration, and distribution of a lesion will vary from patient to patient depending on the energy transferred to the skin. The color and thickness of the lesion as well as a patient's skin type must also be considered in the overall treatment procedure. Lasers used for the treatment of vascular lesions include the argon, flash lamp pulsed dye, copper vapor, KTP (potassium titanyl phosphate)/532 (double frequency Q-switched yttrium-aluminum garnet), and krypton lasers. The laser surgeon's understanding of a particular laser and wavelength, its availability, and the type of vascular lesion will ultimately determine the preferred treatment.

Selective photothermolysis is the targeting of specific chromophores within the skin to absorb laser light selectively within the thermal relaxation time. Thermal relaxation time is the duration required for the heat generated by the absorbed light energy within the chromophores to decrease to 50% of its initial value immediately after exposure to the laser energy [1]. The selectivity for a specific chromophore will allow the majority of the laser energy absorbed by the target structure to be retained and reduce nonspecific thermal damage to surrounding tissue.

## Telangiectasia

Telangiectasias are the most common vascular lesions seen in a dermatology/plastic surgery practice. These lesions can be isolated or diffuse but most frequently are located on the face and neck. They can be simple, arborized, spider, or papular [2]. Spider angiomas are the most difficult to treat and are especially common on the nose and malar areas. More than one treatment may be required to eradicate these lesions.

Diagnosis is easily established by blanching the vessels with gentle pressure and noting refill on release. When the distribution is central facial, it is frequently secondary to acne rosacea. Prior to treating the telangiectasias in acne rosacea it is necessary that the patient's flare-ups are under control. This is best accomplished with oral antibiotics and topical metronidizole cream which will reduce the flushing and inflammation which might result in additional telangiectasias. Patients must be educated to avoid factors that may trigger the development of telangiectasias such as alcohol, spicy foods, hot beverages, temperature change, or excessive exercise.

The use of the flash lamp pulsed dye laser at 585 nm can usually eradicate the telangiectasias in one to two treatments. A fluence of 6.0 to 7.25 $J/cm^2$ with a 5 mm spot size seems to work the best. The area of the vessels are single pulsed with minimal overlap (less than 10%) which results in immediate dark purple purpura and sometimes surrounding erythema (Figure 2-1). The purpura is impressive and can be a drawback to patient acceptance. The purpura will fade over a two-week time period. Postoperative care includes topical antibiotics for crusting lesions and avoidance of sun exposure for the next two months. Ultraviolet light exposure can exacerbate hyperpigmenation due to initial hemosiderin deposition after FLPD treatment. Cosmetics should not be used over the treated areas for one week. All of these factors may affect the eventual outcome.

The KTP/532 laser is a quasi-continuous wave laser that can treat telangiectasias. Although it does not adhere strictly to the principles

**Figure 2-1**
A 36-year-old female with telangiectasias secondary to acne rosacea. Purpura with surrounding erythema noted immediately following treatment with pulsed dye laser. Treatment fluences were 6.75 $J/cm^2$.

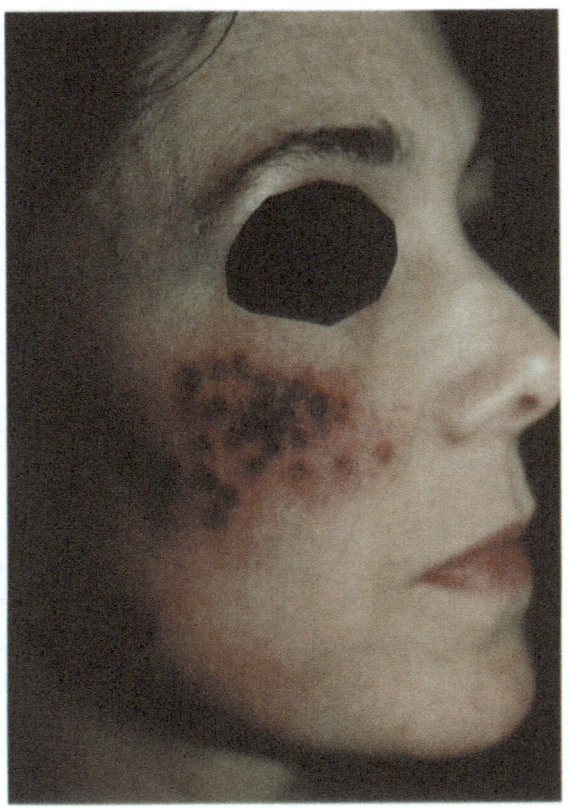

of selective photothermolysis, I find it effective when using a spot diameter smaller than the vessel size. It also has a great affinity for the color red, the color of vascular lesions, and readily passes through water. This results in a relatively confined thermal injury to the vessel. The KTP/532 has multiple hand pieces to achieve target specificity by tracing vessels individually or using a hexagonal scanning device to cover large surface areas. A new KTP laser delivery system, The Star Pulse®, has recently been introduced which has the ability to dial in a variable pulse duration and fluence to achieve selective photothermolysis for superficial vessels 1–15 mm in diameter. Results are encouraging on this new laser [3].

The advantages of this laser over the flash lamp pulsed dye laser are the elimination of the purpura. Treatment with The Star Pulse® results in immediate blanching of vessels with the development of a fine crust which separates in approximately five days (Figure 2-2 A–C). Recurrences can occur requiring additional treatments. Recurrence of telangiectasias may be a result of injury to a vessel which recovers by re-canalization or by recovery of vessel spasm.

**Figure 2-2 A, B**
A) A 69-year-old male with telangiectasias. B) Treatment of vessel with KTP/532 laser. Target vessel is traced with 250 m beam at a fluence of 1.0 watt and 0.2 s pulse duration. The optimal laser settings are obtained with vessel blanching. No purpura noted, but frequently fine crusting will occur.

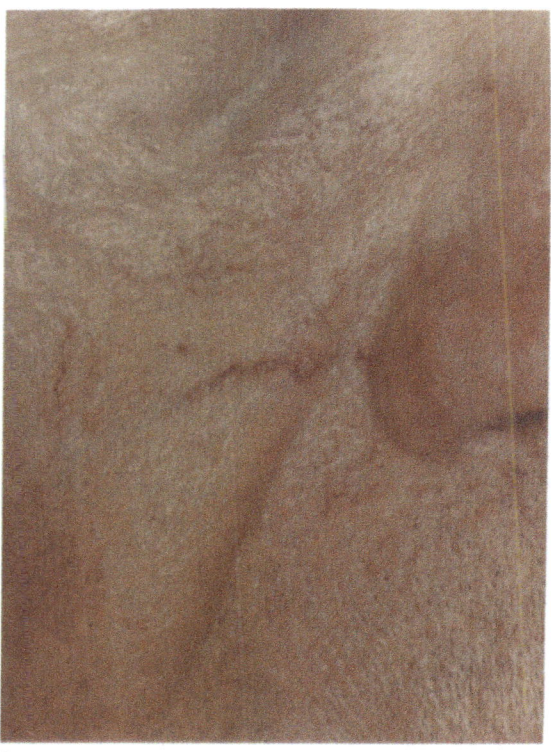

A

B

**Figure 2-2 C**
C) Thirty days following treatment.

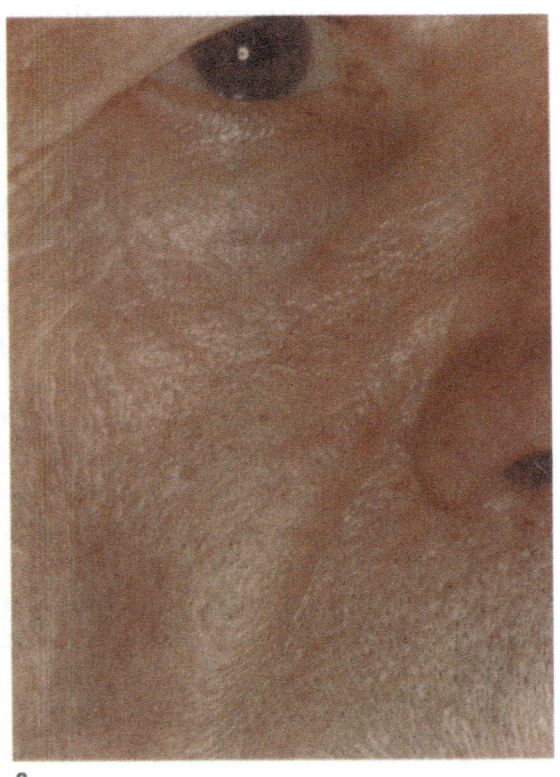

C

**Figure 2-3 A, B**
A) A 34-year-old female with a spider angioma of the nose previously treated twice by electrodesiccation. B) Five weeks post KTP/532 laser treatment using the scanner. Fluence of 16 J/cm$^2$ with a pulse length of 38 ms.

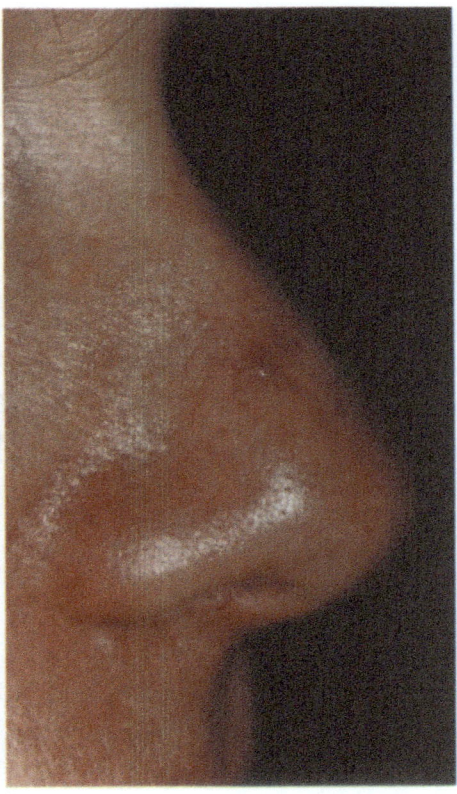

A

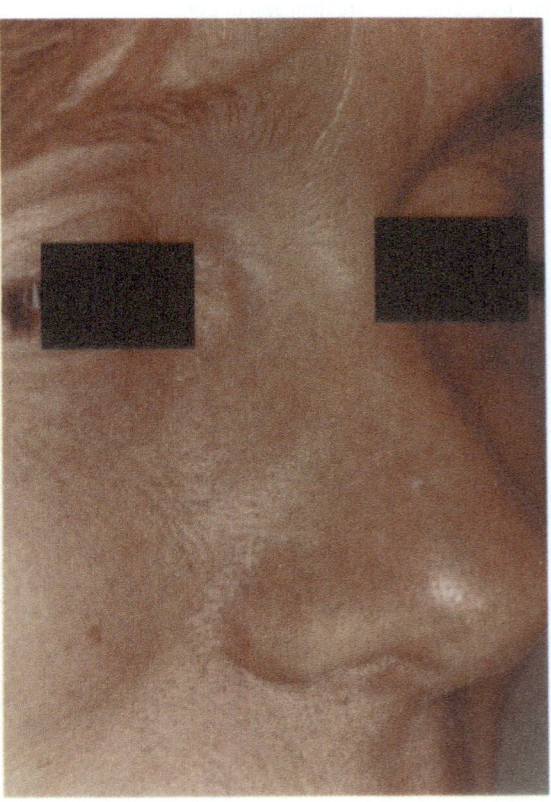

B

Alternative treatments may include electrosurgery for telangiectasias. This is performed with a 30-gauge needle attached to a hyfurcator at low current. Electrosurgery may result in punctate scars, especially after multiple sessions. Laser surgery should be considered after one to two unsuccessful elective treatments (Figure 2-3 A–B).

Another treatment for telangiectasias and venulectases is intense pulsed light therapy. This device is not a laser, uses noncoherent light, and can treat enlarged leg blood vessels up to 3 mm in diameter and 3 mm in depth. Results are encouraging for this new treatment modality.

## Leg Telangiectasia

Laser treatment for leg telangiectasia has recently received Food and Drug Administration (FDA) approval. The long pulsed tunable dye laser is designed to optimize selective photothermolysis with multiple wavelengths of 585 mm, 590 mm, 595 mm, and 600 mm. A pulse duration of 1500 ms and a $2 \times 7$ mm elliptical spot size are utilized. This treatment may complement or replace sclerotherapy. In addition, intense pulsed light therapy is currently being used for leg telangiectasias with good results.

## Port Wine Stains

Just twelve years ago the treatment of port wine stains (PWS) of the face was a risky proposition. Some patients developed scarring and textural changes which often left a patient worse off than before treatment [4]. Due to the advent of the pulsed dye laser and the understanding of selective photothermolysis, the treatment of PWS has been improved. The wavelengths of these lasers correspond to the absorption peaks of oxyhemoglobin, making them more selective. As a result, lateral thermal damage is limited.

Port wine stains are congenital vascular malformations with an incidence of 0.3 to 0.5% in the general population [5]. They are composed of ectatic superficial and dermal capillaries with an average depth of 0.46 mm [6]. Port wine stains most commonly involve the face and neck. When the V1 and V2 divisions of the trigeminal nerve are involved, they often are associated with ocular glaucoma [7]. Opthamology monitoring is essential for these cases. Port wine stains that involve the medial cheek, upper lip, or extremities require an increased number of treatments. In contrast, PWS located on the forehead, lateral face, and neck resolve after fewer treatment sessions [8]. The earlier laser treatment is initiated, the smaller the vessel diameter and, therefore, the greater chance of success. More mature PWS are thicker and therefore the laser light must penetrate significantly deeper which increases the chances of scar formation, texture change, and hypopigmentation.

The pulsed dye laser is the treatment of choice for thin PWS [9] (Figure 2-4 A–C). The settings vary from a fluence of 5.5 to 6.5 J/cm$^2$ with a slight overlap of pulses. Thinner PWSs, require lower energy for treatment. Thicker PWSs, require higher fluences, approaching

6.5 to 8.0 J/cm$^2$. Higher energy settings are necessary for darker skinned individuals since melanin will compete somewhat with light absorption.

Deeper PWS can be treated by a pulsed dye laser or KTP/532 laser or, a combination of the two. The KTP/532 wavelength can penetrate deeper into the skin for thicker vascular malformations. A scanning device can be utilized with the KTP/532 laser to cover large surface areas efficiently and to prevent overlapping of treatments. The scanner is a hexagon shape and the treatment areas are aligned side-by-side like a honeycomb. Rarely is general anesthesia necessary. Most often, topical EMLA cream (ASTRA USA, Inc., Westboro, MA) is utilized. The KTP/532 laser used for deep PWS will result in purpura shortly after treatment and may cause blistering or crusting. Topical antibiotics are useful for wound healing. Repeat treatments are performed at six to eight week intervals, and a total of six to ten treatment sessions may be required (Figure 2-5 A–D).

## Hemangiomas

Hemangiomas are benign vascular malformations that appear in the first few weeks of life [5]. These vascular tumors can grow rapidly in size the first several months of life up to about one year of age and then, in many cases, gradually involute to a fibrous, fatty scar by age twelve [10].

**Figure 2-4 A**
A) An 8-year-old female with thin PWS of the right cheek and neck areas.

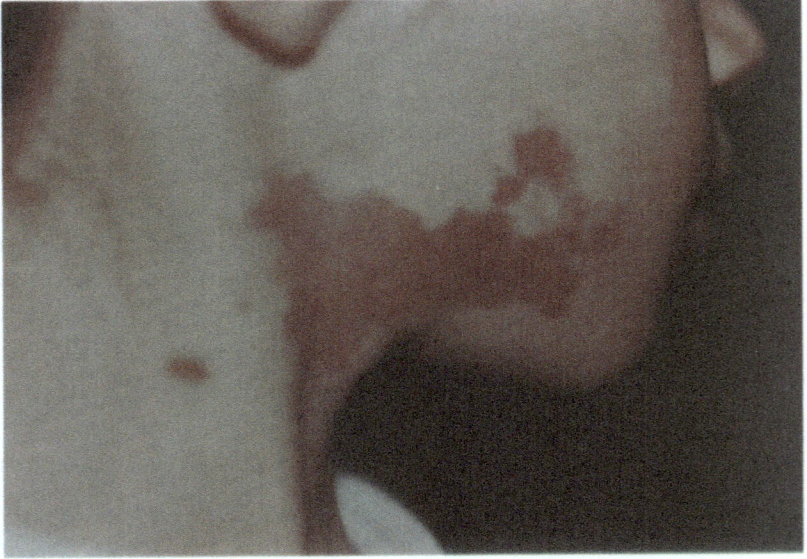

A

**Figure 2-4 B, C**
B) Results after seven treatments using pulsed dye laser at 6.76 J/cm² and a 5 mm hand piece. C) Almost complete resolution of PWS after fifteen treatments.

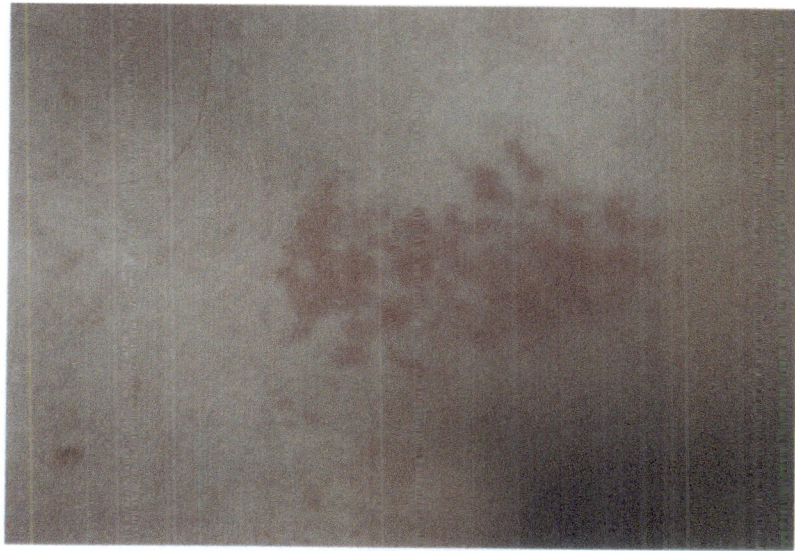

B

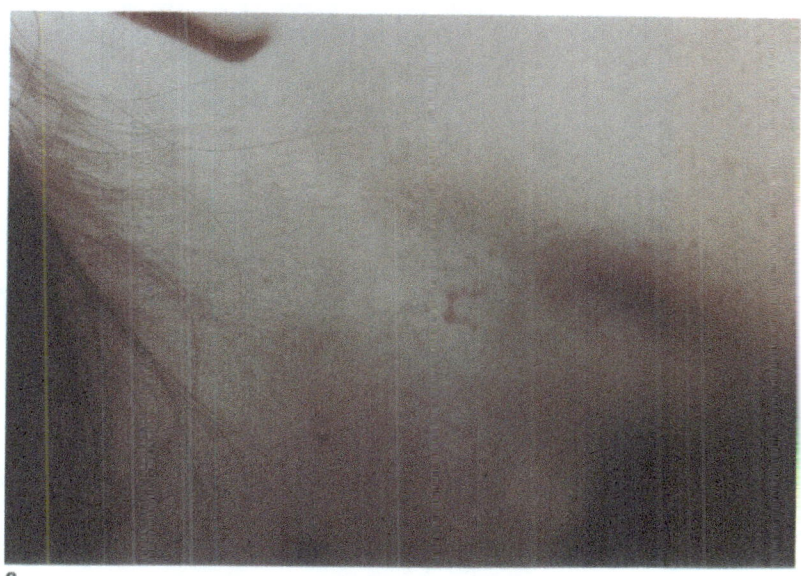

C

**Figure 2-5 A, B**
A) A 71-year-old female with a mature, deep PWS of the right chin and neck areas. Dark hexagonal areas are test patches. B) Results eight weeks following test patch of PWS. Note hexagonal lightening of PWS on neck area. Fluences of 12 to 20 J/cm² were used.

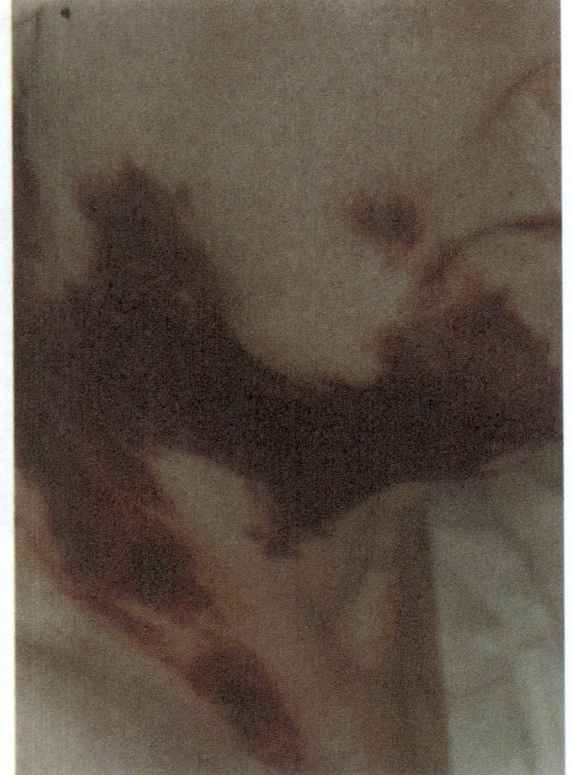

A

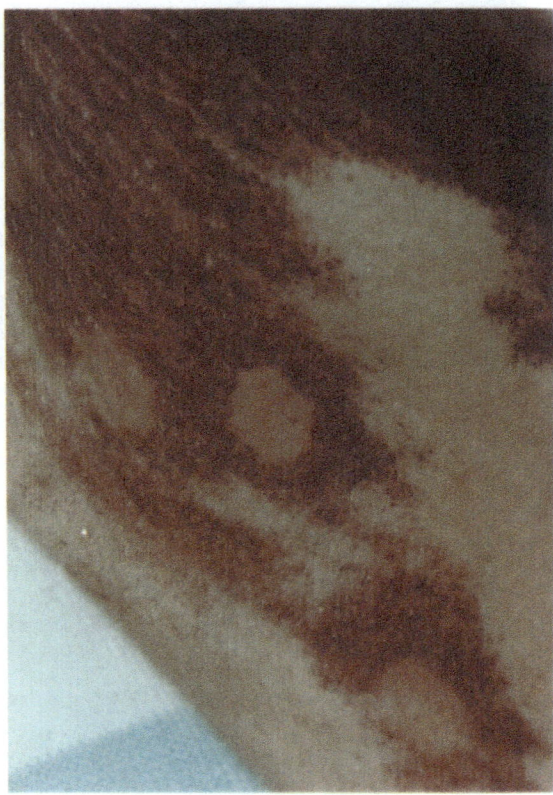

B

**Figure 2-5** C, D
C) Results eight weeks following first treatment at a fluence of 12 J/cm$^2$ and a pulse duration of 30 ms. D) Results following six treatments.

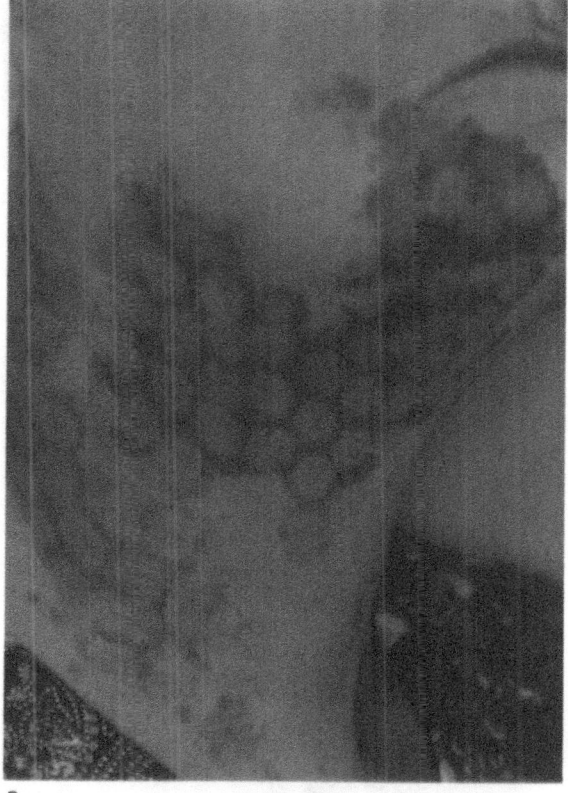

C

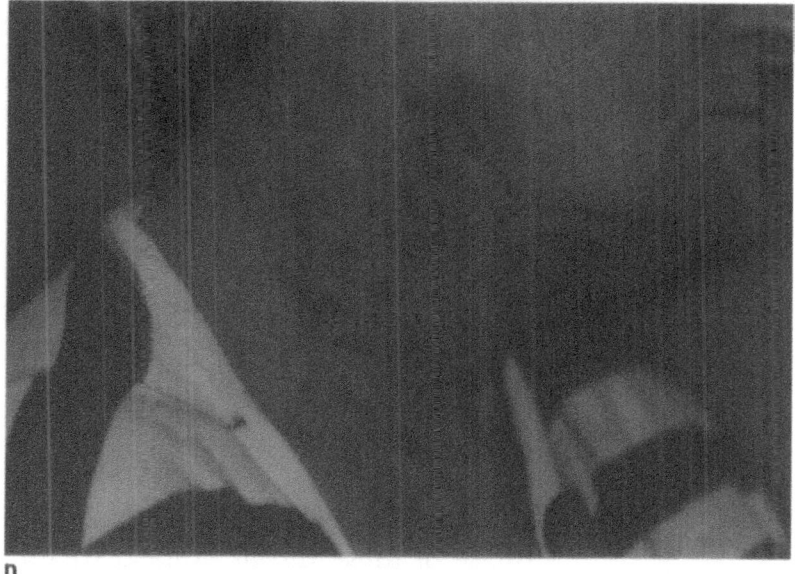

D

The superficial hemangiomas are most responsive and are best treated by pulsed dye laser [11, 12]. Mixed or deep hemangiomas are frequently treated using contact Nd:YAG laser. Scar formation and skin texture change are not uncommon. The elevated lesions can be compressed by a glass slide for easier treatment. Often, the healing of ulcerated mixed or deep hemangiomas can be enhanced by pulsed dye laser treatment of the ulcer, which slows the rapid proliferation

**Figure 2-6 A, B**
A) A 10-month old female with ulcerated hemangioma of the buttocks. B) Complete healing of hemangioma following three treatments with the pulsed dye laser over the ulcerated areas. Fluence was 6.5 J/cm² and double pulsing of ulceration was performed.

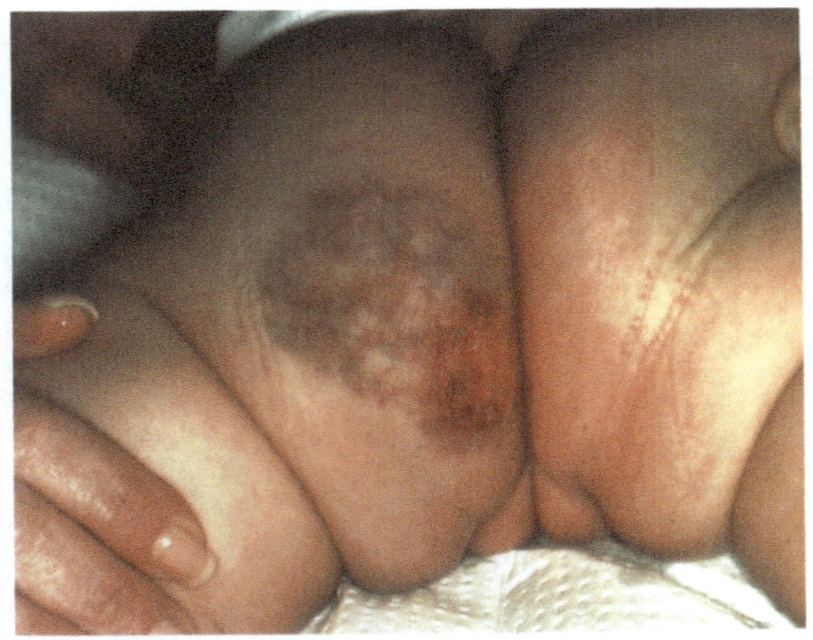

A

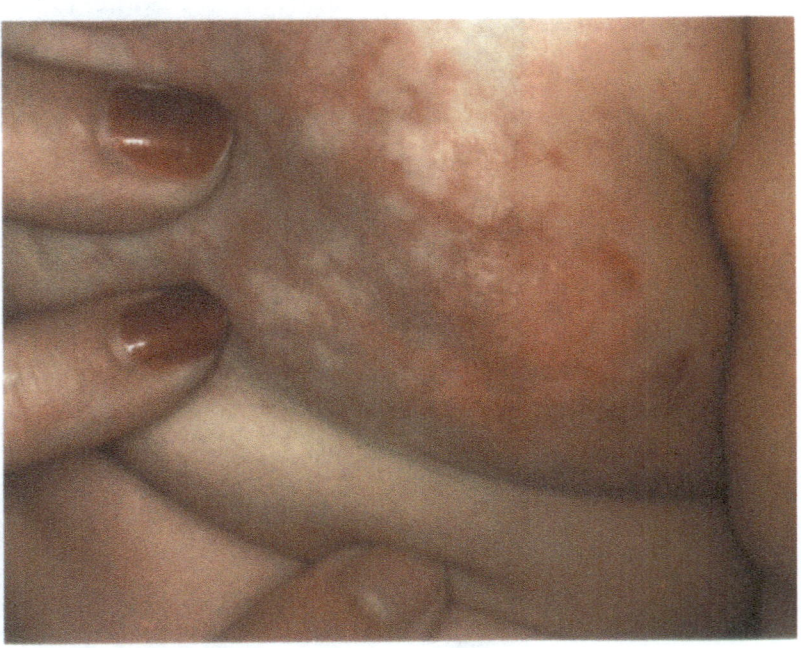

B

phase of these vessels. Repeat treatments are necessary every two to four weeks [13]. A 10-month-old female was treated with the pulsed dye laser. Settings used were 6.0 to 7.5 J/cm² and the lesions were double pulsed (Figure 2-6 A–B).

## Poikiloderma of Civatte

Poikiloderma of Civatte is a result of chronic ultraviolet exposure to the sides of the neck and upper chest area. The anterior aspect of the neck is usually spared. Skin telangiectasias, hyperpigmentation, hypopigmentation, and atrophy are usually present.

**Figure 2-7**

A 56-year-old female with scarring of the neck secondary to treatment of Poikiloderma of Civatte using a krypton laser with a wavelength of 568 nm.

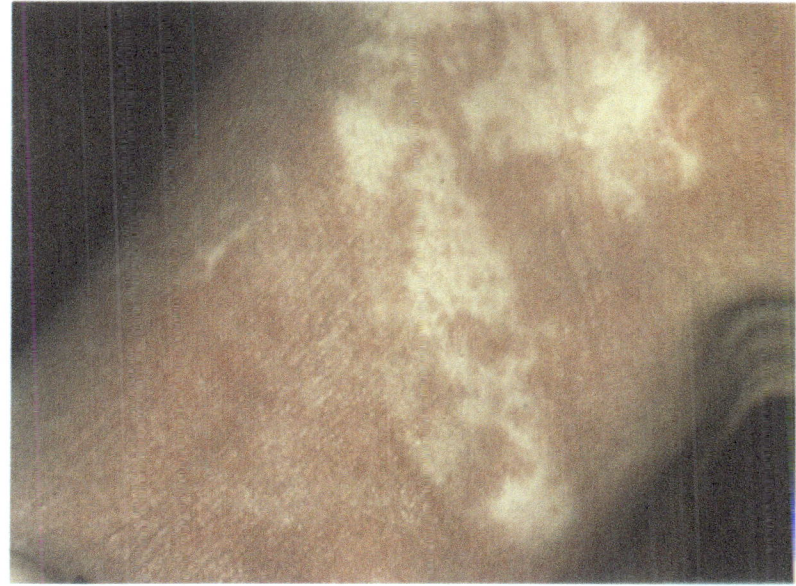

The pulsed dye laser is the treatment of choice for this condition. In my experience, fluences in the range of 6 to 6.75 J/cm² provide optimal clinical results. Multiple treatments are necessary due to the large surface area. Other lasers (krypton) have been used, but scarring can frequently occur on such atrophic skin (Figure 2-7).

## Venous Lakes

Venous lakes are benign, raised, dark blue papular lesions frequently found on the face of elderly patients. They are easily treated with either the pulsed dye laser at 7 to 8 J/cm² with double pulsing or the KTP/532 laser at 18 Joules and 30 ms using a scanning device (Figure 2-8 A–B). Recurrences are rare.

**Figure 2-8 A, B**

A) A 65-year-old female with a venous lake of the lower lip. B) Resolution of lesion after one treatment with the KTP/532 laser with scanner at a fluence of 20 J/cm² and a pulse duration of 42 ms.

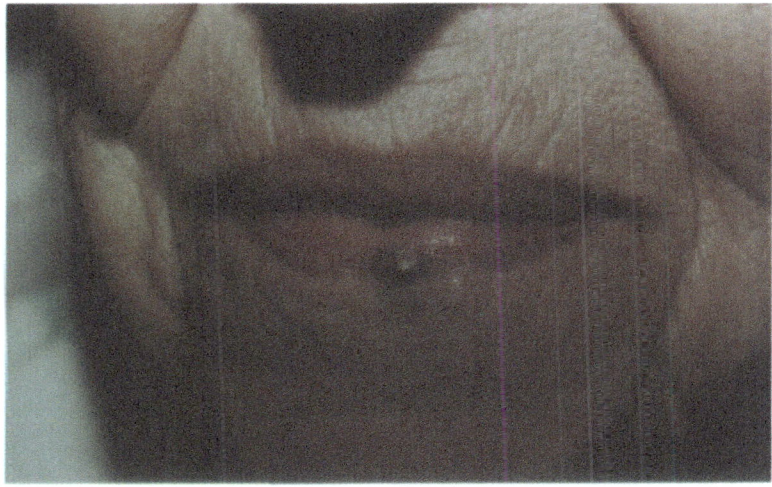

A

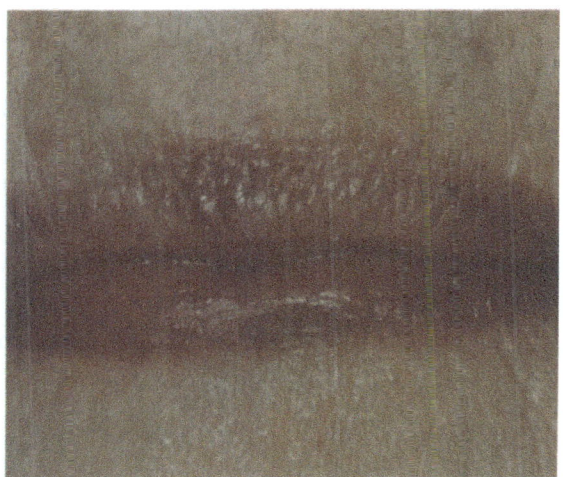

B

## Conclusion

The field of cutaneous laser surgery is very exciting. Over the last decade, great strides have allowed surgeons to treat cutaneous lesions that previously could not be attempted. The ability to access these lasers is the only limiting factor for physicians treating cutaneous vascular lesions. It is essential that physicians have an understanding of laser tissue interactions and that they attend didactic and clinical courses to remain at the forefront of technology. Experimentation with new wavelengths and methods of delivery will continue to advance this treatment alternative and reduce complications.

### References

1. Anderson RR, Parrish JA. Selective photothermolysis: Precise microsurgery by selective absorption of pulsed radiation. *Science* 1983; 220:524–527.

2. Goldman MP, Bennett RG. Treatment of telangiectasia: A review. *J Am Aced Dermatol* 1987;17:167–182.

3. Hruza GJ, Leal-Khouri S. Aesthetic laser surgery. *J Geriatric Dermatol* 1995;3:249–264.

4. Brauner G, Schliftman A, Cosman B. Evaluation of argon laser surgery in children under 13 years of age. *Plast Reconstr Surg* 1991;87:37–43.

5. Jacobs AH, Walton RG. The incidence of birthmarks in the neonate. *Pediatrics* 1976;58:218–222.

6. Batsky SH, Rosen S, Geer D, Noe JM. The nature and evolution of port-wine stains: A computer-assisted study. *J Invest Dermatol* 1980; 74:154–157.

7. Goldman MP, Fitzpatrick RE. Treatment of cutaneous vascular lesions. In *Cutaneous Laser Surgery*. St. Louis: Mosby, 1994;19–105.

8. Tan OT, Sherwood K, Gilchrest BA. Treatment of children with port-wine stains using the flashlamp-pulsed tuneable dye laser. *N Engl J Med* 1989;320:416–421.

9. Ashinoff R, Geronemus RG. Flashlamp-pumped pulsed dye laser for port-wine stains in infancy: Earlier versus later treatment. *J Am Acad Dermatol* 1991;24:467–472.

10. Spicer MS, Goldberg DJ, Janniger CK. Lasers in pediatric dermatology. *Cutis* 1995;55:270–280.

11. Garden JM, Bakus AD, Paller AS. Treatment of cutaneous hemangiomas by the flashlamp-pumped pulsed dye laser: Prospective analysis. *Pediatrics* 1992;120:555–560.

12. Garden JM, Bakus AD. Clinical efficacy of the pulsed dye laser in the treatment of vascular lesions. *J Dermatol Surg Oncol* 1993;19:321–326.

13. Lask GP, Glassberg E. 585 nm Pulsed dye laser for the treatment of cutaneous lesions. *Clinics Dermatol* 1995;13:63–67.

# 3

# Treatment of Vascular & Pigmented Lesions

Donald Groot, *M.D., F.R.C.P.(C), F.A.C.P.*, and
Patricia Johnston, *B.Sc., M.Cl.Sc., M.B.A.*

In the 1960s, a revolution in medicine began. The introduction of lasers as a means of altering tissue created fundamental changes in the way in which medicine has been practiced, particularly in the last decade, and will have a significant impact on the future.

For years aesthetic surgery focused on adjustments to proportion and symmetry to create a more pleasing appearance. Attention was given to the color and texture of the skin through the use of chemical peels and dermabrasion, but the risks associated with these procedures were often high and the results were not always as reliable as one would hope due to issues of control and healing.

Unwanted abnormalities of the skin such as vascular and pigmentary lesions were best left alone. As excision and/or grafting were generally the only treatment options available, the patient had to make a difficult choice between an abnormality and a scar. Decisions were often made on the basis of which was the least psychologically traumatic.

The advances in laser technology have significantly altered the cosmetic surgeon's approach to the treatment of many conditions, including neoplastic, vascular, and pigmentary lesions of the skin. The goal of the dermatologic laser surgeon has been to remove those components of the skin that are abnormal or unwanted without disturbing that which is normal. The applied theory of selective photothermolysis to a large extent has made this possible.

The key variables that make laser systems adaptable to the treatment of a wide variety of cutaneous lesions are wavelength and pulse duration. In the mid-1980s, Parrish and Anderson explained that selective destruction of tissue without damage to adjacent tissue was possible if the correct wavelengths and pulse durations were applied [1]. Different components of the skin preferentially absorb different wavelengths of light, so in order to obtain an optimum response, the targeted tissue must be precisely matched with the wavelength that it is most likely to absorb. To minimize thermal damage to adjacent tissue, the pulse duration of the selected wavelength must be shorter than the thermal relaxation time (TRT) of the targeted component of the skin.

Laser technology for the treatment of dermatologic conditions has taken a new direction based on this theory. The skin has two chromophores, hemoglobin and melanin, that contribute to color in normal and atypical tissue. Each has an affinity for the absorption of certain wavelengths of light. Laser systems with wavelengths concurrent with the color of hemoglobin and melanin were developed to dispense with these chromophores. These lasers have also proven valuable in the removal of foreign material introduced into the skin by accident or on purpose, such as particles of asphalt and dyes [2].

Lasers have been developed for the removal or alteration of nonspecific tissue in the skin. For example, at a wavelength of 510 nm, the flash lamp-pumped pulsed dye laser is effective in the treatment of epidermal pigment, and at 577 to 585 nm, it is useful in the removal of vascular lesions. The Q-switched ruby, Q-switched Alexandrite, and Q-switched double frequency neodymium:yttrium-aluminum-garnet (Nd:YAG) lasers are effective in the removal of epidermal and dermal pigment as well as tattoos. The Q-switched ruby and Q-switched Alexandrite lasers are in the visible light spectrum at wavelengths of 694 nm and 755 nm, respectively. The Q-switched Nd:YAG is in the infrared spectrum and is usually at a wavelength of 1064 nm. This wavelength can be halved to 532 nm by directing the laser beam through a potassium diphosphate crystal. This enables the laser light to be absorbed by pigment in the skin. It is thought that because the Q-switched lasers produce a high power pulsed output measured in nanoseconds, that a photoacoustic response may contribute to the destruction of the melanin or foreign color in the skin. The vibration from the impact of the laser light on the pigment, along with the thermal reaction to the absorption of the light, causes it to explode into minuscule particles. An additional chemical response to the extreme temperatures has also been postulated as an explanation for the breakup of the pigment. The resulting debris is carried away by the macrophage cells of the immune system [2, 3].

The $CO_2$ laser is in the infrared spectrum. At 10,600 nm it targets water. By heating the water in the cells to 100°C it is able vaporize tissue in a defocused mode or cut it in focused mode [3]. The significant breakthrough in $CO_2$ laser technology has been the alteration of the pulse duration to less than the TRT of the skin, thereby allowing the removal or alteration of targeted tissue with minimal peripheral damage.

It is my belief that in order to provide comprehensive care to a patient for the removal of dermatologic skin conditions of a vascular, pigmented, or neoplastic nature, the surgeon must have access to lasers that are specifically targeted to these entities. At the very least this means that the laser surgeon must have at his or her disposal three target-specific lasers. More lasers than this simply increases the specificity with which the same entities are treated. Fewer lasers limits the therapeutic alternatives available to the laser surgeon and their patients.

A further argument for access to an adequate number of cutaneous lasers is the need to use more than one laser to treat the same condition, albeit a condition composed of several components. For example, if you separate a scar into its component parts and treat each of the elements, such as vascularity with a dye laser, hyperpigmentation with a Q-switched ruby laser, and textural irregularity with a $CO_2$ laser, then the results are synergistic. The whole, in terms of the aesthetic goal, is greater than the sum of the parts.

At our laser center we actively utilize a flash lamp-pumped pulsed vascular dye laser (Cynosure™), a Q-switched ruby laser (Laserphotonic™), a continuous wave $CO_2$ laser (Surgilase™), an ultrapulsed $CO_2$ laser (Coherent Ultrapulse™), a potassium titanyl phosphate (KTP) laser (Laserscope™), a long pulsed green Nd:YAG laser (Coherent VersaPulse™), a Q-switched Alexandrite (Coherent VersaPalse™) and a single and double frequency Q-switched Nd:YAG laser (Coherent VersaPulse™). Each of these systems serves a different but useful function. In addition, we have several obsolete systems lying in state in our laser graveyard. This is a warning to the uninitiated laser surgeon that staying current in laser surgery can be a costly experience.

## Pigmented Lesions

### Nevus of Ota

Nevus of Ota, or oculocutaneous melanosis, is an acquired pigmentary disorder which may appear anywhere from early childhood into the early stages of adulthood. It is most commonly found in females of oriental descent and is thought to be a variant of the deep blue nevus [4]. There is a tendency for the lesions to increase in size over time.

Bipolar or stellate melanocytes found in the reticular dermis and around blood vessels, sweat, and sebaceous glands are responsible for the production of a mottled pattern of pigment along the distribution lines of the first and second branches of the trigeminal nerve. The lesions may appear on one or both sides of the face and may extend into the sclera of the eye. The color of these lesions varies, including hues of black, brown, purple, and blue [4, 5].

The long wavelength of the Q-switched ruby laser at 694 nm or the Q-switched Alexandrite laser at 755 nm are effective in reaching into the reticular dermis to eradicate the melanocytes that produce this unique pattern of pigmentation. A pulse duration time of 29 to 100 ns is shorter than the TRT of the melanocytes, thereby containing the thermal damage to the lesion. This significantly reduces the risk of post-procedural scarring or textural changes to the skin. I have observed that after a treatment with the Q-switched ruby or Q-switched Alexandrite laser there is often a short period of crusting and post-inflammatory hyperpigmentation which fades over six to twelve months. This expected delay in lightening is due to the time necessary for the macrophage cells to remove the pigmentary debris gradually. Deeper nevi of Ota may require a deeper penetrating laser with pigment selectivity such as the 1064 nm Q-switched Nd:YAG laser.

Dark skinned patients are less likely to develop dyschromia with this wavelength.

Depending on the depth and intensity of the pigmentation, more than one treatment session is usually necessary to eradicate the lesions. A 100% resolution is difficult to achieve and should not be expected. Many patients require two to seven sessions to achieve a satisfactory result. It is optimal to wait at least six months between treatment sessions in order to observe the extent of fading and to minimize the risk of hypopigmentation. In certain cases, however, in order to expedite the treatment process, sessions are performed at six-week intervals. Preoperative counseling is necessary to ensure that the patient does not become impatient and discouraged with the apparently slow response to treatment.

If the lesion is around the eye, it is very difficult to remove the pigment at the margin of the eyelid. To closely visualize a periocular lesion, it is helpful to insert a protective eye shield. First the eye is anesthetized with eye drops such as Pontocaine™. Eye ointment is then applied to the stainless steel shield and it is inserted over the cornea of the eye.

The first example represents an asian woman, age 36, who was treated with the Q-switched ruby laser at a fluence of 9 joules/cm². Four treatment sessions were required to reach this level of resolution (Figure 3-1 A–B). A second patient, also an asian woman of

**Figure 3-1 A, B**
Nevus of Ota: cheek, asian female, Q-switched ruby laser.

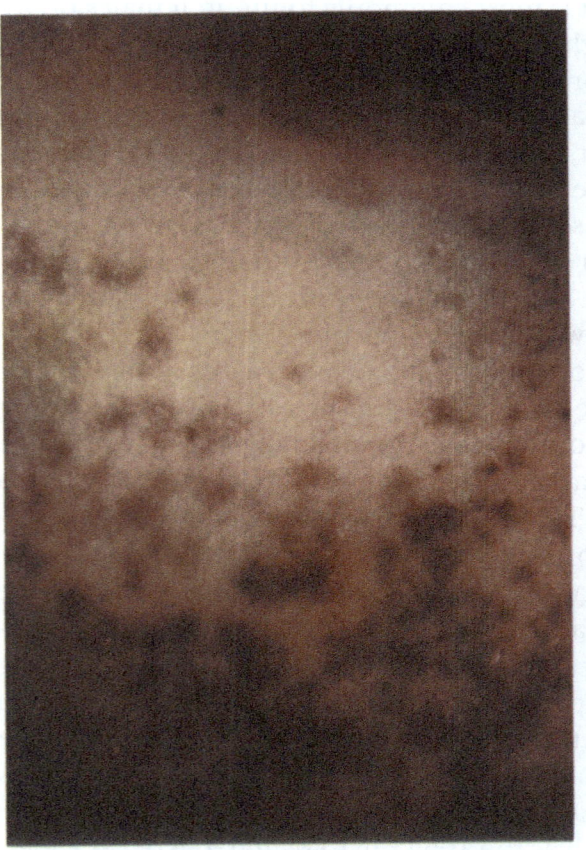

A

B

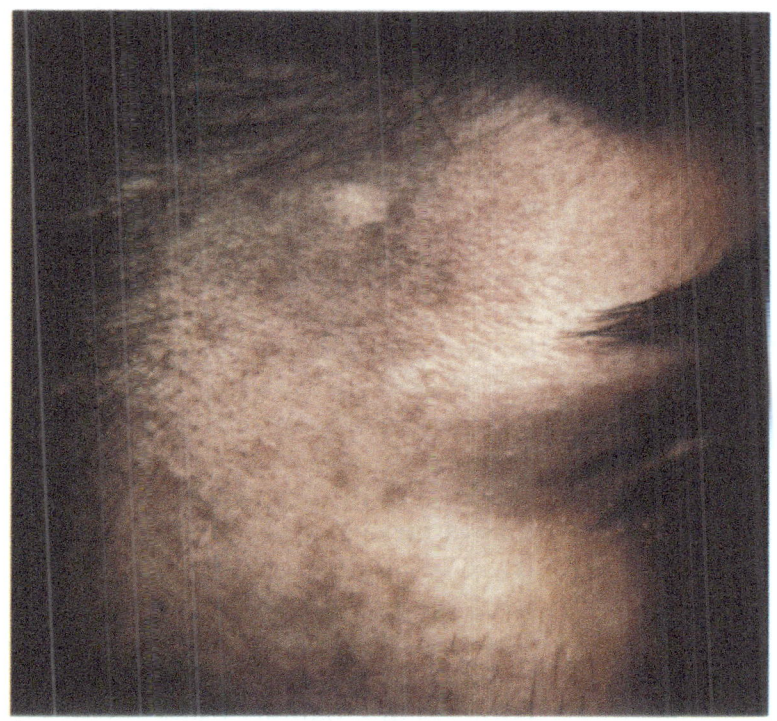

A

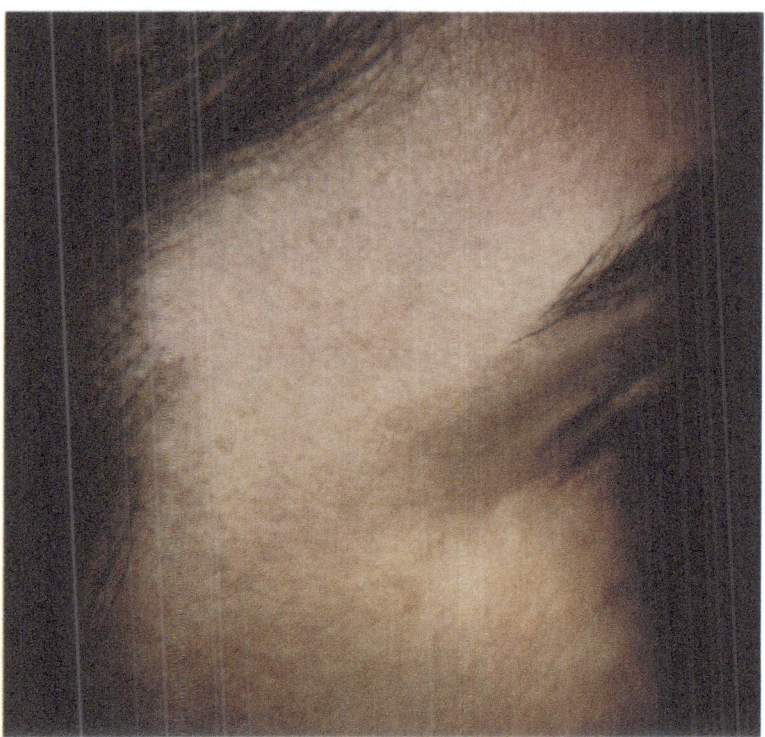

B

39 years of age, responded to treatment with the KTP laser utilizing
the Hexascan at 17 joules/cm$^2$. Six treatment sessions were required
(Figure 3-2 A–B).

In both cases, the skin responded to the laser beam with immediate blanching of the targeted tissue, followed by the formation of
a dark, superficial crust which sloughed off once the top layer of the

skin turned over. The time it takes for the crust to fall away depends on the condition being treated and the area of the body where the lesion occurs. Coherent Lasers Inc. has developed a chilled tip which when adapted to various laser systems is beneficial in protecting the superficial pigmentation and minimize the discomfort experienced by patients during the procedure.

Generally I have found the Q-switched ruby and Q-switched Alexandrite lasers much more reliable for removing nevi of Ota. Test sites are invaluable in determining which laser system is best suited for the treatment of any given lesion.

Due to the fact that nevus of Ota is a deep dermal lesion often seen in individuals with darker skin tones, a balance must be found between the risk of destroying the normal epidermal pigment of the skin in an effort to reach the abnormal pigment in the dermis. This may result in a disharmonious appearance to the treated skin whereby there is residual blue/black pigment below a temporary or permanent depigmentation of the overlying epidermis. The effect is a translucent, bluish-grey color to the skin. To minimize this effect, it is beneficial to perform several test sites with the laser system of choice. For example, using the Q-switched ruby laser, I would select three different fluencies, 5j, 7j, and 9 joules/cm$^2$, and apply them to three different sites on the lesion before proceeding with a complete treatment session.

Another Q-switched laser that has proven effective in the treatment of nevus of Ota is the Q-switched Nd:YAG with wavelengths of 532 and 1064 nm and a pulse duration of 10 to 20 ns [2, 3, 5, 6]. Tse et al. found that treatment of nevus of Ota with the Q-switched ruby laser was superior to the Q-switched Nd:YAG [7].

## Café Au Lait Macule

Single café au lait macules are benign in nature and tend to occur in 10 to 20% of the adult population. The pale beige lesions may be anywhere from 0.5 to 1.5 cm in size and larger in rare instances. They may appear anywhere on the body. When multiple lesions occur they are generally associated with other disease entities such as neurofibromatosis, Albright's syndrome, Westerhof's syndrome, Watson's syndrome, or gastrocutaneous syndrome [4].

Histopathologic examination demonstrates that the number of melanocytes in the epidermis are generally unchanged, however, there is an increase of the amount of melanin in the epidermis [4]. This suggests that the melanocytes are producing more pigment, although the reason for this increased activity is unknown.

Café au lait macules may or may not respond to current laser technology, as is the case with Melasura and Becker's Nevi. In my experience, over half of the café au lait macules I have treated did not respond to laser surgery. As David Goldberg suggests, this may be due to the fact that the lasers have a selective affinity for melanosomes rather than melanocytes which are overactive, as is the case with these lesions [5]. However, since there are no other effective treatment modalities available for people who find these lesions to be cosmetically annoying, a test site with the Q-switched ruby laser or equivalent laser system is certainly warranted.

In some cases more than one treatment session may be required in order to eradicate the lesion, and there is the risk that post-inflammatory hyperpigmentation may occur. In many cases, despite an early hint of success, the treated area may show signs of repigmentation within a six- to twelve-month period.

It is important to counsel the patient as to the limitations of the laser as a treatment modality for café au lait macules, otherwise he or she may become disillusioned with the number of treatment sessions required, the lack of response to the laser therapy, and the tendency for the macules to recur.

In our example, the café au lait macule appeared under a 32-year-old caucasian woman's eye (Figure 3-3 A–B). Confirmation of the diagnosis was made through pathological analysis. We noted that she had similar lesions elsewhere, but there was no associated syndrome. Using 4 joules/cm$^2$, the lesion was successfully removed with the Q-switched ruby laser after three treatment sessions. The lesion has not returned after four years of follow-up observation.

Tse and colleagues concluded that the Q-switched Nd:YAG was similar to the Q-switched ruby laser in the treatment of epidermal pigmented lesions [7]. Fitzpatrick and colleagues found that the flash lamp-pumped pulsed pigment dye laser (510 nm, 300 ns) was effective in the treatment of epidermal lesions [8].

## Nevus Spilus

Nevus spilus, or speckled lentiginous nevus, may be present at birth but more often appears during infancy or in early childhood. A light, brown macular patch (café au lait macule), ranging in size from 1 to 10 cm in diameter, is speckled with darker pigmented lesions (nevi) 1 to 2 mm in diameter. It may be flat or raised. Typically these anomalies appear on the trunk of the body or the extremities, although their presence may be found elsewhere. Lentiginous melanocytic hyperplasia characterizes the darker elements of the lesion, while the light brown background is characterized by a proliferation of melanocytes, and, in some cases, nevus cells [4, 10]. At a glance, the lesions may look like a café au lait patch or a close gathering of nevi depending on which components are most prominent.

It is prudent to perform a shaved biopsy of the lesion prior to proceeding with laser therapy, for there have been some reported cases of dysplastic changes found in these lesions. It has been my experience that dysplasia is more common than has been reported.

**Figure 3-3 A, B**
Café au lait macule: lower eyelid, caucasian female, Q-switched ruby laser.

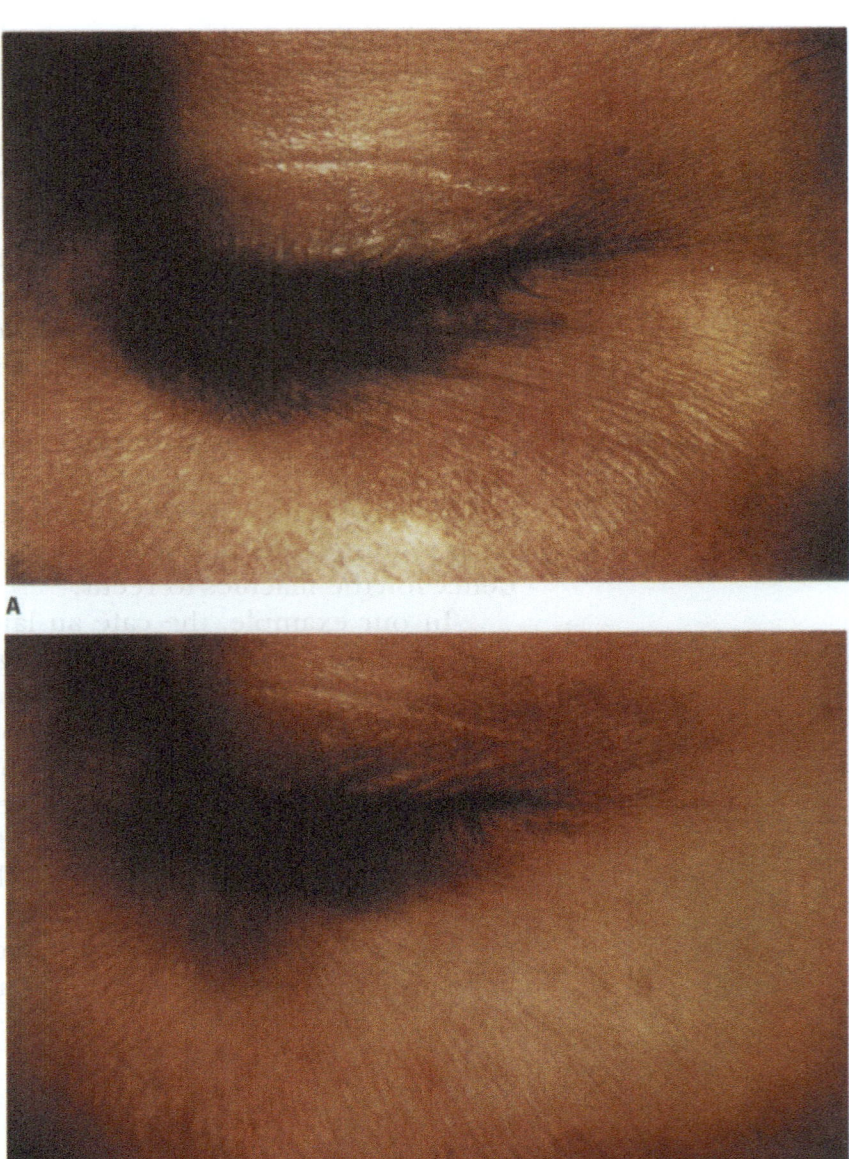

A

B

Our example is that of a 6-year-old caucasian boy who presented with a large nevus spilus on his cheek that had been present for three years (Figure 3-4 A–B). Nevus spilus is composed of two elements: a crop of nevi with a backdrop of a café au lait patch. The laser selected for therapy is dependent on which of the two components is most prominent. In some cases a combination of lasers may provide a better result. Because the speckled darker lesions were very obvious in this young boy and the café au lait patch was hardly noticeable, the nevi were removed with a continuous wave $CO_2$ laser set at 20 watts. After local infiltration with 1% xylocaine with epinephrine, the lesions were removed using a defocused beam at 3 mm and a pulse-like action controlled by the foot pedal. Ice was intermittently applied to cool the skin and to control heat transmission and thermal dam-

**Figure 3-4 A, B**
Nevus spilus: right face, caucasian
male, continuous wave $CO_2$ laser.

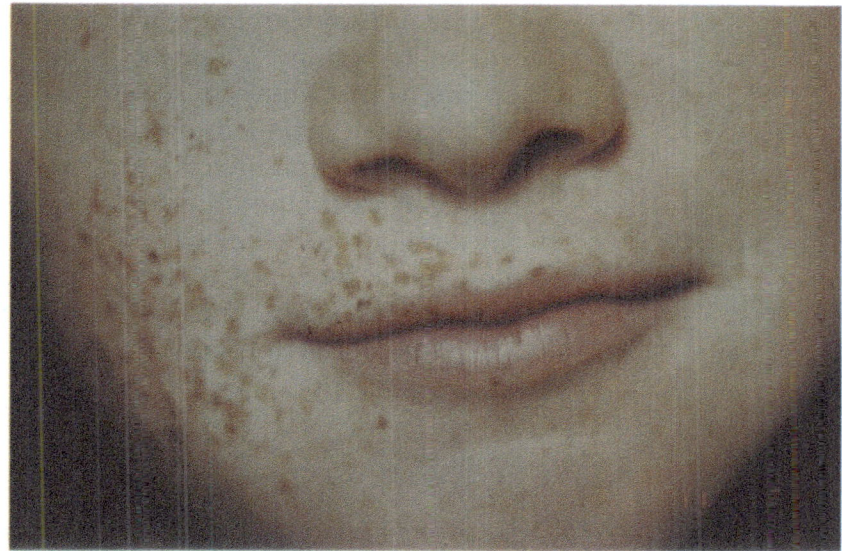

A

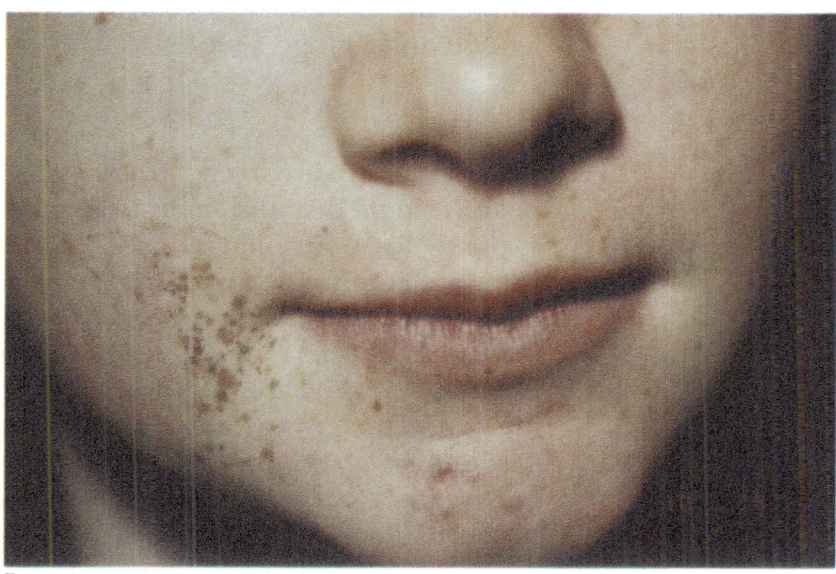

B

age to adjacent tissue. A period of postoperative erythema was expected and resolved within six weeks. Once the nevi were removed, the underlying light brown patch of pigment was of no cosmetic consequence to the patient and was not treated. He was advised to apply a broad spectrum sunscreen over the patch and the face daily in order to prevent the café au lait macule from becoming darker in color. If a patient is concerned about the underlying pigment, it would be treated in a similar fashion to that of a café au lait macule.

The ultrapulsed $CO_2$ laser would be an alternative choice for the treatment of these lesions. Because the duration time of the pulses is lower than the TRT of the skin, transference of heat to the adjacent tissue is minimized. Therefore, icing the skin to control for thermal scatter would not be necessary. The Q-switched ruby, Nd:YAG

[5], and Alexandrite lasers are also alternative forms of therapy for nevus spilus lesions. However, if the pigmented nevi are deep, more than one session may be required to obtain a satisfactory result. As the café au lait macule is often resistant to treatment, test sites of the lesion are recommended before a full therapeutic session is undertaken. The flash lamp-pumped pulsed dye pigmented laser probably would not be sufficient to eradicate this lesion as the shorter wavelength limits its depth of penetration. Laser selection is largely dependent on the depth and color of the nevoid elements and the color of the café au lait component.

## Lentigines

Lentigines are small brown discolorations of the skin that are characterized by a proliferation of melanocytes in the epidermis. Our examples are demonstrative of two common types of lentigines: solar lentigo and lentigo simplex.

### Solar Lentigo

Solar lentigines are irregularly shaped, light brown macules which appear as single or multiple lesions in areas of the body that have been exposed to ultraviolet radiation from the sun or artificial sources. They are commonly found on the face and the dorsum of the hands. Since there is a direct correlation between this condition and age, it is sometimes referred to as *solar lentigo senilis* and *senile lentigines*. However, these terms are not all together accurate, because solar lentigines may appear in younger people depending on the amount of ultraviolet light exposure that they have received [4, 10]. Although benign in nature, many individuals seek to have these lesions removed because of their association with the aging process.

The caucasian gentleman in Figure 3-5 A–B received one session with the Q-switched ruby laser at a fluence of 6 joules/cm$^2$ to remove the solar lentigo on his nose. The example in Figure 3-6 A–B is of a caucasian male who presented with diffuse solar lentigines. He was treated with the Q-switched ruby laser at a fluence of 5 joules/cm$^2$. After three weeks of healing and some obvious residual lentigines, he received a second treatment session leading to a satisfactory resolution of the problem.

The expected response to the laser is an initial blanching followed by a period of crusting. When the crusting is sloughed, the skin is initially pink but gradually returns to the same shade as the surrounding tissue. It is important not disrupt the skin too much. If the skin begins to bubble up, there is a risk of post-surgical scar with postinflammatory hypo- or hyperpigmentation. Postinflammatory hyperpigmentation is common in darker skinned individuals. This potential complication is rare if lower energy levels are applied.

**Figure 3-5 A, B**
Solar lentigo: nose, caucasian male, Q-switched ruby laser.

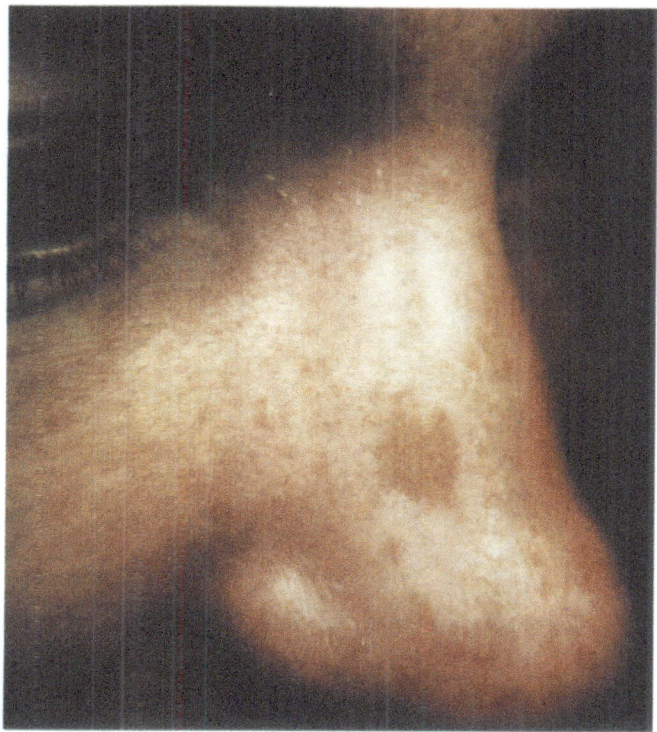

A

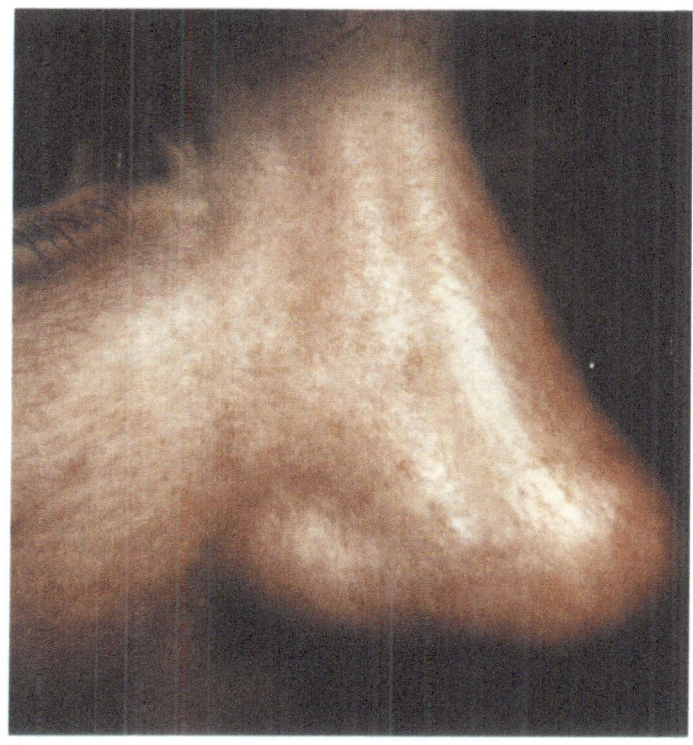

B

**Figure 3-6 A, B**
Solar lentigines: cheek, caucasian
male, Q-switched ruby laser.

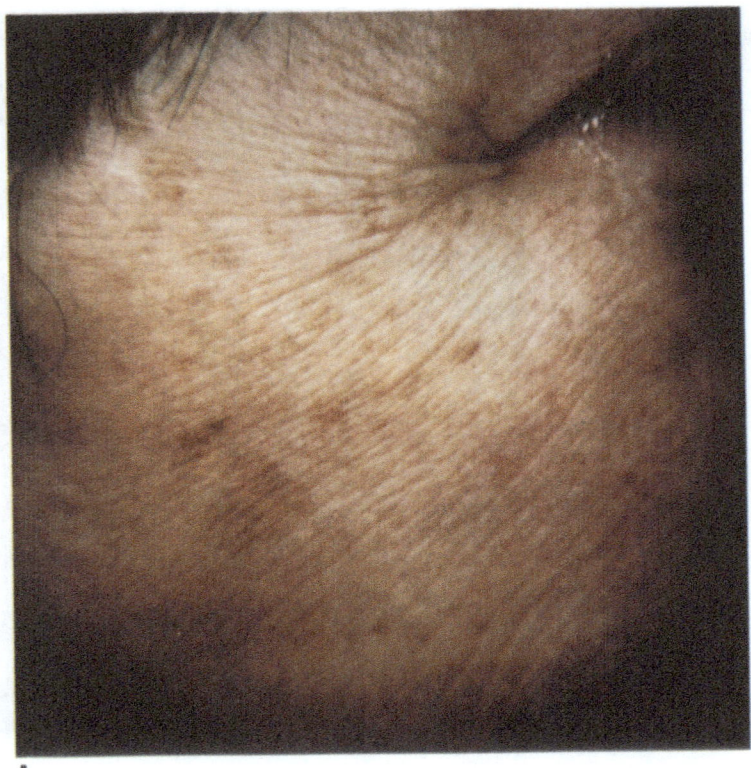

A

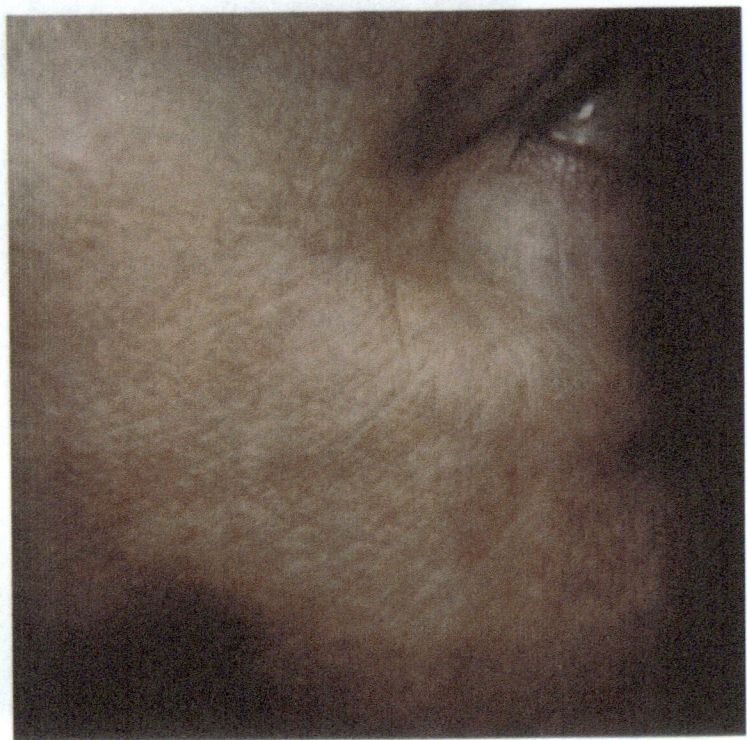

B

## Lentigo Simplex

Lentigo simplex, unlike solar lentigines, is not related to exposure to ultraviolet light. It may appear at any age and may involve the skin, nail bed, or mucous membranes. These lesions tend to be flat, evenly pigmented, isolated, and a few millimeters in diameter. Multiple lentigines may be associated with LEOPARD syndrome, Peutz-Jeghers syndrome, LAMB syndrome, or centrofacial lentiginosis [4, 10].

Benign in appearance, lentigo simplex are generally removed for cosmetic reasons. Otherwise treatment is not required, unless the pigment in the lesion is unusually dark or irregular. Then a biopsy is required to rule out the possibility of atypical melanocytic activity [10].

I have had experience with the use of a double frequency Nd:YAG using a KTP crystal at a wavelength of 532 nm, the Q-switched ruby laser at a wavelength of 694 nm. The Q-switched Alexandrite laser at 755 nm, and the Q-switched single and double frequency Nd: YAG lasers at 1064 nm and 532 nm, respectively for the removal of lentigines. Both of these wavelengths are selectively absorbed by melanosomes in the epidermis and the dermis. The Q-switched ruby laser is set at 6 joules/cm$^2$, the KTP is set at 16 joules/cm$^2$ using a Hexascan, 1 cm$^2$ pulsed mode, the Q-switched Alexandrite laser is set at 4 to 6 joules/cm$^2$, the Q-switched single frequency Nd:YAG is set at 5 joules/cm$^2$ or the Q-switched double frequency Nd:YAG is set at 3 joules/cm$^2$.

The 22-year-old asian female in Figure 3-7 A–B presented with a lentigo simplex on her cheek. The top portion of the lesion was treated with the double frequency KTP Nd:YAG laser and the lower portion with the Q-switched ruby laser. The Q-switched ruby laser was set at 6 joules/cm$^2$, and the KTP was set at 16 joules/cm$^2$ using a Hexascan pattern of 1 cm$^2$ in a pulsed mode. Only one treatment session was required with both lasers. Although the results were comparable, I generally prefer the Q-switched ruby laser, because in my experience it is more reliable in removing lentigines is less likely to leave hypopigmentation and requires fewer sessions.

**Figure 3-7 A, B**
Lentigo simplex: cheek, asian female, KTP and Q-switched ruby lasers.

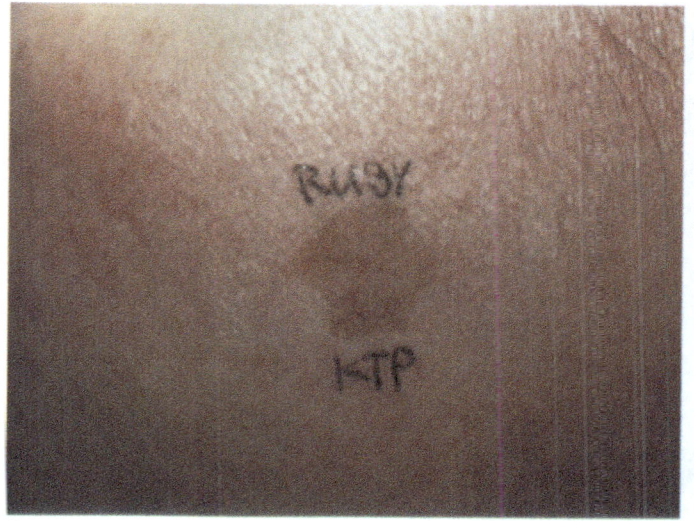

A

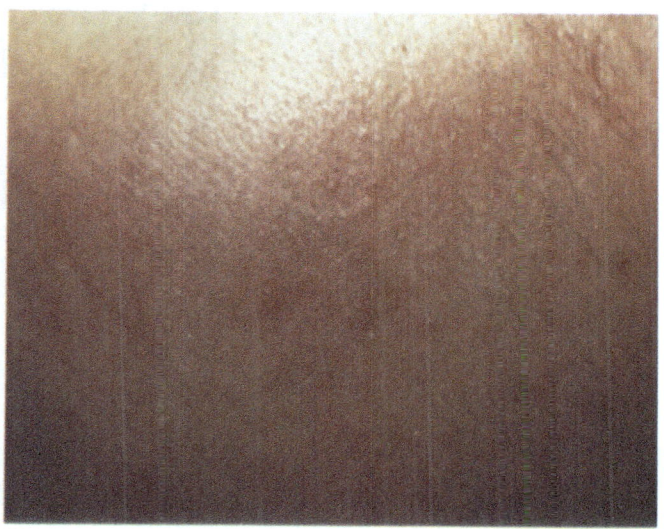

B

Furthermore, the double frequency KTP Nd:YAG laser is not Q-switched. Therefore, the exposure time is longer and the risk of thermal transfer to surrounding tissue is greater, increasing the risk of texture changes in the skin.

The second example is that of a 29-year-old asian female who presented with multiple lentiginous simplex macules on her cheeks (Figure 3-8 A–B). Using the Q-switched ruby laser with a fluence of 4 joules/cm$^2$ the lesion was removed in a single session. No anesthesia was required.

**Figure 3-8 A, B**
Lentigines simplex: cheek, asian female, Q-switched ruby laser.

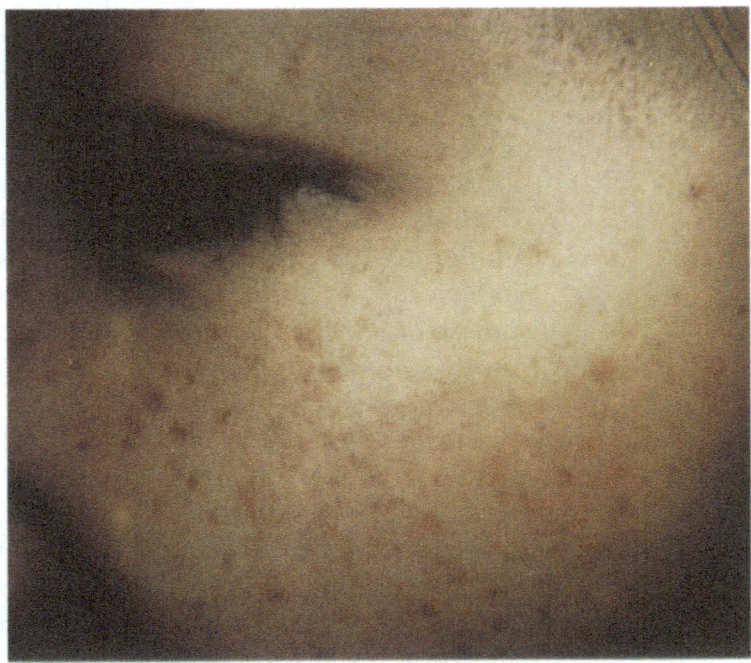

A

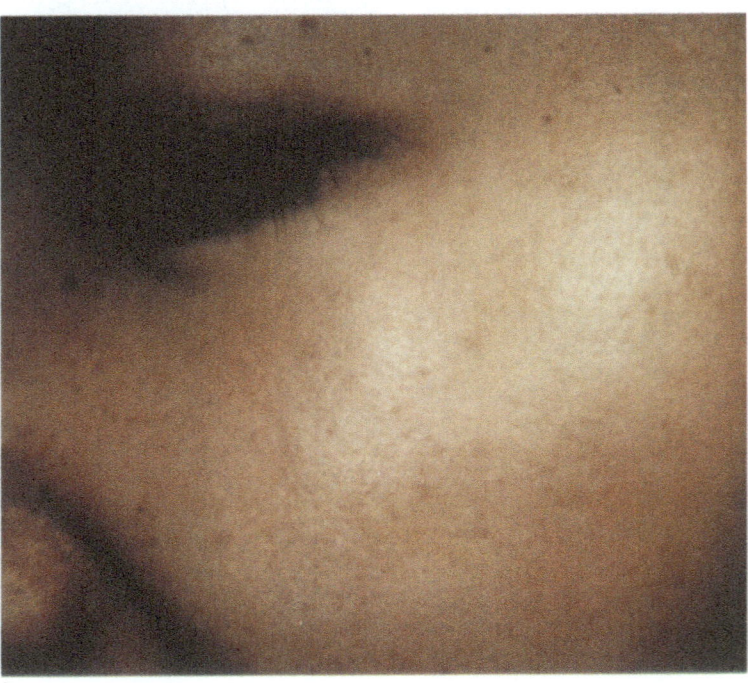

B

Other lasers such as the Q-switched Nd:YAG [7], the Alexandrite [2] lasers, and the flash lamp-pumped pulsed pigmented dye laser [8] may also be used to remove solar lentigines effectively. Some laser surgeons, however, claim that the Q-switched ruby laser provides the best results after one treatment session [5].

Cryotherapy with liquid nitrogen was a common treatment modality for solar lentigines in the past. However, the lack of specificity often resulted in damage to surrounding tissue, resulting in problems with blistering, hypopigmentation, and scarring.

## Melasma

Although melasma is often associated with pregnancy or the use of oral contraceptives in women, its precise pathogenesis is unclear. It is not exclusive to women, there have been occurrences in men. Exposure to ultraviolet light is known to exacerbate the problem [2, 10].

In melasma, light to dark brown pigment changes occur on the face. The pattern of change may simply involve the cheeks or may extend over the nose and into the forehead and mandibular regions. Histopathologic examination demonstrates increased production of melanin in the epidermis, the dermis, or both. Epidermal melasma is most responsive to the popular treatment regimes, which utilize topical bleaching creams containing kojic acid and/or hydroquinone in combination with tretinoin or alpha hydroxy acids, such as glycolic acid, and the regular use of broad spectrum sunscreens. Chemical peels utilizing a variety of acids occasionally work.

The use of lasers to treat this condition has met with varying degrees of success. The use of the Q-switched ruby laser for this condition is most beneficial in fair-skinned individuals, although the results tend to be incomplete and temporary [5].

The woman in Figure 3-9 A–B is a 46-year-old caucasian. The Q-switched ruby laser was used with a fluence of 6 joules/cm$^2$. Only one treatment session was needed to obtain this level of resolution, however, the risk remains that the lesion will recur. To avoid a sharp line of demarcation, the borders of pigmented lesions are blended by decreasing the fluence to 2 joules/cm$^2$ and moving into the normal tissue surrounding the pigment.

I have found the following regime far more beneficial for my patients than the use of laser treatments for melasma. Patients are prescribed a tretinoin cream of a strength best suited to their skin type to be applied in the morning followed by a broad spectrum sunscreen. Prior to bed, they are advised to apply a cream containing an alpha hydroxy acid, specifically glycolic acid, with kojic acid or hydroquinone. The combined use of tretinoin, alpha hydroxy acids, and hydroquinone or kojic acid has a synergistic effect. If the patient is not improving with this regime after six months, a chemical peel is the next alternative used prior to laser therapy. The results of a chemical peel are generally more reliable and cost effective for the patient.

**Figure 3-9 A, B**
Melasma: cheek, caucasian female, Q-switched ruby laser.

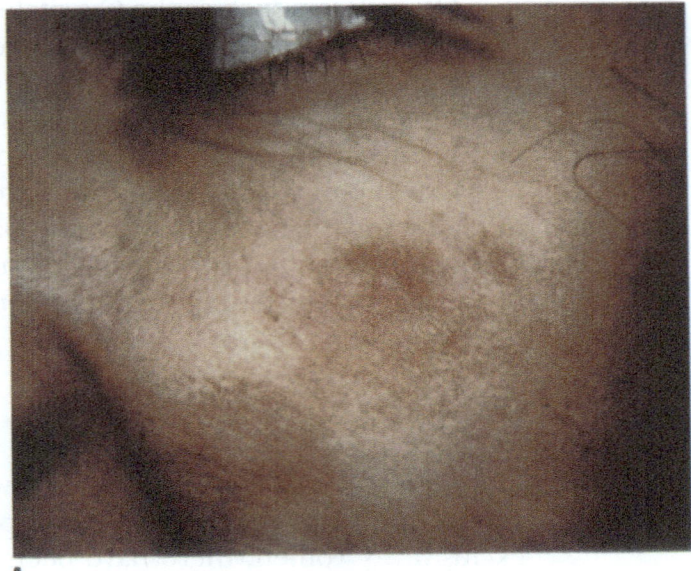

A

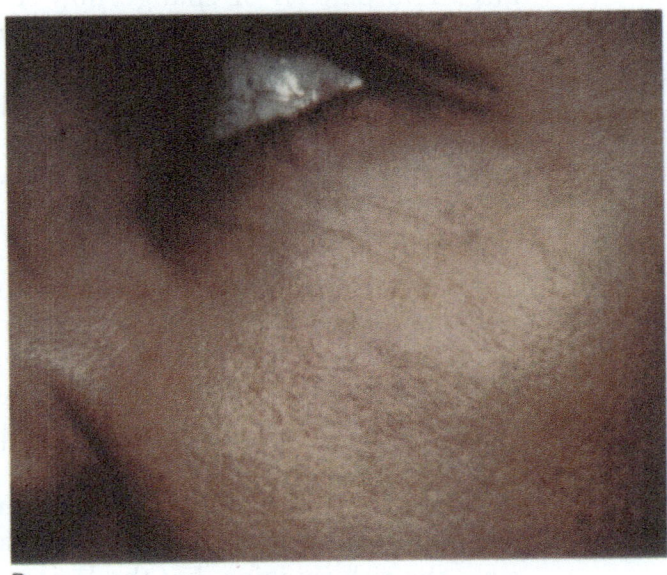

B

I use a Jessner 35% trichloroacetic acid peel or in some cases a series of glycolic acid washes.

## Solar Keratoses

Solar or actinic keratoses are erythematous, scaly lesions which are generally less than 1 cm in diameter. They commonly are found on the skin of fair-skinned individuals in regions that have been exposed to sunlight over long periods of time, most commonly the back of the hands, the face, and the ears. Generally, more than one lesion is present, and it is more often seen in elderly populations, although cases have been reported in young adults in regions where the sun is intense [9, 11].

Solar keratoses are characterized by an atypical squamous cell configuration, which has a tendency to evolve into squamous cell cancer in an estimated 20% of patients with these lesions [9]. Therefore, any lesion that appears visually atypical, that is large and indurated, should be biopsied prior to proceeding with therapy. It is my experience that excision or vaporization with a $CO_2$ laser followed by curettage are both acceptable means of removing a cancerous lesion. However, it is important that adequate tissue be removed beyond the border of the cancer to ensure that unobserved cancerous cells are eliminated. Furthermore, close follow-up must be maintained. As with any treatment modality, aggressive carcinomas may spread distally beyond the surgical site despite the surgeon's efforts to completely eradicate the tumor.

Although most people seek therapy due to concerns over the precancerous nature of the lesions, they are also pleased to have them removed because of their cosmetically unappealing appearance.

In our example, a 65-year-old caucasian male presented with several solar keratoses on the dorsum of his hands (Figure 3-10 A–B). The area was first locally infiltrated with 1% xylocaine with epinepherine. The ultrapulsed $CO_2$ laser was used at 300 millijoules, 60 ms pulse width and 12 pulses per second to vaporize these lesions. A double pass over the keratoses was made. The lesion turned white and the debris was wiped away with a saline soaked gauze. The underlying skin had a chamois-like appearance. Crusting was sloughed off after ten days. The skin was pink for several months after surgery.

Other surgical options include excision, curettage, and cryotherapy. Of these alternatives, curettage is the better of the three. Excision leaves an unnecessary scar, and cryotherapy bears the risk of hypopigmentation. For cosmetic purposes, the laser is probably the best surgical alternative.

Chemical ablation may also be used. The patient applies a topical preparation of 5% fluorouracil solution (Efudex™ cream) twice daily over the entire sun-damaged area for a period of two to three weeks, depending on the extent of the lesion. The advantage of this method is that precancerous areas that are not visually evident are covered by the treatment. The disadvantage is that irritation and al-

**Figure 3-10 A, B**
Solar keratoses: hands, caucàsian male ultrapulsed $CO_2$ laser.

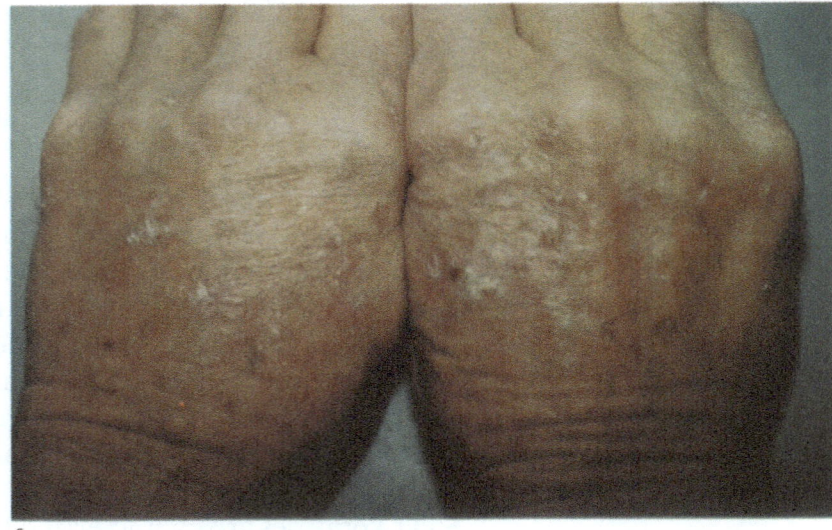

A

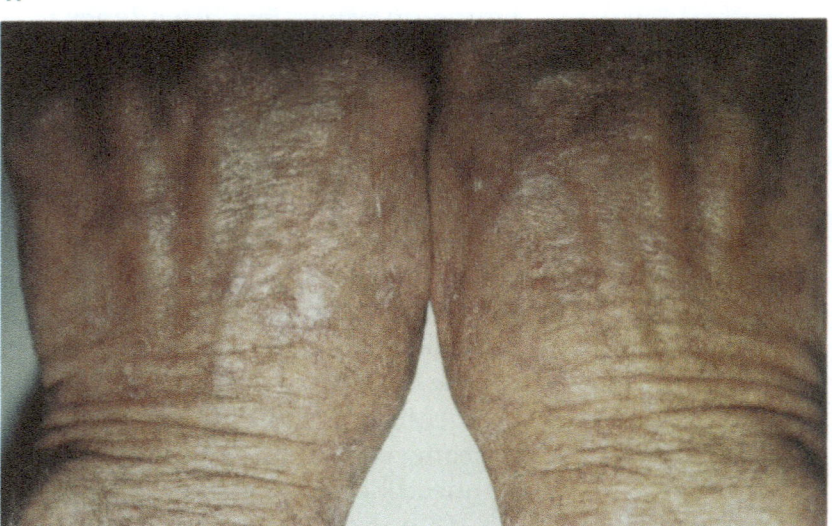

B

lergic reactions are frequent and thicker lesions do not respond to this therapy. Chemical peels using trichloroacetic acid are an alternative form of chemical ablation and are effective for more superficial lesions. Thicker lesions are best treated by vaporization with a $CO_2$ laser. With the advent of the ultrapulsed $CO_2$ laser and its accompanying computerized scanning technology, solar keratoses and sun-damaged skin may be resurfaced in a controlled manner. Resurfacing not only eradicates the solar keratoses but also diminishes other signs of photo injury, including texture and pigment changes. [12, 13]

## Solar Cheilitis

Solar cheilitis, or leukoplakia, is essentially solar keratosis of the lower lip. Atypical epidermal cells are located in the squamous mucosa of the vermilion border of the lip. This area tends to get a lot of un-protected sun exposure in individuals who work out of doors, such as farmers. The signs of solar cheilitis may include chronically chapped lips, cracking, bleeding, and/or a thick leathery texture [13]. The normally pink lip is usually overlaid with a layer of white or brown discoloration. As with solar keratoses, it is prudent to perform a biopsy prior to proceeding with surgical laser therapy [14].

Our example is that of a 57-year-old male farmer (Figure 3-11 A–B). A combination of a bimental nerve block and local infiltration with 1% xylocaine with epinephrine was used to anesthetize the area. The expansion from the infiltration helps to stretch out the creases in the lip. Wet gauze was placed between the lower lip and the teeth in order to keep the lip extended during surgery. Using the ultrapulsed $CO_2$ laser without the computerized scanner, the following parameters were selected: an energy setting of 300 millijoules/pulse, a pulse width of 60 ms at 12 pulses/second and a spot size of 3 mm. Two passes were made over the entire lower lip in a similar fashion

**Figure 3-11 A, B**
Solar cheilitis (leukoplakia): lower lip, caucasian male, ultrapulsed $CO_2$ laser.

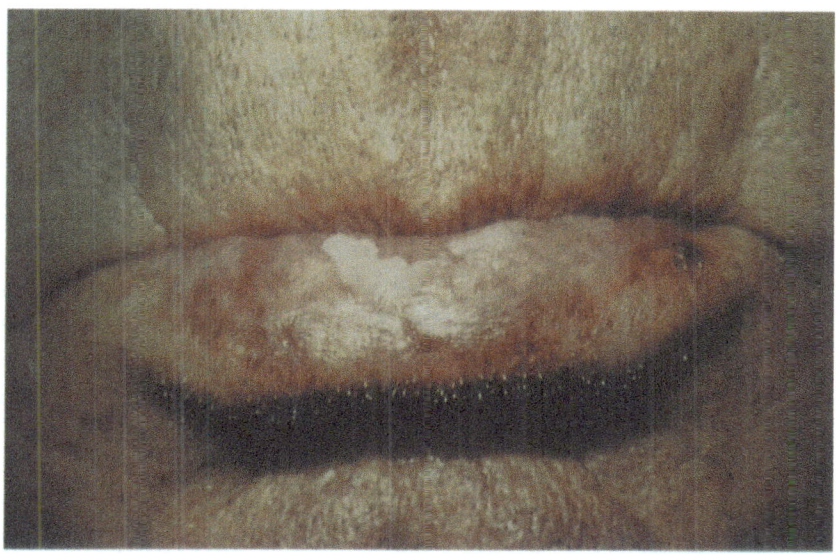

A

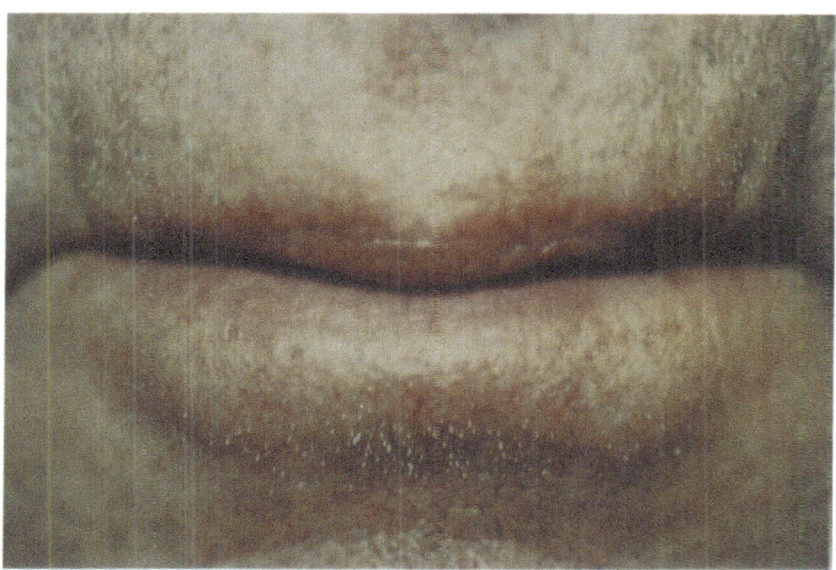

B

to a wash on a water-color painting. The mucosa turned white and was largely char free. This film of debris was wiped away with gauze soaked in saline. Saline is preferable to hydrogen peroxide (the latter causes a stark white discoloration, making observation of the tissue response to the laser difficult). The remaining submucosal tissue is pink in appearance, as compared to the skin which is chamois-like in appearance after a similar treatment with the laser. Following the surgery, the patient will experience a period of crusting, which will slough within seven to twenty-one days. The complications are few with this procedure, and the cosmetic results are excellent. Recurrence is rare.

I prefer to use the handpiece rather than the computerized scanner in this procedure, because at the vermilion cutaneous junction a more sharply defined border can be achieved. Solar cheilitis is often thicker in some areas than others. Therefore, by using the handpiece, I am able to pulse more than once over those areas where more depth is required. If the computerized scanner is used, I select the following parameters: 300 millijoules, 100 watts, 2.5 mm spot size, pattern 14, density of 7. In a similar manner to the free-hand application of the laser light, I make two passes over the lower lip unless the keratosis is very thick.

A continuous wave $CO_2$ laser may also be used to treat solar cheilitis effectively, which can take up to eight weeks to heal. The ultrapulsed laser offers high pulsed energy and a short pulse width. Therefore, better control is achieved, and there is less risk of thermal damage. Some clinicians have reported that healing time is reduced on average to two weeks. I find, however, that it takes closer to three or four weeks before the healing process is complete. This, however, is variable depending on the depth of surgery. The healing process may take one week or, in some cases, up to five weeks.

Other treatment alternatives for solar cheilitis, including topical application of 5% fluorouracil, vermilionectomy with an advanced mucosal flap, cryotherapy, and electrodesiccation, have lost their appeal, because treatment with the $CO_2$ laser is superior in terms of cosmetic result, speed of recovery, fewer complications, and rate of recurrence [13, 14, 15].

## Seborrheic Keratoses

Seborrheic keratoses are superficial lesions of the skin that tend to appear in the fifth decade in life, particularly in the caucasian population. These raised lesions combined with an oval and circumscribed border give the impression that the lesion is stuck to the skin. Ranging in size from a millimeter to several centimeters, these lesions often appear in crops and increase in number with advancing age. The distinguishing features of these lesions are the fine, patterned fissures and keratotic plugs around the follicular openings of the lesion. This gives the surface of the lesion an uneven wart-like or verruca appearance. Seborrheic keratoses present with varying shades of brown discoloration, and the surface is dull due to a layer of greasy keratin on the surface. Although they may appear on any part of the body, they are most common on the torso and the face. In some cases, the seborrheic keratoses may become pedunculated. When irritated, these lesions become inflamed and itchy and may be accompanied by bleeding, swelling, and crusting [8, 9].

Biopsies confirming the presence of immature keratinocytes in the epidermis are valuable for distinguishing these lesions from others, which based on clinical examination alone may present a similar appearance. These lesions are not precancerous [8, 9].

For multiple lesions on the torso, the spots are anesthetized with 1% xylocaine with epinepherine, and the lesions are removed with cryotherapy, curettage, or laser surgery with a $CO_2$ laser. I have had excellent results using a continuous wave $CO_2$ laser at 20 watts of energy in a defocused mode, manually pulsing the beam with a foot pedal. This creates enough heat to encourage a separation between the seborrheic keratoses and the underlying dermis. A light gray, raised edematous appearance occurs after pulsing over the lesion. Generally, the lesion will wipe off with a saline-soaked gauze, although in some cases, it may need to be gently curetted to ease it away from the underlying skin.

Our example is that of a seborrheic keratosis that was removed using an ultrapulsed $CO_2$ laser where the amount of heat transference is controlled and the lesion was simply vaporized away (Figure 3-12 A–B). This 80-year-old caucasian female presented with a single seborrheic keratosis over her right eyelid. A biopsy confirmed that there was no abnormal pathology, however, the woman wanted the lesion removed for cosmetic reasons. The area was infiltrated with 1% xylocaine with epinepherine. The parameters using the ultrapulsed $CO_2$ laser with the computerized scanner were: 300 millijoules, 100 watts, 2.5 mm spot size, and a density of 7. Utilizing a large hexagon pattern number, the seborrheic keratosis was vaporized with overlapping pulses applied in a continuous field. Three passes were made over the entire area, with an additional six passes over thicker areas. The resulting debris was removed with a saline-soaked gauze, and the underlying normal pink dermal skin was noted. It took approximately ten days for the post-surgical crusting to slough and four months for the residual erythema to fade.

If the lesions are superficial and darkly pigmented, the Q-switched ruby, Nd:YAG, or Alexandrite lasers or the flash lamp-pumped pulsed pigmented dye laser can be used. A higher density such as 9 joules/$cm^2$ is required when treating seborrheic keratosis with a Q-switched ruby laser as compared to the treatment of a solar lentigo at 4 joules/$cm^2$. When a seborrheic keratosis is superficial, it can be difficult to distinguish clinically from a solar lentigo which is flat. Even so, it does require a higher fluence to remove the keratotic lesion with a Q-switched laser successfully, and in thicker areas, overlapped pulses to the same area may be necessary.

**Figure 3-12 A, B**
Seborrheic keratosis: eyelid, caucasian
female, ultrapulsed $CO_2$ laser

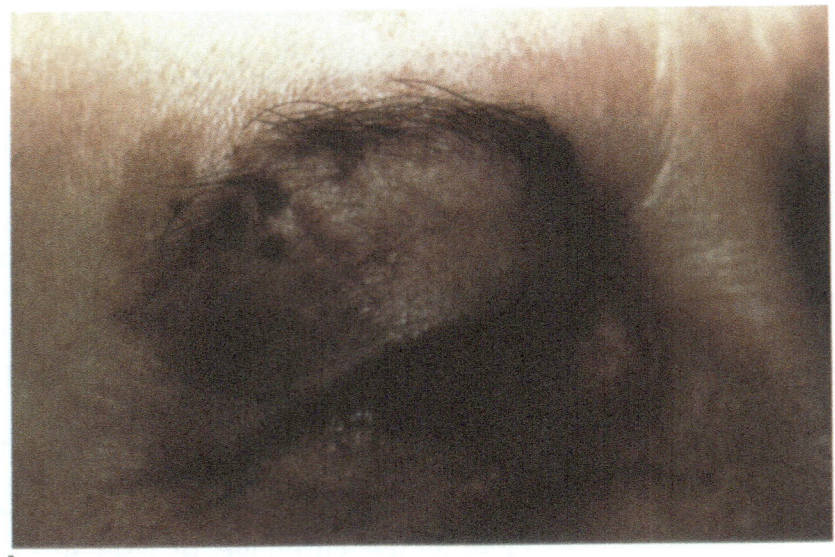

A

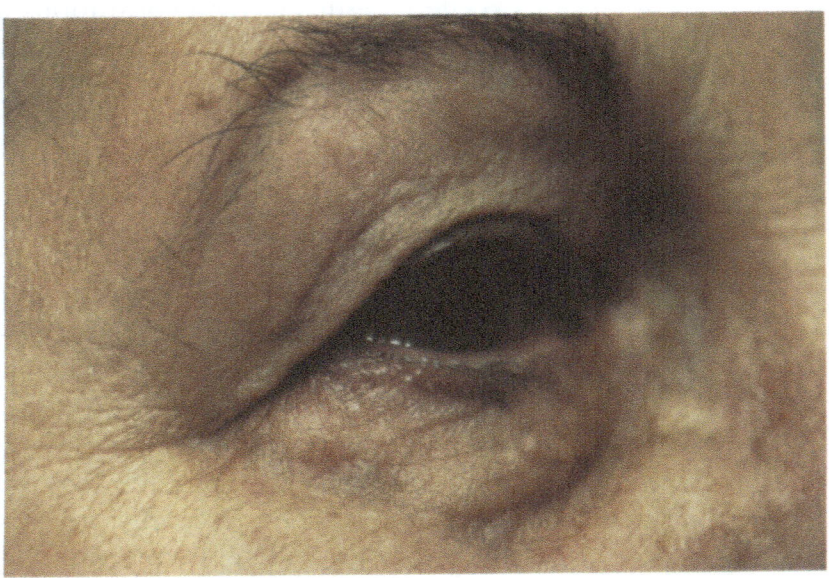

B

The advantages of laser surgery over cryotherapy or curettage
are that there is more control and the results are more predictable.

### Postinflammatory Hyperpigmentation

Postinflammatory hyperpigmentation is self-explanatory. An increase
of pigment occurs following an episode of inflammation, resulting in
a patch that varies in color from light to dark brown. The hyperpigmented area tends to follow the pattern of the inflamed area, although the margins tend to be indistinct. This reaction is more common in darker skinned individuals [4].

This 57-year-old caucasian female developed postinflammatory
hyperpigmentation after the use of cryotherapy for the treatment of
lentigines (Figure 3-13 A–B). The initial preferred course of treat-

**Figure 3-13 A, B**
Postinflammatory (cryotherapy) hyper-pigmentation: cheek, caucasian female, Q-switched ruby laser.

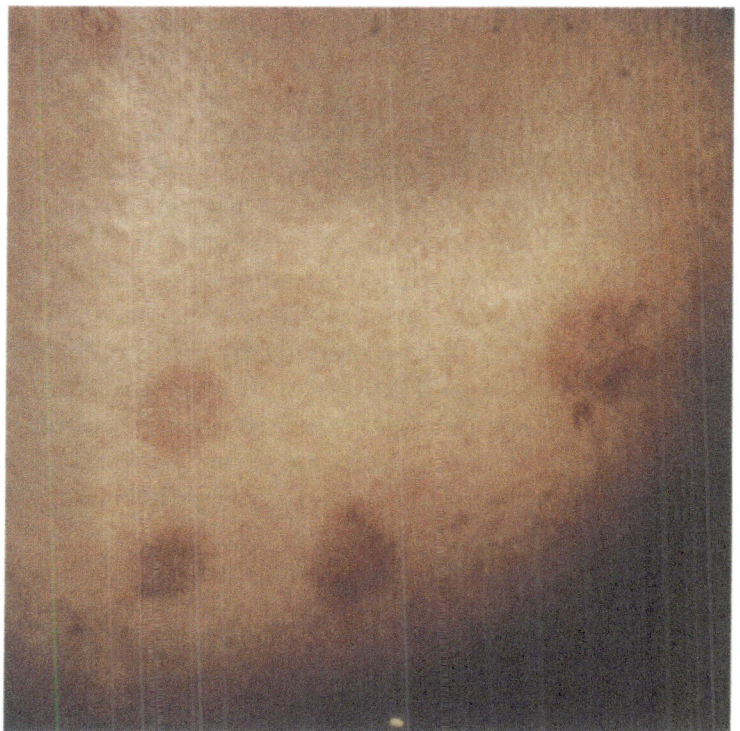

A

B

ment for postinflammatory hyperpigmentation is the regular alternating application of tretinoin and 2 to 4% hydroquinone or kojic acid with or without glycolic acid, along with the diligent use of a broad spectrum sunscreen. Some patients, however, are resistant to this form of therapy, as was the case with this patient. Therefore, we opted to try the Q-switched ruby laser. One session at 4 joules/cm² was adequate to eradicate the lesion. It is important to advise all patients who are treated for pigmentary problems to use a broad spectrum sunscreen after treatment for a prolonged period of time.

Post-traumatic hyperpigmentation occurred on the face of a 27-year-old caucasian female following an abrasion caused by a fall on artificial turf during a sports match (Figure 3-14 A–B). One session was required using the Q-switched ruby laser at 6 joules/cm² to remove the melanin from the traumatized site.

Sclerotherapy for leg veins may cause a unique postinflammatory hyperpigmentation of the skin due to a combination of hemosiderin and melanin. In many cases, this reaction responds well to treatment with the Q-switched lasers.

**Figure 3-14 A, B**
Postinflammatory (trauma-induced) hyperpigmentation: cheek, caucasian female, Q-switched ruby laser.

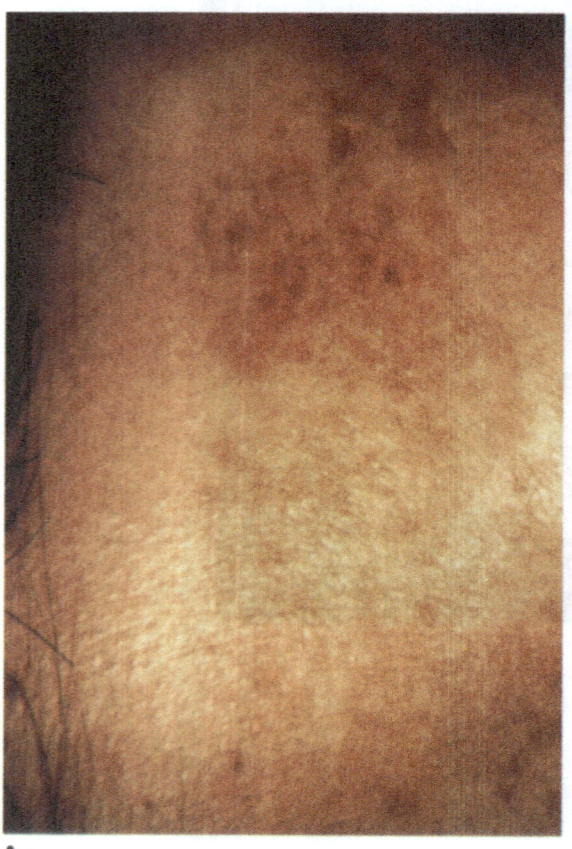

A

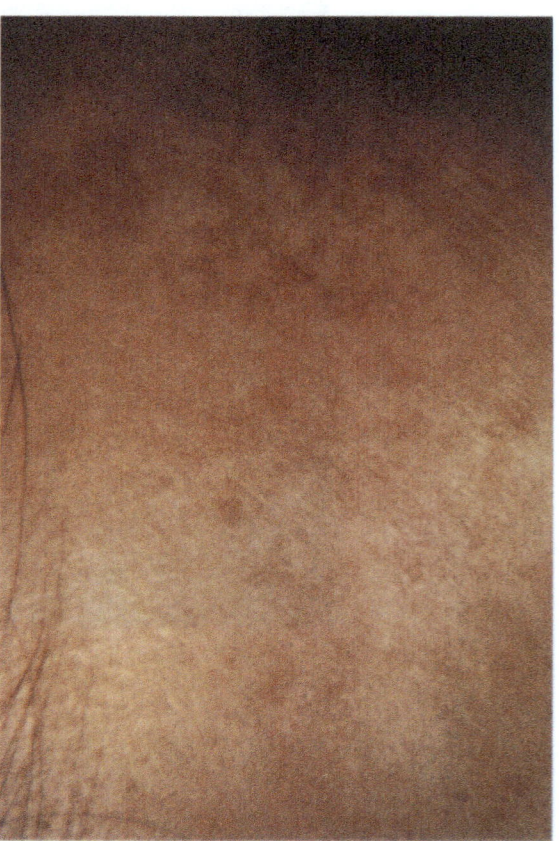

B

## Epidermal Nevus

Epidermal nevus, also referred to a cutaneous epithelial nevi or verrucous nevi, is a papillomatous, hyperkerotic, acanthotic papule [10]. These lesions may be present at birth or may appear in childhood or early adulthood. They may be located anywhere on the body but are commonly found on the torso and limbs. Their shape may vary depending on where they are located. For example, they may be linear on the limbs and oval on the torso of the body. The lesions vary in color from a skin tone to a yellowish brown hue. At first they tend to be flat and velvety in texture, transforming into raised, granular papules with a verruca-like appearance. These lesions are generally asymptomatic when they are isolated, but in larger numbers, they may be indicative of skeletal or central nervous system disorders [10, 17]. Epidermal lesions originate from the dermis, which is probably why it is so difficult to remove them surgically without some disturbance to the dermis [17].

Our example is that of an 18-year-old caucasian male with a congenital epidermal nevus on the left thigh (Figure 3-15 A–B) It is necessary that a biopsy be performed on these lesions, because although they are generally removed for cosmetic purposes, a variety of benign or malignant tumor formations may develop within the lesion. There is a trade-off between the lesion and the potential for hypopigmentation, depigmentation, or scar at the site. For this reason, a test site is particulary useful to confirm that a cosmetically acceptable result is possible. The area was locally infiltrated with 1% xylocaine with epinephrine. After shaving the elevated portion flush to the skin with a scalpel, a continuous wave $CO_2$ laser was used at 20 watts in a defocused mode combined with gentle curetting. The laser beam was delivered in a pulsed fashion by manually tapping the foot pedal. Saline-soaked gauzes were used to constantly wipe away the char in order to observe the laser's progress. When the chamois-like color of underlying skin appeared, surgery was terminated to minimize the likelihood of an unacceptable scar, even if some residual pigment remained visible. The surgical site was covered with a topical antibiotic such as Bactroban™ or Fucidin™ ointment and covered with a dressing. The patient was instructed to remove the dressing and to wash the treatment site with lukewarm water and a mild soap such a Neutrogena™. In addition, the patient was told to reapply the topical antibiotic after cleansing the site twice daily for a period of one week. Further occlusion with a dressing was not necessary. The treatment site re-epithelialized within three months.

Because an epidermal nevus may have various components, such as the involvement of sebaceous glands, it often has invaginations penetrating deep into the dermis. Therefore, removal of the entire lesion without scar formation is a challenge.

An ultrapulsed $CO_2$ would have been a better choice for the removal of these lesions rather than a continuous wave $CO_2$ laser because of the limited thermal damage that results from the controlled

**Figure 3-15 A, B**
Epidermal nevus (test site): thigh, caucasian male, continuous wave $CO_2$ laser.

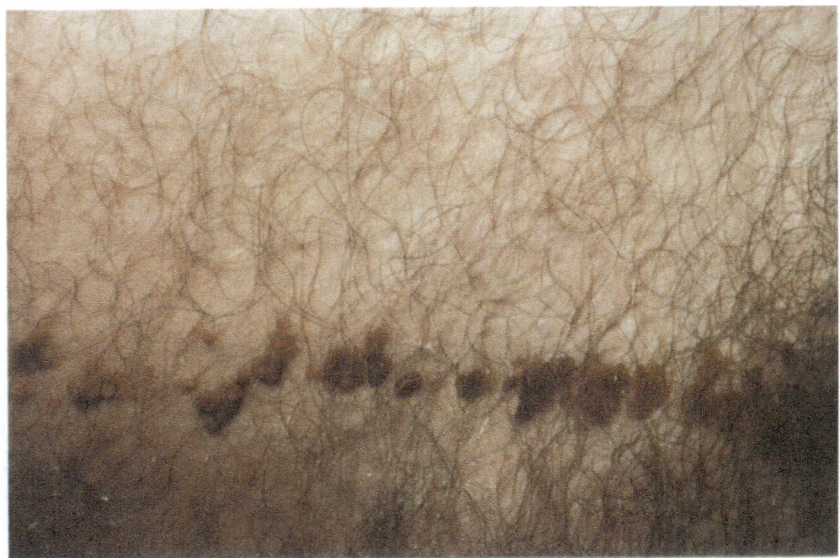

A

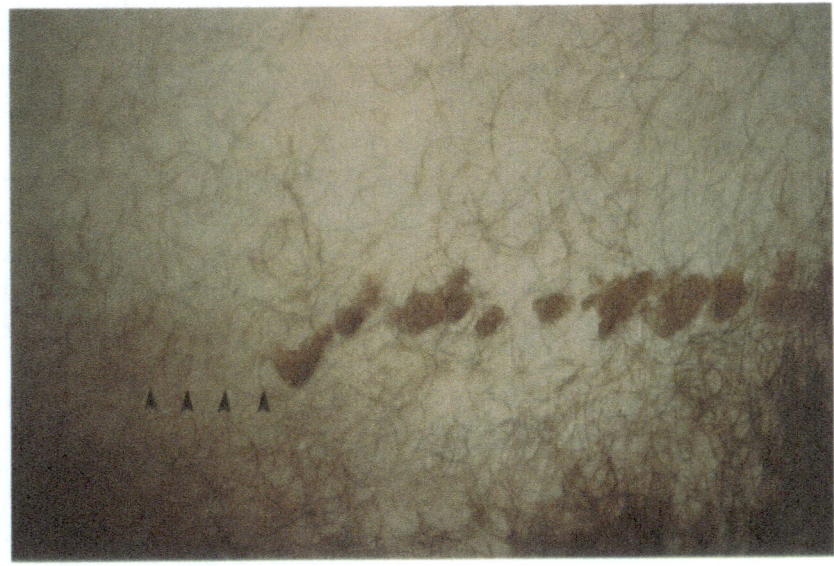

B

delivery of shorter pulse duration times. Thus, the risk of scarring and hypopigmentation is reduced. If the epidermal lesion is linear, a simple excision provides acceptable results.

Another alternative for the treatment of deep pigmented epidermal nevi is the Q-switched Nd:YAG laser set at 12 joules/cm$^2$. Three to six sessions are usually required to completely eradicate the lesions with minimal dyschromic and texture change.

## Benign Melanocytic Nevus

Benign melanocytic nevi vary in appearance, but the common characteristic which classifies them as nevi is the clustering of melanocytes at different levels of the skin with no dendritic processes [10]. Benign melanocytic nevi may be found anywhere on the skin or the mucous membranes. They appear in childhood, increase in adolescence, and plateau during the adult years. Unlike congenital melanocytic nevi, acquired nevi are usually less than 1.5 cm in diameter. The three most common classifications of benign melanocytic nevus are junctional, compound, and intradermal. Two unique variants have been identified and are known as congenital melanocytic nevi and spitz nevi.

### Junctional Nevus

Junctional nevi are usually flat, pigmented lesions with a smooth surface. The color of each lesion may vary from light to dark brown. The color of any given lesion may be dark in the center, fading toward the edges. Melanocytic cells gather in clusters at the junction of the epidermis and the dermis. These lesions are generally only found in children, as they represent the early stages of compound nevi. The exception is their occurrence on the palms of the hands, soles of the feet, and genitalia. In these cases, they may be found in all ages [10, 17].

### Compound Nevus

Compound nevi are raised, pigmented lesions. Some are papillomatous. Circular or elliptical in shape, the most common type rises gently from the borders of the lesion to a central pinnacle. These lesions often become darker and thicker and may increase in number over time. The color at the margins has an indistinct smeared appearance, which is lighter than the center of the lesion. Melanocytic cells are found in the basal layer of the epidermis and dermis [10, 17].

The 43-year-old caucasian male in our example had two benign compound melanocytic nevi on the forehead (Figure 3-16 A–B). The nevi were removed with the Q-switched ruby laser at a fluence of 9 joules/cm$^2$. Residual pigment after the first session was successfully removed with one more treatment. The advantage of the Q-switched ruby laser is that it seldom leaves a scar, although the potential

**Figure 3-16 A, B**
Melanocytic nevi: forehead, caucasian
male, Q-switched ruby laser.

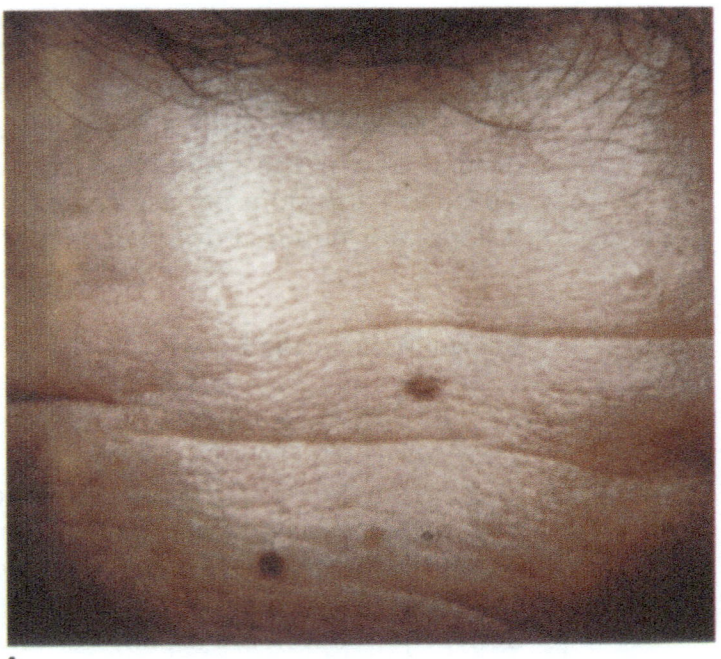

A

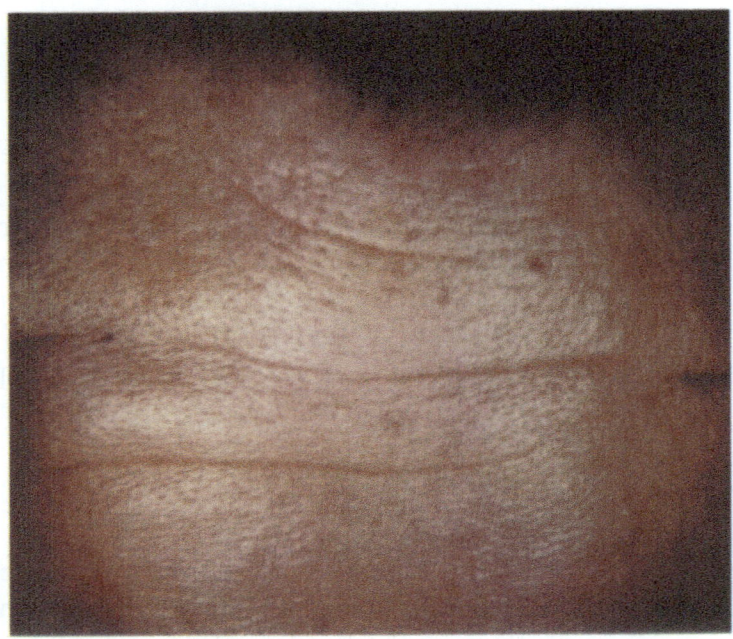

B

for hypopigmentation exists. The Q-switched Nd:YAG laser at 12 joules/cm$^2$, three pulses per treatment area is also effective. Excision of these lesions on the forehead would invariably result in a scar that might not be cosmetically acceptable to the patient. Given the nature of pigmented lesions, it is important to be certain clinically that the lesion is benign before proceeding with removal using a target specific laser. You are always walking a tight rope between selecting the most cosmetically acceptable means of removing a pigmented lesion and the need for pathological confirmation that it is a benign lesion. This is where clinical experience and knowledge becomes essential. The general rule for pigmented lesions is: When in doubt, get a second opinion and/or do a biopsy. The Q-switched double frequency Nd:YAG or Alexandrite lasers could also be used to remove these benign lesions. The flash lamp-pumped pulsed pigmented dye laser probably would not be able to reach the depths necessary to eradicate the dermal components of compound melanocytic nevi.

## Intradermal Nevus

Intradermal nevi vary in shape, size, and color. They may be papillomatous, domed, or pedunculated in shape. Some are smooth and others are wart-like in texture. In some cases, coarse hair grows from the center of the lesion. Generally, they have very little color, as melanocytic cells are sparse. Fat cells may or may not be present [10, 17].

The 36-year-old caucasian female in our example had an intradermal nevus removed from her face in two stages (Figure 3-17 A–B). The nevus was first outlined with permanent ink, and then the area was anesthetized with 1% xylocaine with epinephrine. Although the lesion is pigmented, ink markings demarcate the edges distorted by the local anesthetic. Using a scalpel, the raised portion of the lesion was shaved flush with the skin. Then the ultrapulsed CO$_2$ laser was used at 300 millijoules and 60 ms to resurface the lesion and feather the borders into the surrounding normal skin. The purpose here is to achieve a cosmetically acceptable result, not necessarily to reach deep into the dermis to obliterate the entire lesion. The patient was counseled that there may be islands of nevus cells below the surgical site, but that removal of the entire lesion would probably leave an unacceptable scar. As a result, the nevus may push past the surface of the skin again as time passes. After laser removal, antibiotic ointment should be applied to the treatment site to prevent infection and promote healing. As with the junctional melanocytic nevus, the Q-switched ruby laser at 9 joules/cm$^2$ was used to eradicate the deeper pigment.

## Congenital Melanocytic Nevus

One percent of children are born with a congenital melanocytic nevus. They may vary in size from 1.5 cm in diameter to lesions that cover large areas of the body and are over 20 cm in diameter. The

---

**Figure 3-17 A, B**
Benign melanocytic intradermal nevus: cheek, caucasian female, combined laser therapy with the ultrapulsed CO₂ laser and the Q-switched ruby laser.

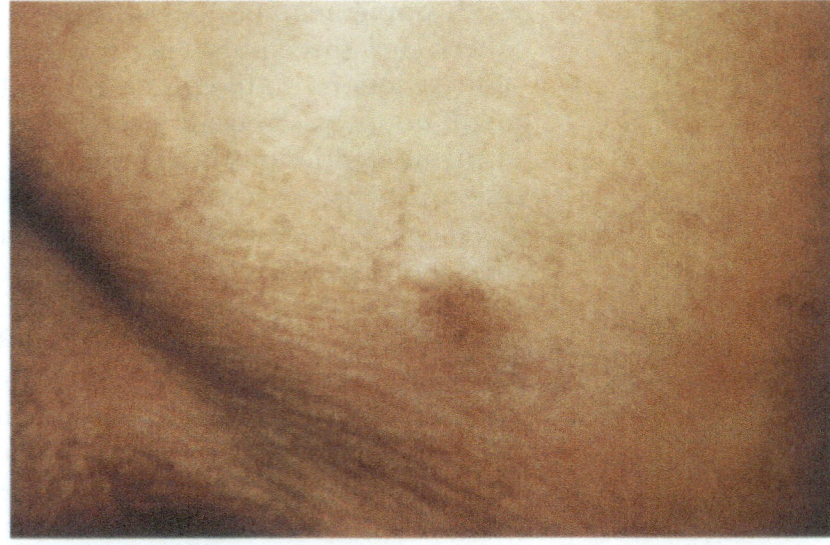

A

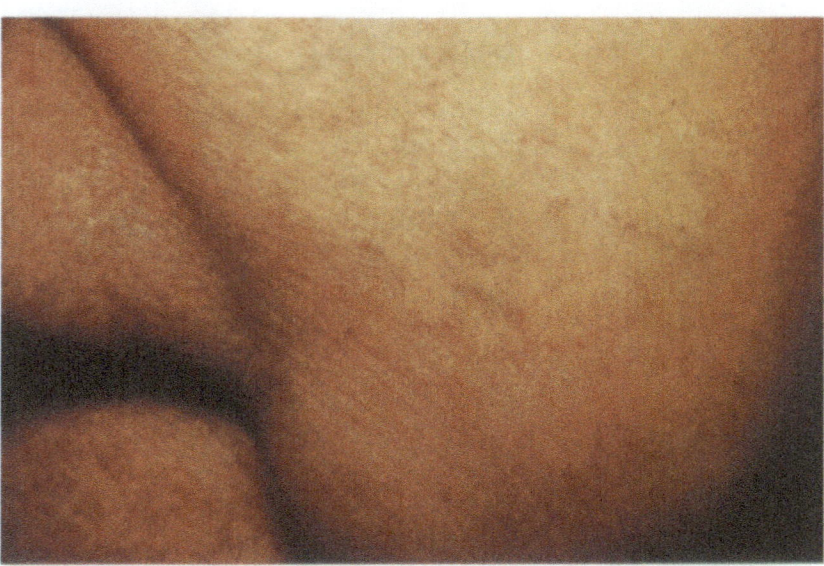

B

smaller lesions develop into malignant melanomas in less than 1% of cases, whereas the extensive lesions have an incidence of 12%. The raised lesions have a distinct irregular border. They tend to be dark brown in color and are characterized by the growth of a moderate amount of coarse dark hair. As the lesion matures, it tends to become thicker and the surface takes on a verucca-like appearance. Nodules may also develop [10, 17].

Prior to three months of age, atypical melanocytes clump together at the junction of the epidermis and dermis. As the lesion matures, clusters and columns of nevus cells reach deep into the reticular dermis and, in many cases, into the subcutaneous fat. The nevus cells may be found between the collagen bundles of the dermis, in proximity to cutaneous appendages, and within sweat ducts and glands, sebaceous glands, hair follicles, blood vessel walls, and the perineurium of nerves [10].

If the lesion is large, thick, and hairy, it usually requires some form of deep excisional removal. The particular technique will depend on the size, depth, and location of the lesion. The ultrapulsed $CO_2$ laser is generally not used to vaporize lesions with these clinical manifestations, because the depth required to eradicate them would leave an unacceptable scar. The ultrapulsed $CO_2$ laser is better used as a resurfacing tool to improve the appearance of scars from excision removal and grafting techniques. Because of the inclination for these lesions to develop into malignant melanomas, a biopsy and early removal is recommended.

Our example is that of a 24-year-old asian female who presented with a small, congenital melanocytic nevus on her upper lip (Figure 3-18 A–B). Due to the size, location, and stability of the lesion, we opted

**Figure 3-18 A, B**
Congenital melanocytic nevus: upper lip, oriental female, Q-switched ruby laser.

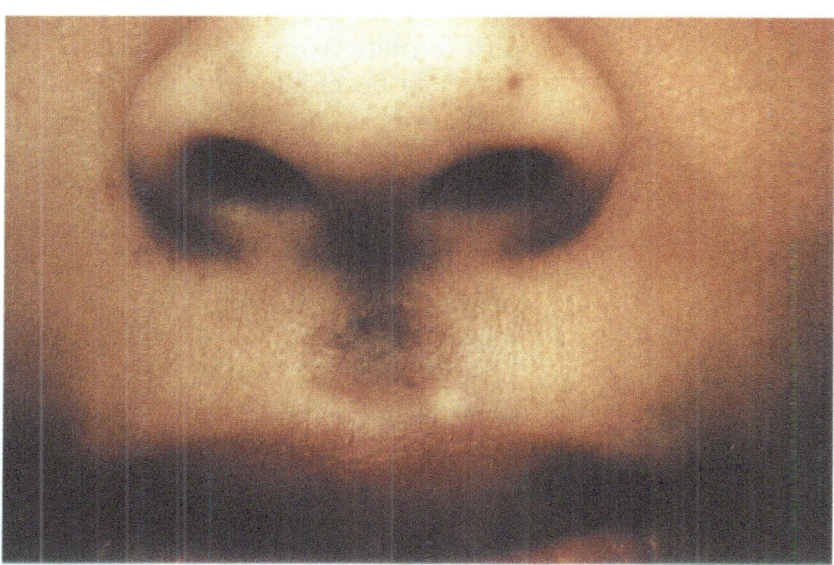

A

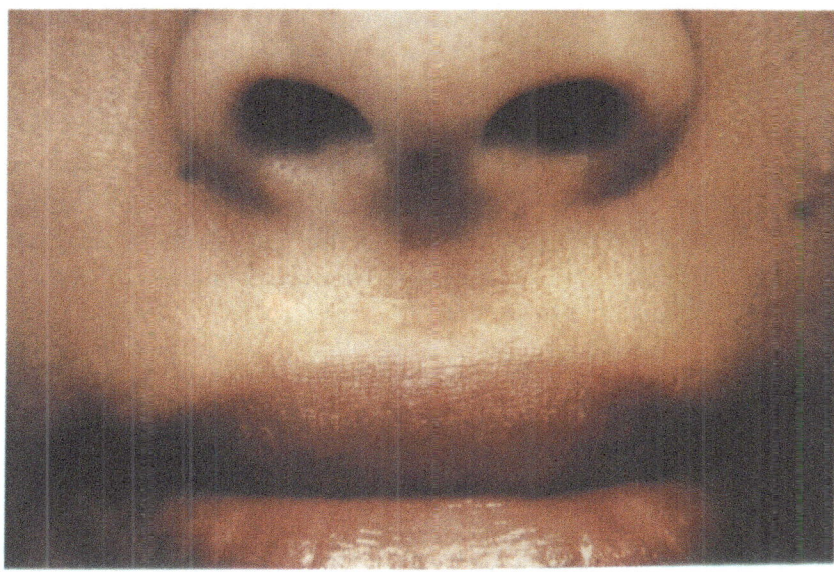

B

to remove it with the Q-switched ruby laser set at 8 joules/cm$^2$. A layer by layer removal requiring eight sessions was necessary because of the depth of the lesion. Regular follow-up visits were scheduled to watch for recurrence or any suspicious changes in the area.

### Spitz Nevus

Spitz nevus, also known as a benign juvenile melanoma or a spindle epitheloid cell nevus, generally occurs in children. However 25% of reported cases occur in adults. These dome-shaped nodular tumors are usually reddish-pink in color and less than 1 cm in size. However, they may be varying shades of brown or black and can reach 2 cm in diameter. The variation in color is due to a vascular and a pigmented component of the nevus. They tend to appear suddenly and grow rapidly. Most often they are located on the face or appendages but are not exclusive to these areas [17, 18].

Due to the variability in color and size, they can be difficult to differentiate from other lesions of the skin. Microscopic examination may also be challenging as the cellular configuration is very similar to that of a malignant melanoma. The best course of treatment is excision, followed by pathological evaluation, preferably by a dermatopathologist.

The lesion shown in our example is that of a rapidly growing, black nodular tumor located on the buttock of a four-year-old caucasian female (Figure 3-19 A–B). A general anesthetic was administered because of the necessity to keep the child still during surgery. The skin incision was made with a scalpel, as it is my experience that healing takes longer and there is a greater tendency for the development of an unacceptable scar when the laser is used to cut the skin. The KPT laser in an excisional mode at 8 watts was then used to remove the tumor. A tapered contact tip provided valuable tactile feedback. The hemostatic property of laser excision provided a clear visual field, which in this location was extremely valuable because of the number of large blood vessels in the region.

I have noted that when an excision is performed with a laser, the healing time is longer. This is probably due to the sealed blood vessels. Generally speaking, unless I feel a clear visual field is necessary or the surgery is extensive, I perform most excisions with a scalpel. The results are the same, and the healing time is less. An exception is the use of the $CO^2$ laser in a focused mode when performing laser associated blepharoplasties as swelling and bruising are substantially reduced.

**Figure 3-19 A, B**
Spitz nevus: buttock, caucasian female,
KTP laser excision

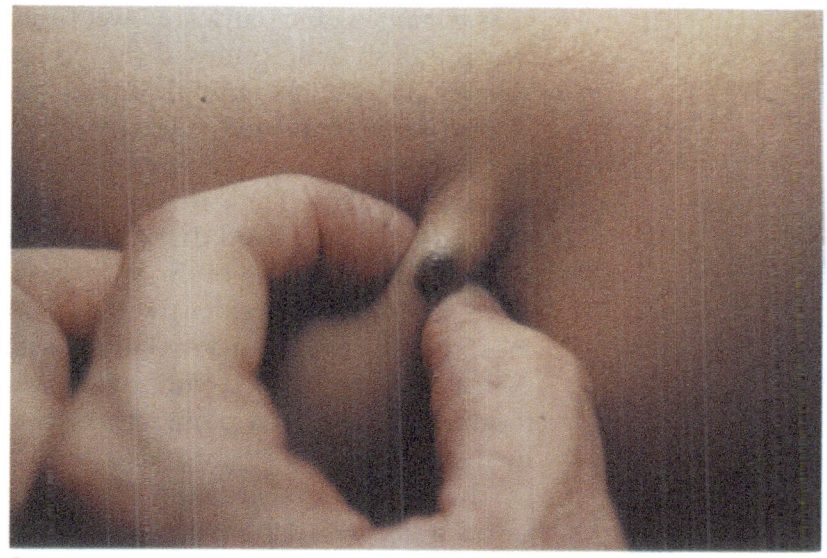

A

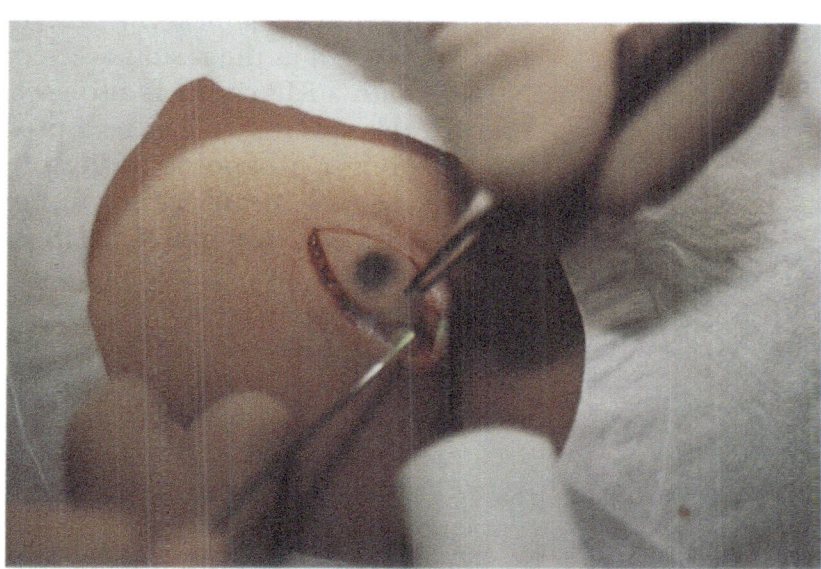

B

## Vascular Lesions

### Port Wine Hemangioma

Port wine hemangiomas, or port wine stains, are benign vascular malformations that are present at birth. They may appear on any part of the skin surface and can range in size from a few centimeters squared to large areas of the skin's surface. Port wine hemangiomas do not tend to become larger or involuted, although exceptions do occur. In some cases, a lesion may show signs of regression with time [19]. The lesion is generally flat at birth, and the color may vary from light pink to a deep burgundy shade depending on the depth and extent of the vascular malformation. As time progresses, a lesion may become darker in color and may show signs of thickening and nodularity, as a result of vascular ectasia [19]. This is commonly referred to as *vegetations*. Fitzpatrick, Lowe, Goldman, and colleagues recognized that the flash lamp-pumped pulsed vascular dye laser (577 or 585 nm wavelength, 450 ms pulse duration) was very effective in the treatment of port wine stains and, therefore, conducted a study to define prognostic factors in determining the success of dye laser treatment for hemangiomas [20]. Their findings concurred with those of several other researchers, who found that the number of treatment sessions affected the ultimate outcome of the surgery. The greater the number of treatment sessions, the greater the resolution of the problem. However, the most significant response occurred with the first treatment session, and the returns diminished with further sessions [23, 24, 25, 26, 27]. I have found that there is a point at which the lesion reaches a plateau and further treatment sessions with the flash lamp-pumped pulsed vascular dye laser are of no avail. In these instances, I have used two other vascular lasers to achieve deeper penetration and therefore greater resolution of the problem. The Versapulse™ variable pulse width (VPW) vascular laser at 9.5 joules/cm², 10 msec and 4mm spotsize is the laser I use most often as the results are very reliable. The double frequency Nd:YAG with a KIP crystal is also useful for this purpose although the thermal relaxation time can be a problem.

Color is a prognostic indicator in the treatment of port wine stains. Lesions that are lighter in hue tend to demonstrate a better response to laser removal than those that are darker [2, 20, 23]. I have found that purple lesions rather than pink port wine stains are more responsive to treatment.

The depth of the lesion is also a factor in determining the success of therapy. For example, it is easier to predict excellent results when the port wine stain is superficial and nodular, even though more treatment sessions may be required than if the lesion is deep and flat [20]. The flash lamp-pumped pulsed dye laser is not always powerful enough to penetrate through the layers of blood vessels of nodular lesions. In this case, I use the VPW green 532 nm Nd:YAG laser, the double frequency Nd:YAG with a KTP crystal laser, or the ultrapulsed $CO_2$ laser to pare down the nodularity. Then, I proceed with treatments using the flash lamp-pumped pulsed dye laser.

Darker skinned individuals do not respond as quickly to treatments with the flash lamp-pumped pulsed dye laser as their fair-skinned counterparts. Fitzpatrick et al. postulated that this was due to the fact that the capillary malformations must compete with the epidermal melanin of darker skinned individuals for absorption of the light [20].

Port wine stains in children respond much better to treatment than those in adults, often requiring fewer treatment sessions [20, 21, 23, 25]. There are, however, exceptions. The treatment sessions required for children may be more than anticipated because of the progressive growth and ectasia of residual blood vessels following each treatment [18].

The location of the lesion on the body is also an important factor in prognosis. The extremities are not as responsive to treatment as the head, neck, and trunk of the body. The farther the lesion is away from the core of the body the greater the likelihood of a poor response or certainly the need for more treatment sessions [20]. I find this particularly the case with vascular lesions, including port wine hemangiomas, on the legs and have assumed that this is because of hydrostatic pressure.

The woman in our first example is a 46-year-old caucasian with a deep, flat dermal port wine stain on her right cheek (Figure 3-20 A–B). She received seven treatment sessions with the flash lamp-pumped pulsed vascular dye laser at 4 joules/cm$^2$. As can be seen, her response is incomplete. After each treatment session she endured a period of deep purple purpura, which faded over a period of ten days.

I have had good results using the VPW pulsed Nd:YAG laser at 532 nm at 10 ms with a number of adult port wine hemangiomas where a plateau has been reached using the flash lamp-pumped pulsed dye laser. The VPW green Nd:YAG laser often breaks through this recalcitrant erythema and further lightens the port wine hemangioma. The addition of a chilled tip to this laser helps to extend

**Figure 3-20 A, B**
Port wine hemangioma: cheek, caucasian female, flash lamp-pumped pulsed vascular dye laser

A

B

the TRT of the tissue and protects the more superficial layers of the skin, particularly the pigment. The chilled tip pumps cold water at 4°C between two lenses. The laser beam is directed through these lenses and into the skin.

Our second example is that of a 22-year-old caucasian female with a small congenital telangiectatic port wine hemangioma (Figure 3-21 A–B). She was treated solely with the VPW green Nd:YAG laser at a peak power of 250 watts, a pulse width of 5 ms, and a spot size of 4 mm. One session was necessary to remove the lesion. With vessels that are smaller, as is the case in younger port wine hemangiomas, a relatively short pulse width is most effective. However, I have found that in older port wine hemangiomas with larger vessels, a longer pulse duration, such as 10 ms, provides a better result. The visual endpoint in the treatment of small vessels is the disappearance of the vessel itself. On the other hand, with larger vessels, faint whitening or

**Figure 3-21 A, B**
Congenital telangiectatic port wine hemangioma: cheek, caucasian female, VPW green laser.

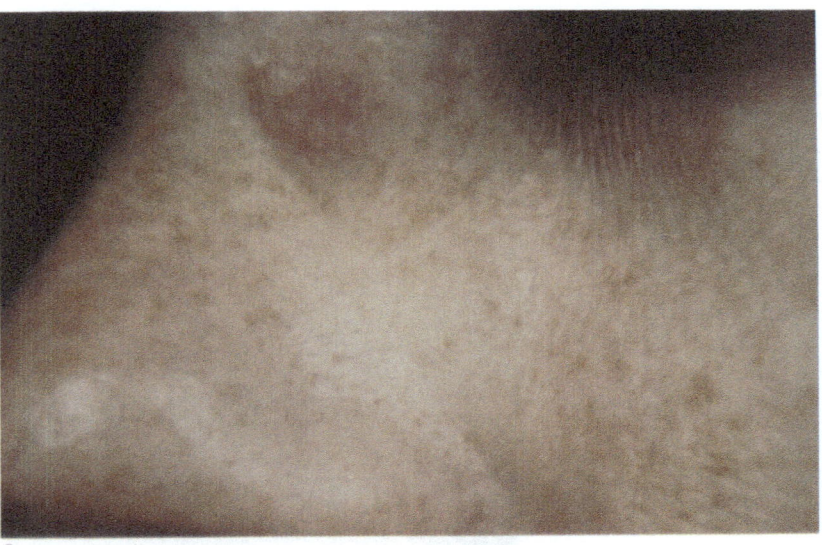

A

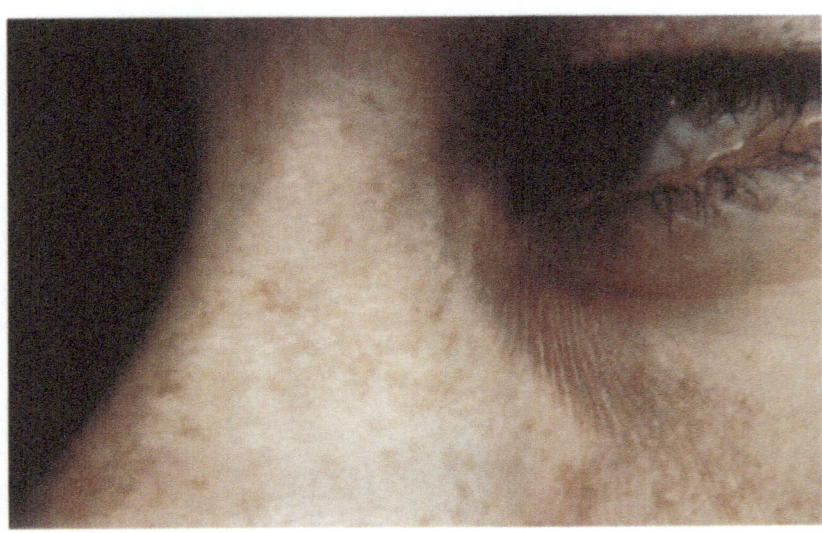

B

Chapter Three   **Treatment of Vascular and Pigmented Lesions**

graying of the tissue suggests greater thermal damage. This is necessary to eradicate larger vessels and leads to faint crusting for up to ten days. Excessive thermal damage may lead to scarring and pigment changes in exceptional circumstances.

When crusting occurs, we recommend that patients apply a topical antibiotic ointment such as Fucidin™ or Bactrobar™ until the crusting is resolved. Fitzpatrick et al. found that 51% of the patients they followed experienced crusting. This was related to the depth of color and to the level of energy emitted during treatment [20]. It is important to keep in mind that excessive crusting is associated with too much absorption of heat, which can result in pigment or texture changes and possibly scarring. I have succumbed to the seduction of higher powers to hasten the resolution of port wine hemangiomas only to be faced with the complication of hypopigmentation in some cases. The four other lasers currently being used for the treatment of port wine stains are the copper vapor, copper bromide, krypton, and Nd:YAG [2, 3].

Generally speaking, most adults tolerate the discomfort experienced with each pulse of the laser well. Children, however, usually do not tolerate discomfort and some form of anesthesia is required, either topical, sedation, or general anesthesia, depending on the location and extent of the lesion. Topical anesthetics such as EMLA™ cream are used by some laser surgeons. My experience has been that topical anesthetics, although useful in some circumstances, tend to prolong the number of treatment sessions. The fading of the port wine hemangioma is lessened because the vasoconstriction caused by the anesthetic lessens the hemoglobin available for the absorption of the laser light.


## Telangiectasia

Telangiectasia is a general term, which refers to the permanent dilation of small blood vessels, including capillaries, venules, and arterioles. They may be nodular, stellate, arborized, or linear in appearance and are varying shades of red, depending somewhat on whether or not they are venous or arterial in nature [10].

The pathogeneses of telangiectasia are many and varied. They may be due to a hereditary disposition, a systemic disorder, or exposure to environmental hazards such as radiation therapy, and sun exposure. It is important to understand the possible etiologies of telangiectasia before preceding with removal with a laser as they may provide an important diagnostic indicator of systemic disorders that need medical attention beyond the removal of an annoying cosmetic condition [10].

The flash lamp-pumped pulsed dye laser (yellow light), the double frequency Nd:YAG with a KTP crystal (green light), and the VPW green pulsed 532 nm Nd:YAG lasers are effective for the treatment of these vascular lesions. I have found that the flash lamp-pumped pulsed dye laser causes significant purpura. Although I have preferred this laser for the treatment of most vascular lesions because of its index of safety. I am using the relatively new Versapulse™ variable pulse width (VPW) green 532 nm Nd:YAG laser frequently. The KTP laser was beneficial in the past in cases where the telangiectatic vessels are very large or the patient is very sensitive about post-therapy cosmesis. However, I no longer use this laser as the VPW with the chilled tip offers the same benefits with less risk of scar hypopigmentation and less pain during the surgery.

According to Wheeland, all of the green light lasers are comparable with regard to outcome when used for the treatment of vascular lesions [3]. Wheeland suggests that by using green light lasers to remove larger vessels followed by the use of yellow laser light the best results are obtained with the least number of complications. The addition of a chilled tip to the VPW laser has significantly expanded the TRT, allowing for greater penetration and the effective treatment of fine, coarse, and coalescent vascular lesions.

Warner et al. compared the copper vapor, a green light laser, and the flash lamp-pumped pulsed dye laser for the treatment of facial telangiectasia and found the three lasers to be equivalent in their ultimate results [27]. However, the copper vapor laser was preferred because patients found it to be less painful. In addition, post-surgical healing-time was shorter and there was no purpura and less swelling. The argon tunable dye laser is also used for the treatment of facial telangiectasia. Broska et al. found that the flash lamp-pumped pulsed vascular dye laser is preferable to the argon tunable dye laser, except in cases where there are fewer telangiectasia and the patient is particularly concerned with post-surgical cosmetic disability [28]. The examples described below have different etiologies and were treated with different laser systems.

### Actinic Telangiectasia

The first example is that of a 56-year-old caucasian female with actinic telangiectasia on her cheeks as a direct result of long-term exposure to ultraviolet light (Figure 3-22 A–B). The flash lamp-pumped pulsed vascular dye laser was used at 4 joules/cm², and the problem was successfully resolved after a single treatment session.

### Diffuse Telangiectasia Due to Topical Steroids

The second example is that of a 62-year-old caucasian female with diffuse, superficial, facial telangiectasia over her entire face (Figure 3-23 A–B). This condition appeared following the long-term use of a topical steroid. As the flash lamp-pumped pulsed dye laser was not available at the time, the continuous wave $CO_2$ laser was used. To control for thermal damage, the laser beam was pulsed using the on/off mechanism of the foot pedal. To maintain a defocused mode, the wand was held at a distance of 12 inches from the skin. A blanching of the skin was sought. Following the procedure the site was very swollen for two to three days, and there was period of superficial crusting.

**Figure 3-22 A, B**
Actinic telangiectasia: cheek, caucasian female, flash lamp-pumped pulsed vascular dye laser.

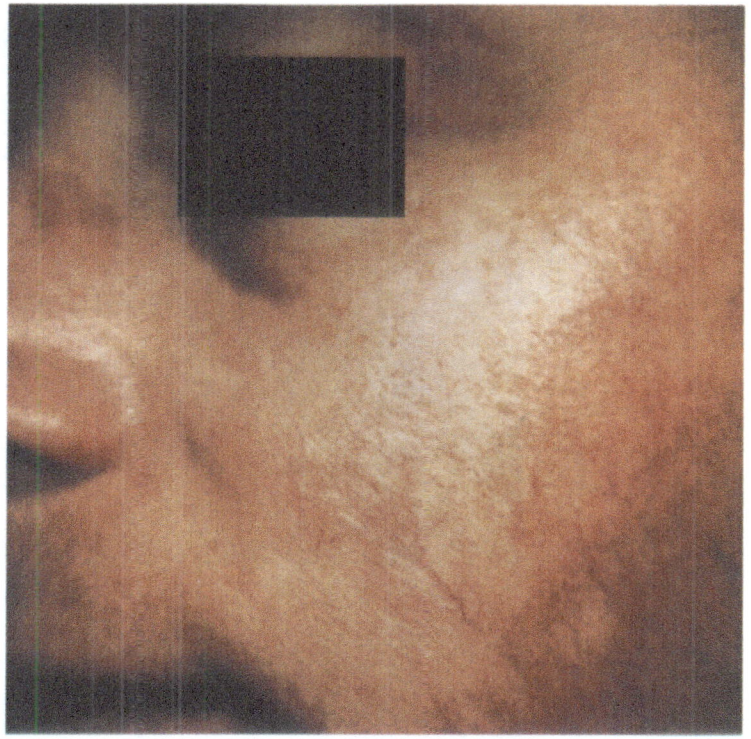

A

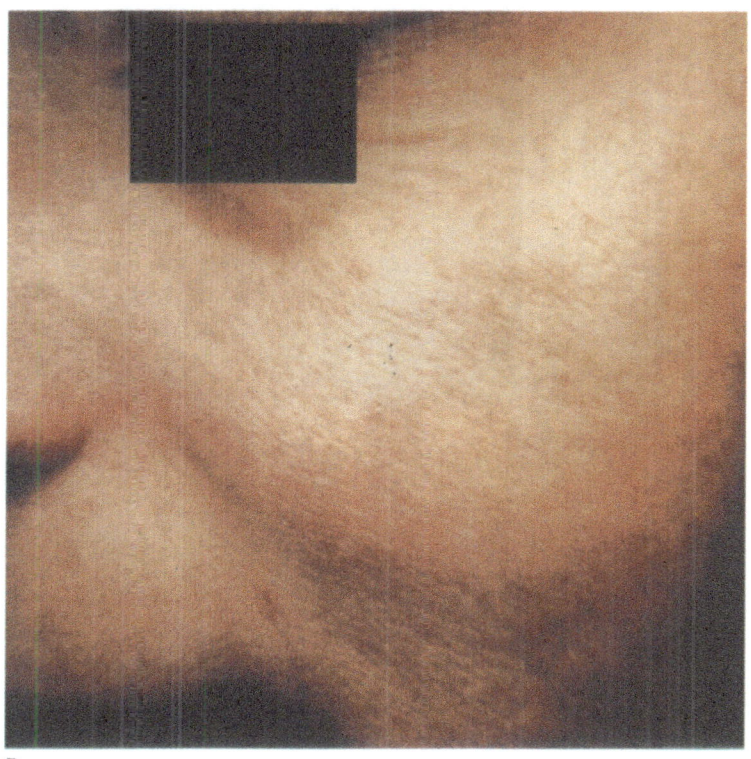

B

**Figure 3-23 A, B**
Steroid atrophy telangiectasia: cheek, caucasian female, flash lamp-pumped pulsed vascular dye laser.

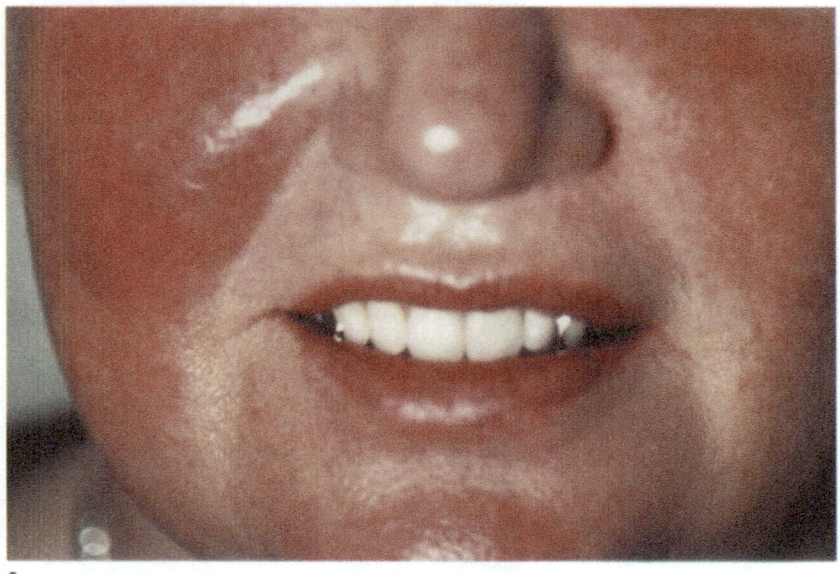

A

B

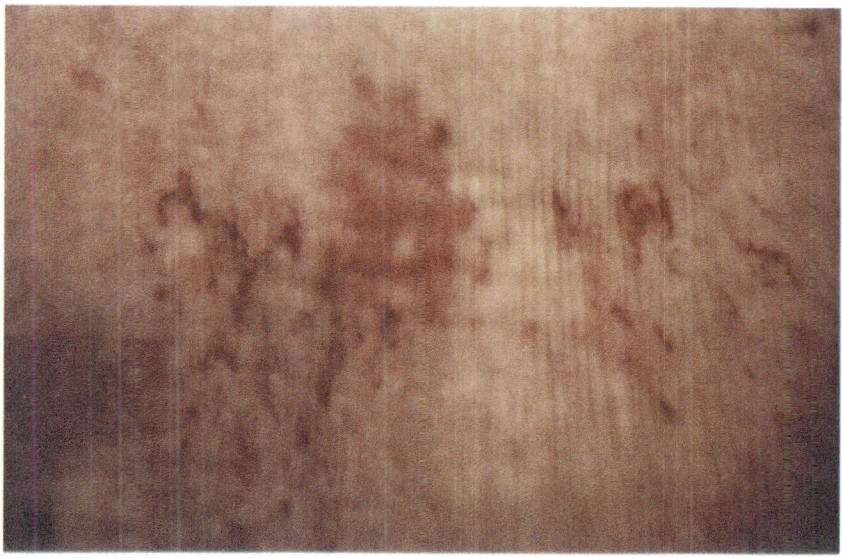

A

B

The results proved to be satisfactory. However, with the new target specific lasers such as the flash lamp-pumped pulsed dye or VPW 532 nm Nd:YAG laser, this procedure would probably now be considered risky and not indicated for fine vessels, particularly in a patient with an element of cortisone atrophy of the skin. When using the flash lamp-pumped pulsed dye laser, I use a lower power, because the skin is often so thin and fragile from the atrophy that crusting and blistering can easily occur at higher powers.

Radiation Telangiectasia

In this example, a 72-year-old caucasian female received radiation therapy following a mastectomy for the treatment of breast cancer (Figure 3-24 A–B). The post-radiation therapy on and above her breast presented her with a cosmetic problem as she was uncomfortable wearing open-neck blouses and dresses. Two treatments with the double frequency Nd:YAG with a KTP crystal laser and the computerized scanner at 12 joules/cm$^2$ improved the appearance of the telangiectasia by 75%, which was a satisfactory result for the patient. In cases of sensitive skin, such as post-radiation telangiectasia, lower fluences are preferable, even if more sessions are necessary, to remove the dilated blood vessels safely. The KTP was used to avoid the post-surgical purpura that accompanies treatment with the flash lamp-pumped pulsed vascular dye laser.

Other treatment options for telangiectasia on parts of the body other than the legs include electrodesiccation, although the results are often unpredictable. Electrodesiccation causes a higher risk of depigmentation and pitted or troughed scarring. Discomfort may be considerable.

### Telangiectasia of the Legs

Small superficial vessels on the legs have traditionally been treated with sclerosants, and in my experience, this is still the treatment of choice. However, fine blush-like vessels may respond to the flash lamp-pumped pulsed vascular dye laser, and slightly larger vessels may respond to the green light laser systems in selected instances. Larger vessels, particularly those with high hydrostatic pressure such as those in the legs, have a tendency to recanalize despite aggressive photothermal treatments with various lasers. Hypopigmentation and scar are common if excessive amounts of energy are used. I have found the use of the VPW green Nd:YAG laser with its chilled tip to be the most promising of all systems thus far, but further research is necessary.

Our example demonstrates the removal of vessels over the ankle in a 52-year-old caucasian female (Figure 3-25 A–B). She was resistant to treatment with sclerosants and the flash lamp-pumped pulsed vascular dye laser. Therefore, the KTP laser set at 2 watts and a spot size of 250 microns was pulsed at a duration of 0.1 s with 0.1 s between each pulse. One session diminished the appearance of the vessels. Postoperative pressure dressings were used to control for recanalization.

## Cherry Hemangioma

Cherry hemangiomas are bright red, benign, raised capillary lesions of the skin. They generally occur on the trunk of adults of advancing years, although they may be found on other parts of the body and in younger individuals. The lesions tend to increase in number with time and vary in size from less than a millimeter to several millimeters in diameter. They generally do not get much larger than a size of a drop of water [10]. In the early stages, these lesions tend to be an aggre-

**Figure 3-25 A, B**
Leg veins: ankle, caucasian female,
KTP laser.

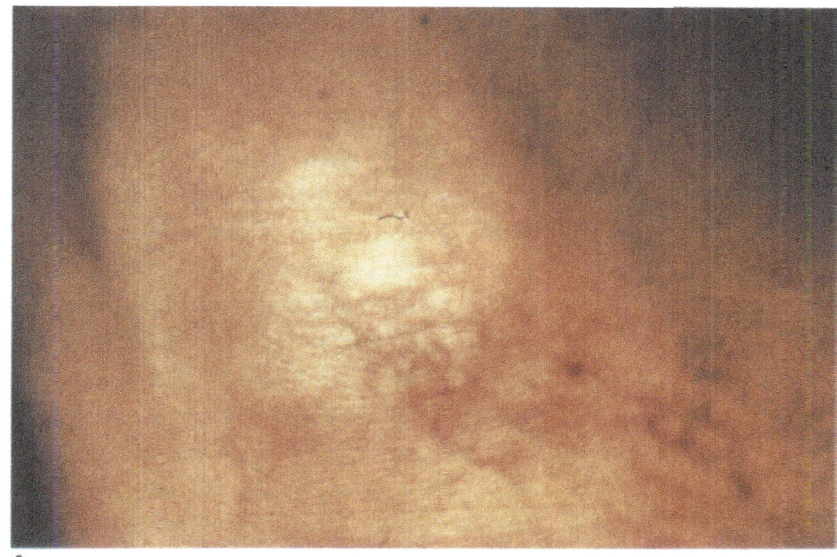

A

B

gate of newly formed capillaries which become dilated with the passage of time. A thinned epidermis wraps itself over the lesion [10].

Many individuals are not concerned with these lesions as they are often hidden under their clothing. However, in others they are cosmetically annoying, therefore they seek to have them removed. Cherry hemangiomas lend themselves very well to removal with the flash lamp-pumped pulsed vascular dye laser or the VPW green 532 nm Nd:YAG laser because of their moderately superficial nature. Multiple pulses with the flash lamp-pumped pulsed vascular dye laser are necessary when the cherry hemangiomas are large, therefore crusting can be expected. If the lesions are very thick, it is preferable to plan a series of treatments to minimize the risk of scarring.

Both of our examples are of cherry hemangiomas on the face of two younger individuals. The diagnosis was based on color, size, and texture. The first example is that of a cherry angioma on an 8-year-old caucasian boy's face (Figure 3-26 A–B). Using the flash lamp-pumped dye laser with a fluence of 7 joules/cm$^2$ the lesion was removed with three pulses of the laser. The expected purpura was noted and faded over the course of twelve days.

The second example is that of a cherry angioma on the forehead of a 19-year-old caucasian female (Figure 3-27 A–B). The VPW green 532 nm Nd:YAG laser with a chilled tip was used at a peak power of 250 watts, a spot size of 4 mm, and a pulse duration of 5 ms. Slight graying was observed immediately after application of the laser beam

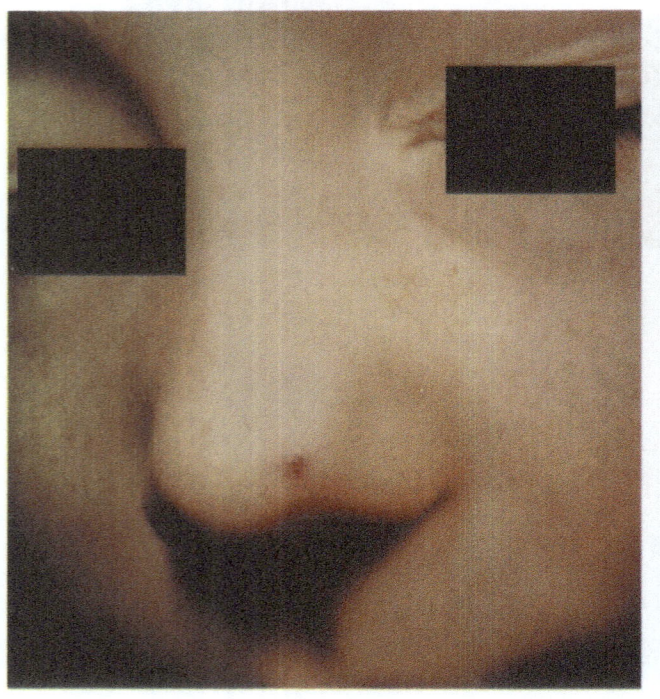

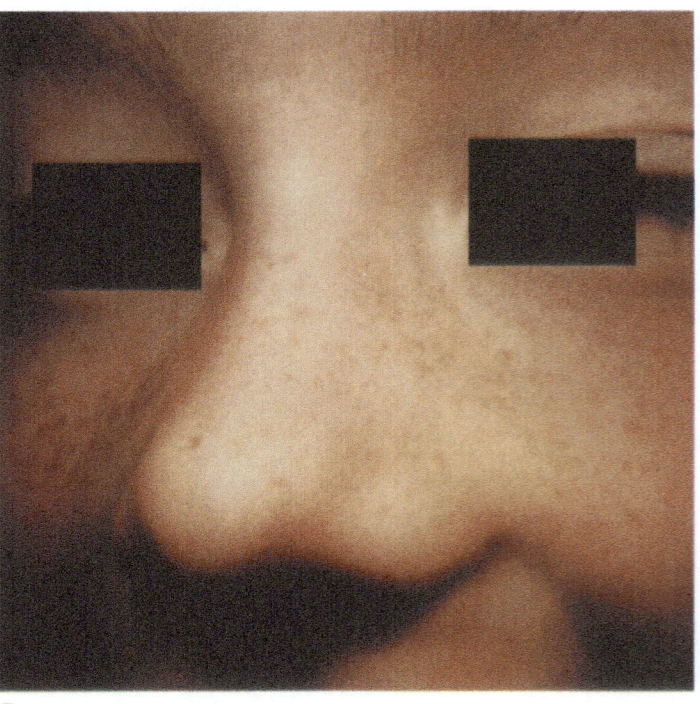

A                                                    B

**Figure 3-26 A, B**
Cherry angioma: nose, caucasian male, flash lamp-pumped pulsed vascular dye laser.

**Figure 3-27**
Cherry angioma: forehead, caucasian
female, VPW green double frequency
Nd:YAG laser.

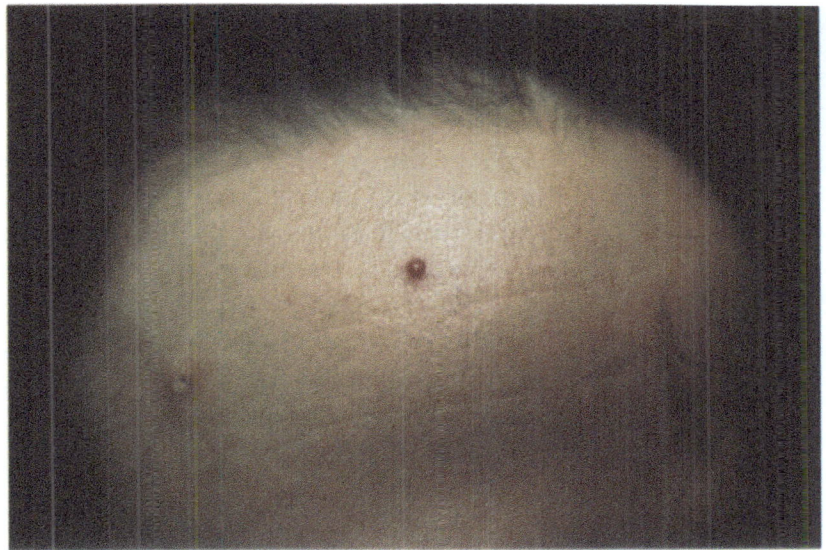

A

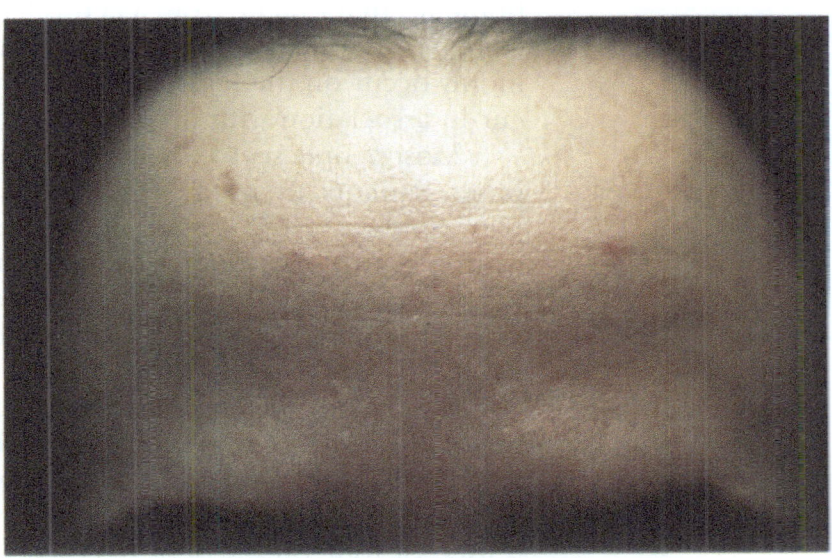

B

to the lesion, followed by a crusting which was sloughed off in nine days. Post-surgical erythema lasted several weeks.

In my experience, the flash lamp-pumped pulsed vascular dye laser and the VPW green 532 nm Nd:YAG laser give comparable results in the treatment of cherry hemangiomas. The VPW green 532 nm Nd:YAG laser is, however, more operator dependent. It is logical to conclude that other yellow or green light lasers would also be effective in the treatment of cherry angiomas.

Electrodesiccation is an alternative treatment option. With the advent of target specific lasers, the risk of scarring has been significantly reduced as a result of decreased thermal damage. This degree of control is not possible with electrodesiccation. Therefore, the element of risk is higher.

## Spider Nevus

A spider nevus, or nevus araneus, is characterized by dilated arterial branches that radiate from a central, red punctum. The source of the center is the dilated end of an ascending artery. These lesions commonly occur on the face. Usually, they are asymptomatic but may occur in association with pregnancy or liver disease [10].

Most people seek to have these lesions removed for cosmetic purposes. Patients often state that at a glance these lesions look like pimples. Spider nevus are bright red and are difficult to camouflage with makeup. In the past, excision and electrodesiccation were common methods of removal. However, the target specific lasers provide far superior cosmetic results and are the obvious treatment of choice.

Two spider nevi on this 8-year-old caucasian male appeared suddenly and were removed for cosmetic purposes (Figure 3-28 A–B). The flash lamp-pumped pulsed dye laser was used at 4 joules/cm$^2$ to remove the lesion in one session. No anesthetic was required as only a total of four pulses were necessary. Over a period of ten days the purpura gradually faded to normal skin color.

This 27-year-old caucasian female presented with an isolated, thick telangiectasia on the forehead of unknown etiology (Figure 3-29 A–B). I elected to use the double frequency Nd:YAG with a KTP crystal laser to remove the vessel because of its thickness. At 4 watts, the laser beam was directed through a blunt tipped contact probe utilizing a foot pedal-controlled pulsing technique. The vessel turned gray and then disappeared. Crusting occurred one day after the procedure and was sloughed off within six days. One session was required to remove the lesion.

In many cases, particulary in adults, the punctum may be quite thick, requiring several pulses of the flash lamp-pumped pulsed dye vascular laser to eliminate the lesion. In some cases, I use the double frequency Nd:YAG (KTP) laser, the VPW green 532 nm Nd:YAG laser, or the ultrapulsed $CO_2$ laser to treat the center of the lesion. I then

**Figure 3-28 A, B**
Spider angioma: cheek, caucasian male, flash lamp-pumped pulsed vascular dye laser.

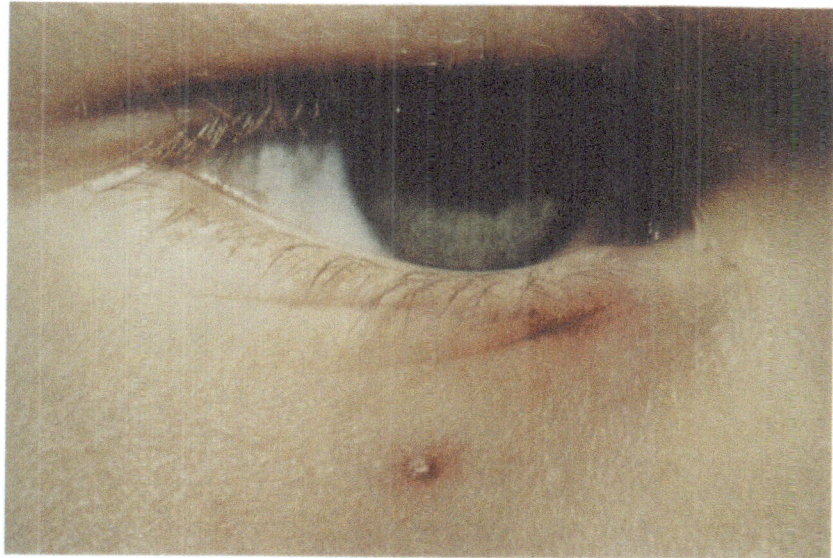

A

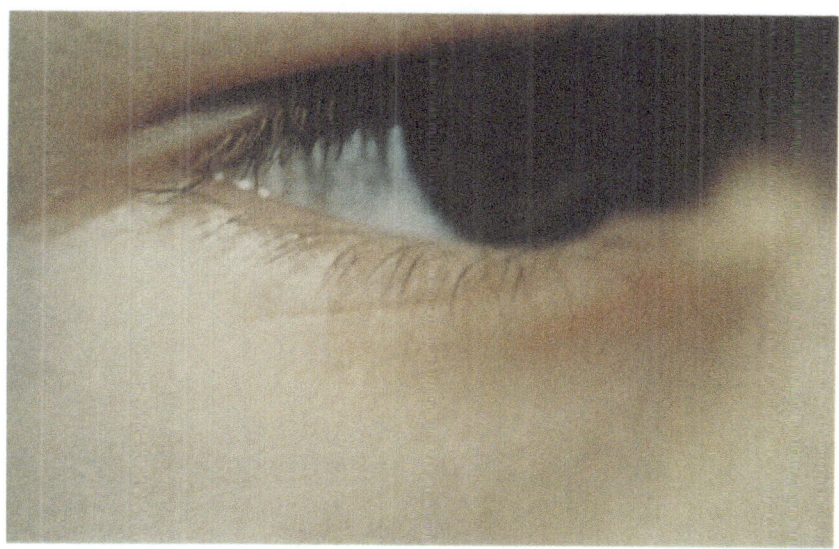

B

**Figure 3-29 A, B**
Large spider angioma: forehead, caucasian female, KTP laser.

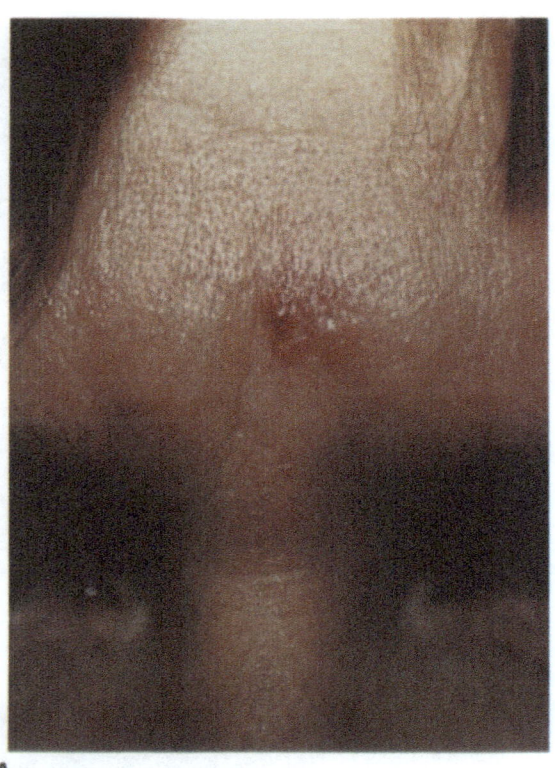

A

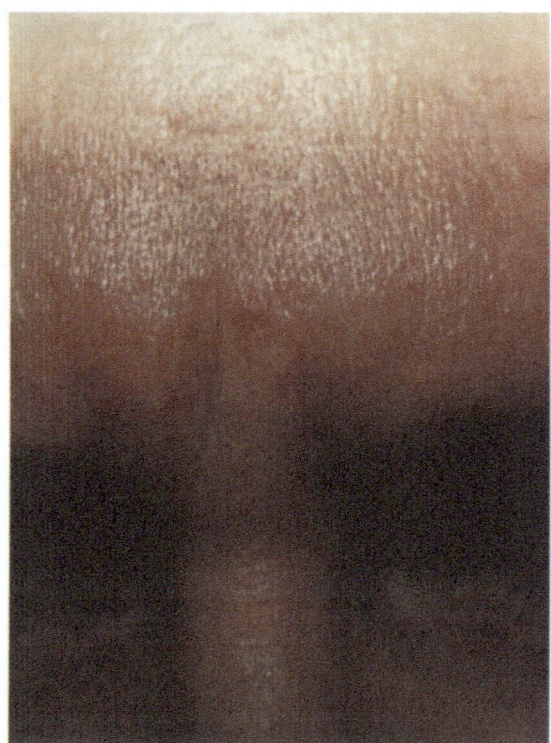

B

use the flash lamp-pumped pulsed dye laser around the periphery to remove the smaller radiating vessels. Occasionally, I quietly confess, that I have regressed to utilizing electrocautery on a particularly thick central vascular puncta.

## Sebaceous Hyperplasia

Usually sebaceous hyperplasia occur on the forehead and cheeks of people past middle age and are characterized by lobules of enlarged sebaceous glands centered around an enlarged sebaceous duct. They are yellowish in appearance and asymptomatic. People generally seek to have these lesions removed for cosmetic purposes [10].

Our example is that of a 47-year-old caucasian female who was referred for treatment for a scar resulting from a vertical furrow excision on her forehead (Figure 3-30 A–B). At the same time she requested treatment for the bumps that were in the vicinity of the scar.

**Figure 3-30 A, B**
Sebaceous hyperplasia superimposed on old laceration scar: forehead, caucasian female, ultrapulsed $CO_2$ laser.

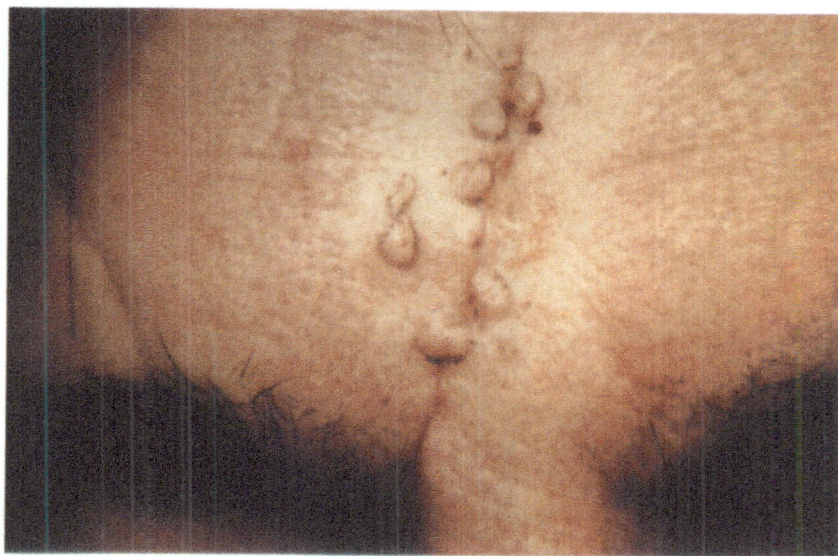

A

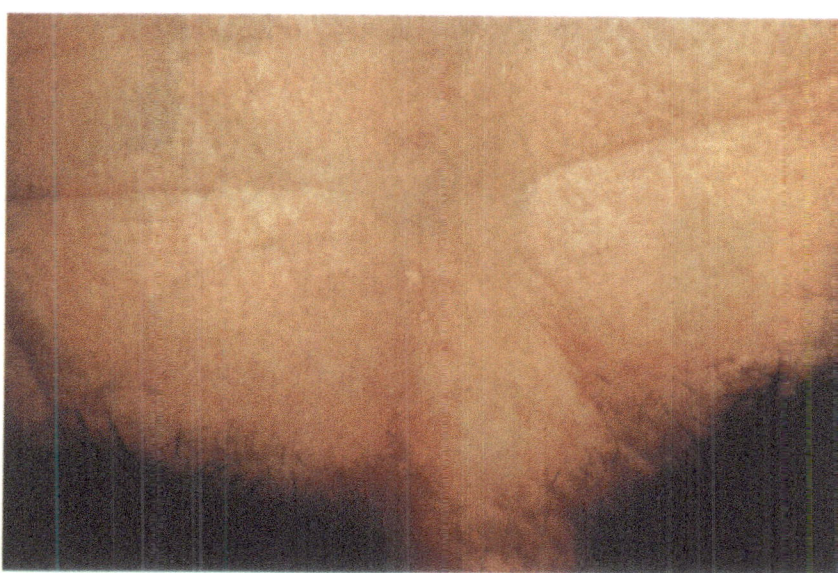

B

The bumps were diagnosed as sebaceous hyperplasia and were vaporized away at the same time that the scar was resurfaced. To accomplish this, I used the ultrapulsed $CO_2$ laser at an energy level of 300 millijoules, a pulse width of 60 ms, and a 3 mm spot size. The sebaceous hyperplasia were vaporized until they were flush with the skin.

A similar technique is used in the treatment of other hamartomas, such as syringomas. Our example is that of a 24-year-old caucasian male with recently developed syringomas on the lower eyelids (Figure 3-31 A–B). The ultrapulsed $CO_2$ laser at an energy level of 300 millijoules, a pulse width of 60 ms, and a 3 mm spot size was used to vaporize the syringomas until they were flush with the skin. This may only take a single pulse or may require several pulses in succession.

**Figure 3-31 A, B**
Syringomas: lower eyelid, caucasian male, ultrapulsed $CO_2$ laser.

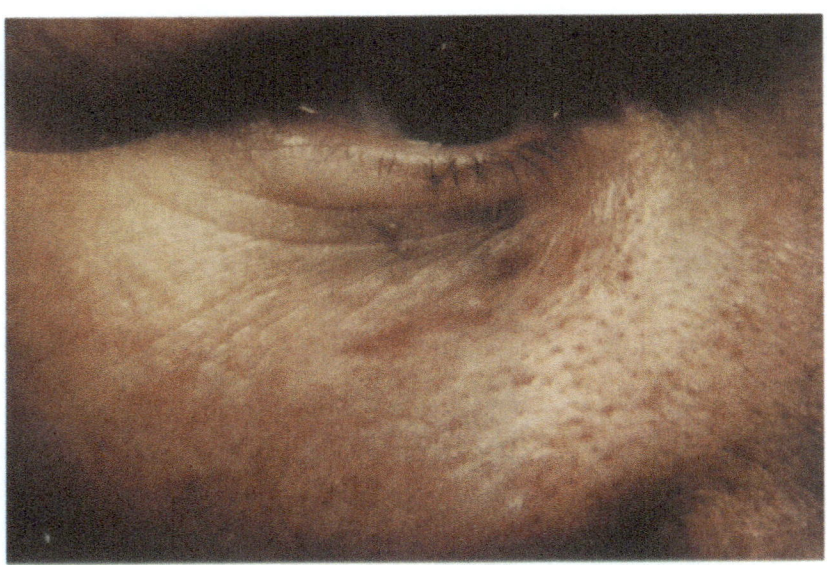

A

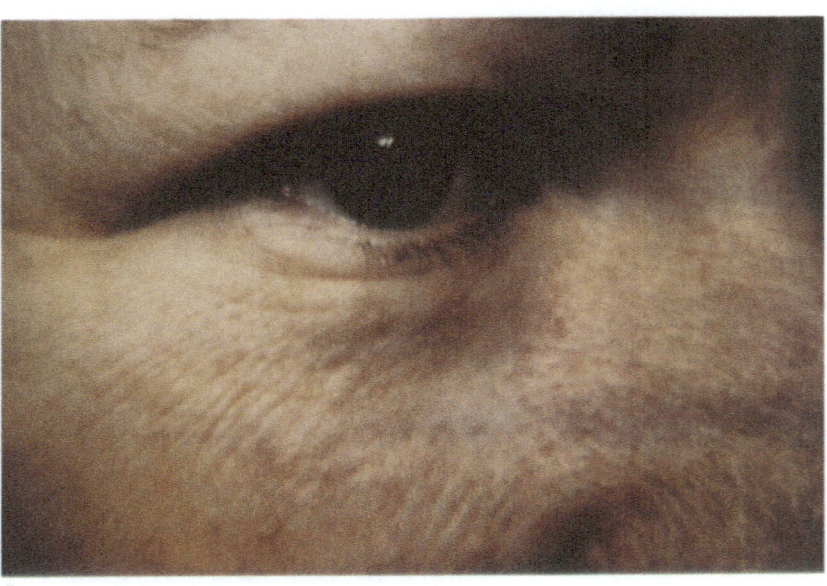

B

In both examples, the patients were instructed to keep the resulting crust moist and free from infection with the use of an antibiotic cream (Fucidin™ or Bactroban™) to be applied after washing gently twice a day. This routine was repeated until the crusts were sloughed in nine days. Some patients find the antibiotic ointment to be quite irritating. In these instances, they are instructed to discontinue the antibiotic ointment and to apply Vaseline™ to the crust until it has been sloughed off.

Syringomas and other lesions of the skin are often in very close proximity to the eye. In this case, we place a stainless steel eye shield onto the cornea. First the eye is anesthetized with Pontocaine™ eye drops. The shield is coated with Polysporin™ eye ointment to protect the eye against abrasion and infection. The shield is then placed over the cornea. Patients are informed that they will experience a feeling of fullness under their eyelids but no discomfort.

Rhynophyma is a form of sebaceous hyperplasia of the nose. In the case of a rhynophyma there are no lobules, the sebaceous glands and ducts are simply enlarged. When a large number of sebaceous glands occur over the nose, they give a nodular, yellowish, enlarged appearance to it. Although of no medical consequence, most people are anxious to improve the cosmetic appearance of these lesions. A social stigma is associated with this condition as one that is caused by the use of alcohol. This condition and alcohol consumption, however, are unrelated.

I have used the KTP, the continuous wave $CO_2$, and ultrapulsed $CO_2$ lasers to pare down the enlarged sebaceous glands of rhynophyma. The first example is that of a 78-year-old caucasian male with rosacea who developed rhynophyma over a period of twenty-five years (Figure 3-32 A–B). The nose was anesthetized with local infiltration of 1% xylocaine with epinephrine. Using the tapered contact tip on the KTP (double frequency Nd:YAG) laser, a power setting of 6 watts was selected. To control the transfer of heat to adjacent tissue, the nose was chilled before, during, and after surgery with an artificial ice pack. I vaporized the irregular lesions and reshaped the nose layer by layer.

The second example is that of a 62-year-old caucasian male who developed rhynophyma over the last two decades (Figure 3-33 A–B). Using a combination of a nerve block and infiltration of 1% xylocaine with epinephrine, the nose was anesthetized. First, for reasons of speed, the bulk of the lesion was pared down by removing the superficial layers with a scalpel. Hemostasis was achieved by gentle desiccation and the application of topical ferrous subsulphate (Monsel's solution). Then the ultrapulsed $CO_2$ laser with the computerized scanner was used to remove and resurface the deeper layers of the lesion. The following parameters were selected: 300 millijoules, 10 watts, 2.5 mm spot size, pattern 14 (small hexagon), density 7. The higher power setting was selected to expedite the surgical process.

Regardless of which system you use, it is important to place a gloved finger inside the nares and exert pressure outwards intermit-

**Figure 3-32 A, B**
Rhynophyma: nose, caucasian male,
KTP laser.

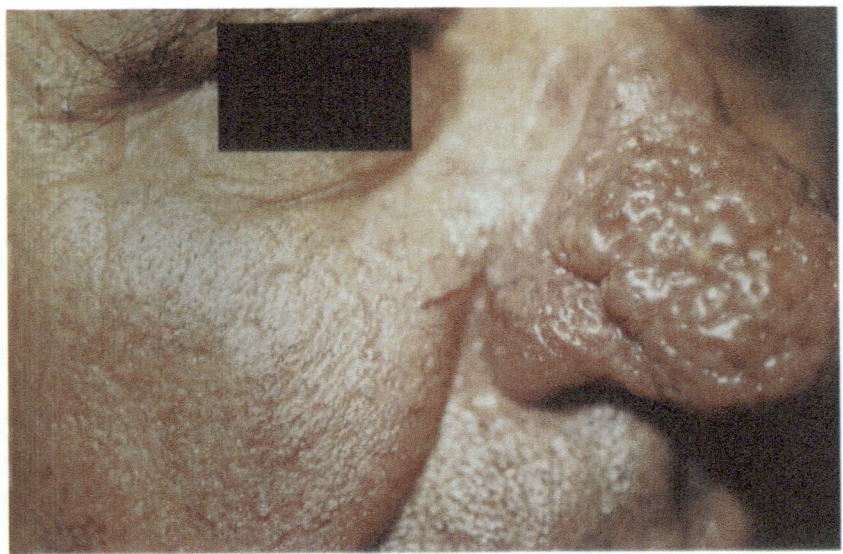

A

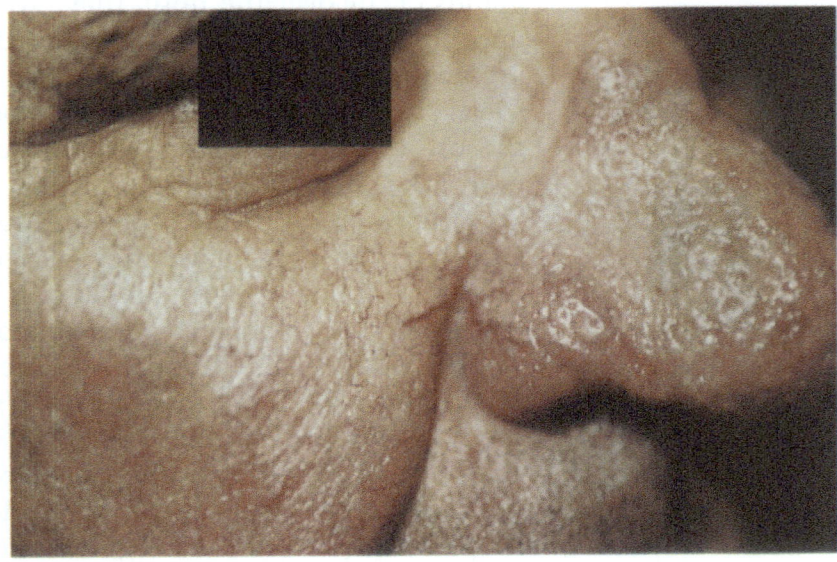

B

**Figure 3-33 A, B**
Rhynophyma: nose, caucasian male, scalpel and ultrapulsed $CO_2$ laser.

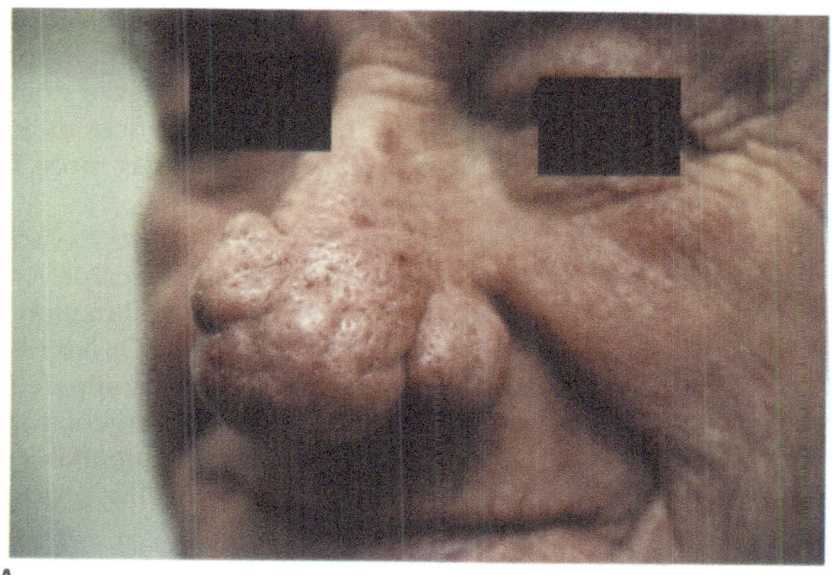

A

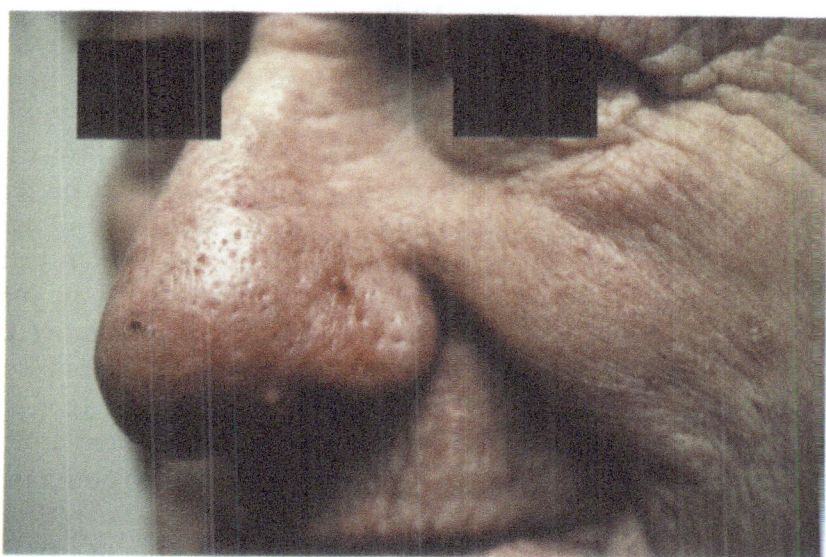

B

tently. As long as sebaceous secretions come out of the pores you can be assured of rapid re-epithelialization over a three to six week period. Damage to the openings of ducts will inhibit re-epithelialization from the pilosebaceous orifices and will tend to occur on the sides of the overall wound. This is more likely to result in the formation of scar tissue.

Other treatment alternatives include the paring down of the sebaceous overgrowths with a scalpel or electrodesiccation in solo. I believe, however, that the combination of scalpel debulking and resurfacing with the ultrapulsed $CO_2$ laser is a far superior and more efficient method of surgical removal compared to the singular use of any of the other options. It allows the surgeon to take into consideration the shape of the nose, not simply the debulking process. In addition, there is also less vascularity and the healing process is not as painful.

## Tattoos

Since Goldman first used a ruby laser that was not Q-switched to remove tattoo pigment from the skin in 1965, the literature has strongly supported the use of the Q-switched ruby, Q-switched Alexandrite, and Q-switched Nd:YAG for the removal of tattoos with little or no scarring. Since each of these lasers produce slightly different wavelengths of light, they are each better suited to remove certain pigment colors from the skin. The Q-switched ruby laser is effective for removing blue, black, brown, and green color from the skin. The Nd:YAG has the advantage of an infrared wavelength at 1064 nm, which when Q-switched can remove black, yellow, and blue pigment at peaked energies with short pulse durations to minimize thermal dispersement throughout the tissue. When passed through a KTP crystal, the frequency is doubled and the wavelength is halved to 532 nm. This green wavelength is effective for absorbing red color. The Q-switched Alexandrite in the red visible light spectrum at a wavelength of 755 nm is also effective in removing black, blue, and green pigments from the skin [2, 3, 12].

It would appear from this discussion that one would need to have at least two of these lasers in order to remove tattoos effectively. I have found that the Q-switched ruby laser is useful in removing most of the amateur, professional, and traumatic tattoos that I have treated in their entirety. Even though colors such as red, orange, and yellow are more resistant to treatment with the Q-switched ruby laser, they generally do fade after several treatments. Lowe et al. appear to agree with this observation [29].

Key variables other than the kind of laser used that impact the removal of tattoos include the type of tattoo (traumatic, amateur decorative, professional decorative), size, location, and age. Traumatic tattoos are easier to remove than decorative tattoos; whereas, amateur decorative tattoos are easier to remove than professional tattoos. This generally relates to the number and types of colors used, the depth at which the color is implanted, and the complexity of the chemicals used to mix the colors. Older tattoos are easier to remove than new tattoos. The larger the size of the tattoo, the longer it takes to remove.

Laser removal of tattoos is not without potential complications. Hypopigmentation is more common with the Q-switched ruby laser because the wavelength (694 nm) is absorbed by melanin. Allergic reactions to the pigment once it has been fragmented may occur [30]. Most pigments used for cosmetic enhancement purposes on the eyebrows, eyelids, and lips can be removed with a laser. Red ferric oxide, however, may oxidize into a black ferrous oxide when in contact with the laser light, which is very resistant to removal [31].

My first example is that of a 33-year-old caucasian female who fell off her bicycle onto a shale path, embedding fragments of foreign material into her skin (Figure 3-34 A–B). Normally, under local

**Figure 3-34 A, B**
Dirt tattoo (asphalt fall), caucasian female, Q-switched ruby laser.

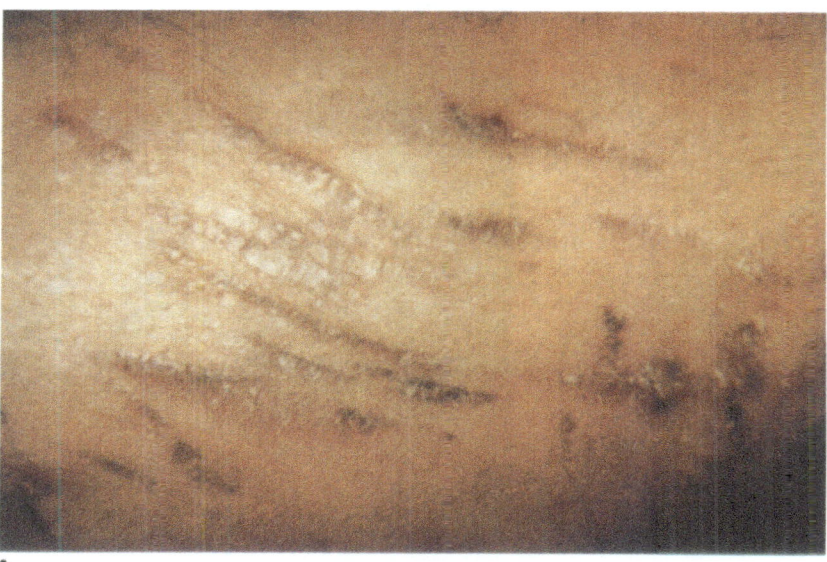

A

B

anesthetic, a wound of this nature would be vigorously scrubbed with a disposable sterile surgical brush containing an antiseptic cleansing solution to remove the debris and the necrosed tissue would be debrided. In this case, despite cleansing, some of the foreign matter remained. To remove this debris and the subsequent discoloration from the skin, the Q-switched ruby laser was used at 9 joules/cm$^2$ on four separate occasions at six-week intervals. An antibiotic ointment (Bactroban™ or Fucidin™) was applied immediately after the surgery, and the patient was instructed to continue to use the ointment twice daily after gently washing the site until the superficial crust disappeared in approximately eight days.

Another example is that of an amateur tattoo on a 13-year-old caucasian female who tattooed her boyfriend's initials and overlapping hearts into her arm with india ink and sewing needles (Figure 3-35 A–B). She requested removal when she was no longer dating this

**Figure 3-35 A, B**
Amateur indian ink tattoo, caucasian female, Q-switched ruby laser.

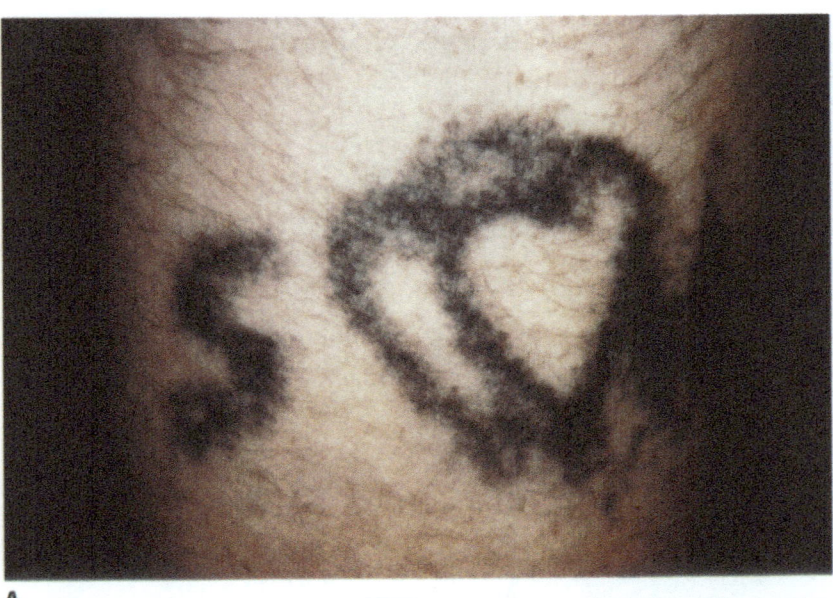

A

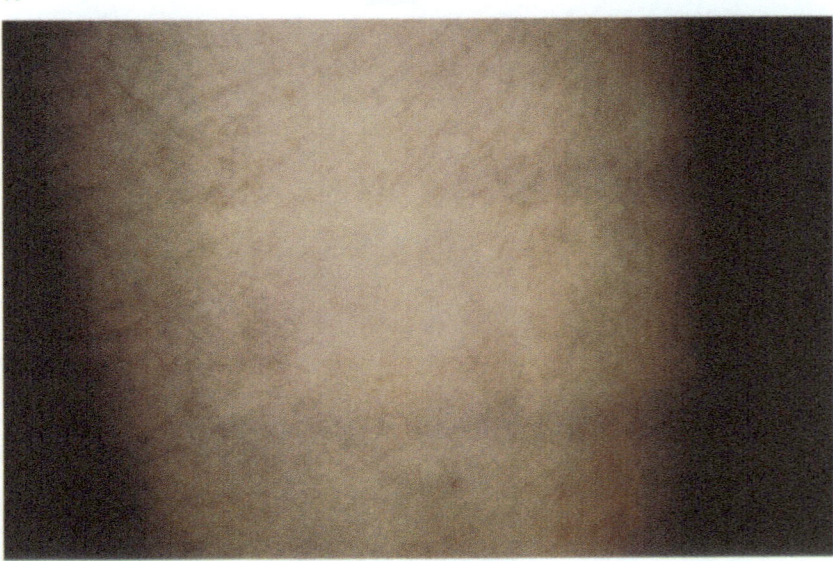

B

young man. The Q-switched ruby laser was used at 9 joules/cm$^2$. It took five sessions three weeks apart to remove all the ink successfully. The same postoperative regime as in our first tattoo example was used.

## Conclusion

Many lasers with various applications are available for the cosmetic surgeon's use. The question remains, "Which one will give the best value in terms of results, ease of use, and cost?"

Laser surgery is not for dabblers. The surgeon must be committed or should not pursue the field. Training is essential, and experience is invaluable in obtaining results that will satisfy both the patient and the surgeon.

When dealing with conditions of a dermatologic nature, it is important to know what you are treating. When in doubt, biopsy, especially those lesions that are pigmented. If possible, have the slides read by a dermatopathologist. It is essential that each stage of diagnosis and therapy be thought out carefully and acted on meticulously.

### References

1. Anderson R, Parrish J. Selective photothermolysis: Precise microsurgery by selective absorption of pulsed radiation. *Science* 1983;220: 524–527.

2. Spicer MS, Goldberg DJ. Lasers in dermatology. *J Am Acad Derm* 1996;31:1–25.

3. Wheeland RG. Clinical uses of lasers in dermatology. *Lasers Surg Med* 1995;16:2–23.

4. Mosher DB, Fitzpatrick TB, Ortonne JP, Hori Y. Disorders of pigmentation. In: Fitzpatrick TB, Eisen AZ, Wolff K, Freedberg IM, Austen KF, editors. *Dermatology in General Medicine.* New York: McGraw-Hill Book Co., 1987:794–876.

5. Goldberg DJ. Benign pigmented lesion of the skin: Treatment with the Q-switched ruby laser. *J Derm Surg Oncol* 1993;19:376–379.

6. Alster TS, Williams CM. Treatment of Nevus of Ota by the Q-switched Alexandrite laser. *J Derm Surg Oncol* 1995;21:592–596.

7. Tse Y, Levine VJ, McClain SA. et al. The removal of cutaneous pigmented lesions with the Q-switched ruby laser and the Q-switched neodymium:yttrium-aluminum-garnet laser: A comparative study. *J Derm Surg Oncol* 1994;20:795–800.

8. Fitzpatrick RE, Goldman MP, Arza JR. Laser treatment of benign pigmented epidermal lesions using a 300 ns pulse and 510 nm wavelength. *J Derm Surg Oncol* 1993;19:341–347.

9. MacKie RA. Tumours of the skin. In Rook A, Wilkinson DS, Ebling FJG, et al., ed. *Textbook of Dermatology.* Oxford: Blackwell Scientific Publications, 1986:2375–2478.

10. Lever WF, Schaumburg-Lever G. *Histopathology of the Skin, 6th ed.* Philadelphia: J.B. Lippincott Co., 1983.

11. Rhodes AR. Neoplasms: Benign neoplasias, hyperplasias, and dysplasias of melanocytes. In: Fitzpatrick TB, Eisen AZ, Wolff K, Freedberg IM, Austen KF, eds. *Dermatology in General Medicine.* New York: McGraw-Hill Book Co., 1987:877–966.

12. Geronemus RG. Laser surgery 1995. *J Derm Surg* 1995;21:399–403.

13. Schwartz RA, Stoll HL. Epithelial precancerous lesions. In: Fitzpatrick TB, Eisen AZ, Wolff K, Freedberg IM, Austen KF, eds. *Dermatology in General Medicine.* New York: McGraw-Hill Book Co., 1987:733–746.

14. Whitaker DC. Microscopically proven cure of actinic cheilitis by $CO_2$ laser. *Lasers Surg Med* 1987;7:520–523.

15. Zelickson BD, Roenigk RK. Actinic cheilitis. Treatment with the carbon dioxide laser. *Cancer* 1990;65:1307–1311.

16. Olbright SM. Use of the carbon dioxide laser in dermatologic surgery: Clinically relevant update for 1993. *J Dermatol Surg Oncol* 19:364–369.

17. Atherton DJ, Rook A. Naevi and other developmental defects. In Rook A, Wilkinson DS, Ebling FJG, et al., eds. *Textbook of Dermatology.* Oxford: Blackwell Scientific Publications, 1986:167–227.

18. From L, Assaad D. Vascular neoplasms, pseudoneoplasms, and hyperplasias. In: Fitzpatrick TB, Eisen AZ, Wolff K, Freedberg IM, Austen KF, eds. *Dermatology in General Medicine.* New York: McGraw-Hill Book Co., 1987:1059–1077.

19. Geroneumus RG, Ashinoff R. The medical necessity of evaluation and treatment of port-wine stains. *J Dermatol Surg Oncol* 1991;17:76–79.

20. Fitzpatrick RE, Lowe NJ, Goldman MP, et al. Flashlamp-pumped pulsed dye laser treatment of port-wine stains. *J Dermatol Surg Oncol* 1994;20:743–748.

21. Tan OT, Sherwood K, Gilchrest B. The treatment of children with port wine stains using flash pump dye laser. *N Engl J Med* 1989;320:416–421.

22. Garden JM, Polla LL, Tan OT. The treatment of port-wine stains by the pulsed dye laser. *Arch Dermatol* 1988;124:889–896.

23. Ashinoff R, Geronemus RG. Flashlamp-pumped pulsed dye laser for port-wine stains in infancy: Early versus later treatment. *J Am Acad Dermatol* 1991;24:467–472.

24. Renfro L, Geronemus RG. Anatomical differences of port-wine stains in response to treatment with the pulsed dye laser. *Arch Dermatol* 1993;129:182–188.

25. Goldman MP, Fitzpatrick RE, Ruiz-Esparza J. Treatment of port-wine stains (capillary malformation) with the flashlamp-pumped pulsed dye laser. *J Pediatr* 1993;122:71–77.

26. Alster TS, Wilson F. Treatment of port-wine stains with the flashlamp-pumped dye laser: Extended clinical experience in children and adults. *Ann Plas Surg* 1994;32:478–484.

27. Warner MW, Dinehart SM, Wilson MB, et al. A comparison of copper vapor and flashlamp pumped dye lasers in the treatment of facial telangiectasia. *J Dermatol Surg Oncol* 1993;19:992–998.

28. Broska P, Martinho E, Goodman MM. Comparison of the argon tunable dye laser with the flashlamp pulsed dye laser in treatment of facial telangiectasia. *J Dermatol Surg Oncol* 1994;20:749–753.

29. Lowe NJ, Luftman D, Sawcer D. Q-switched ruby laser: Further observations on treatment of professional tattoos. *J Dermatol Surg Oncol* 1994;20:307–311.

30. Ashinoff R, Levine VJ, Soter NA. Allergic reactions to tattoo pigment after laser surgery. *Dermatol Surg* 1995;21:291–294.

31. Anderson RR, Geronemus R, Kilmer SL, et al. Cosmetic tattoo ink darkening: A complication of Q-switched and pulsed-laser treatment. *Arch Dermatol* 1993;129:1010–1014.

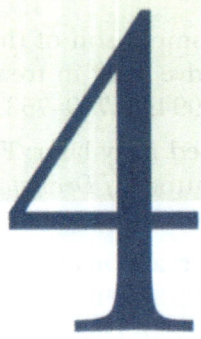

# Aesthetic Laser Surgery

Michael I. Kulick, *M.D., D.D.S.,* and
David B. Apfelberg, *M.D.*

## Introduction

Many lasers are available for aesthetic laser surgery. Due to the number of systems available, this chapter will reflect the combined experiences of Dr. Apfelberg and myself. I will discuss the Laserscope potassium titanyl phosphate (KTP) and Sharplan carbon dioxide ($CO_2$) laser systems, and Dr. David Apfelberg will report on his experience with the Heraeus yttrium-aluminum-garnet (YAG) and Coherent $CO_2$ devices. Each of these systems has proven effective for aesthetic surgery and has reduced postoperative morbidity when used properly.

The ability to cut and coagulate simultaneously without incidental nerve injury is afforded by the use of lasers in surgical procedures. The goal is to reduce postoperative bruising, pain, and swelling, thus shortening the patient's initial recovery period. In addition, patients under intravenous anesthesia experience less discomfort during laser surgery when compared with the use of electrocautery for hemostasis while operating in areas difficult to anesthetize, e.g., resecting the medial fat pocket during blepharoplasty or when the effect of the injected local anesthetic fades.

Achievement of these potential benefits requires a basic understanding of the delivery systems available and the properties of the various wavelengths. The wavelength one selects affects the speed of dissection, depth of penetration beyond the beam–tissue contact area, and the presence or absence of tactile feedback while performing surgery. The YAG wavelength (1064 nm) is an excellent hemostatic tool, and the delivery system affords the surgeon tactile feedback during surgery. However, the potential for deep tissue penetration exists which can also increase postoperative swelling. The KTP wavelength (532 nm) also affords the surgeon tactile feedback, has less tissue penetration than the YAG, and is more selectively absorbed by hemoglobin. This wavelength's attraction to red pigment, however, makes it less effective when cutting into subcutaneous tissue. In contrast, the $CO_2$ wavelength (10,600 nm) is readily absorbed by water and cuts rapidly through subcutaneous tissue. The surgeon must adjust his or her technique and speed of dissection, however, to avoid division of blood vessels prior to sealing, and there is a lack of tactile feedback as he or she dissects. Thus, the "perfect" wavelength and delivery which allows the surgeon to divide all types of tissue with absolute hemostasis, regardless of vessel size or pulse pressure, without heating or damaging tissue beyond the point of division, does not currently exist.

## Review of the Literature

### by David Apfelberg, M.D.

Cosmetic surgery of the face has greatly improved as a result of lasers. Studies have clearly demonstrated that bruising and swelling are present for a shorter period of time when the laser is used as a scalpel. In addition, pain and discomfort are lessened. In 1984, Baker and colleagues [1] first demonstrated that the use of the $CO_2$ laser for blepharoplasty provided less intraoperative hemorrhage and improved postoperative ecchymosis and edema. David and Sanders, in 1987 [2], in contralateral blepharoplasty comparison studies reported better results on the side treated with the $CO_2$ laser than on the side treated with a scalpel/cautery procedure. $CO_2$ laser techniques, including the transconjunctival approach, were further described by David [3], Trelles et al. [4], and Spadoni and Cain [5]. Morrow and Morrow [6] compared laser blepharoplasty to conventional techniques in a contralateral study of ten patients and concluded that the laser decreased operative time, bleeding, bruising, and postoperative pain. Beeson et al. [7] came to similar conclusions in a contralateral study using a superpulsed $CO_2$ laser. Mittelman and Apfelberg [8] were unable to validate such results in their contralateral study; however, the laser was not used exclusively during their procedure. Morrow and Morrow [9] also reported less bruising and swelling in 110 facelifts in which the $CO_2$ laser was used. Apfelberg has reported improved results in facelift and eyelid surgery using the Ultrapulse $CO_2$ laser [10, 11, 12].

Several reports have detailed the use of the contact YAG laser in facial cosmetic surgery. In 1990, Putterman [13] reported the results of a three-year study of eighteen oculoplastic patients, ten of whom underwent contralateral procedures comparing laser to conventional surgery. The laser side demonstrated less bleeding, operative time, and pain during fat resection, but postoperative ecchymosis and edema were not significantly different from that resulting from scalpel surgery. The advantage of the YAG laser in plastic surgery has best been documented for the removal of hemangiomas and other tumors. In 1989, Apfelberg et al. [14] described the use of sapphire tip technology for YAG laser excisions of hemangioma, lymphangiomas, neurofibromas, and hamartomas with excellent hemostasis. More recently, Apfelberg [15] has reported his experience with nine facelift and nineteen blepharoplasty patients using the YAG laser with contact sapphire tips. Bleeding, bruising and swelling were diminished by one third (average of eleven days for laser versus seventeen days for conventional surgery) in the contralateral study cases with an estimated blood loss of only 7.7 cc in blepharoplasty patients.

Keller [16] documented less bleeding and greater visualization during surgery, as well as reduced bruising and swelling during recovery following use of the KTP frequency-doubled YAG laser for face, eye, and forehead lifts. In a study of forty sequential patients undergoing aesthetic procedures of the face, Kulick [17] demonstrated reduced postoperative morbidity. These patients were followed longitudinally and demonstrated a significant reduction in postoperative bruising and swelling when compared to patients undergoing similar procedures with scissor dissection and electrocautery for hemostasis. Patients with a laser assisted procedure also required less prescribed analgesics postoperatively. A prospective eye safety study demonstrated no ophthalmologic complications associated with KTP laser use during eyelid blepharoplasty [18]. Patients were examined by an independent ophthalmologist before and after surgery.

An understanding of the wavelength properties and the color and water density of the tissue being divided will allow the surgeon to benefit from the use of lasers during surgical procedures. These benefits must outweigh the additional cost, time spent learning how to operate with the laser, and the case load required to perfect one's technique.

## Surgical Technique

**by Michael I. Kulick, M.D., D.D.S.**

The goal of aesthetic laser surgery is to try and produce the best possible result, capitalizing on one's experience and harnessing the potential benefits from the laser. This surgical tool, in and of itself, will not make one a better surgeon nor will it guarantee a shorter recovery period with less intra- and postoperative morbidity. However, when used properly, the laser will afford the surgeon less intra-operative bleeding and greater visualization of structures, which may result in greater accuracy and completeness of dissection. When used properly, the advantages of laser surgery for the patient include less bruising, swelling, and pain, and a shorter recovery time. To realize these potential benefits, the surgeon must use the least amount of energy necessary for the surgery and proceed at a speed that keeps the surgeon's intra-operative anxiety to a minimum. High power suction must be used to evacuate the laser plume. When first starting to operate with the laser, it is advisable to keep your surgical technique the same as for conventional procedures. Once you have become comfortable with your laser and how it cuts different types of tissue, modifications in surgical technique will be less frustrating.

Regardless of the wavelength, tissue dissection proceeds with greater ease and there is optimal hemostasis when coursing along normal tissue planes. Prior to the advent of the current delivery systems, the $CO_2$ laser enabled me to perform a rapid, essentially bloodless dissection. However, I frequently divided vessels and had to either focus additional laser energy on the site or utilize electrocautery. This, combined with the char residue created by the dissection, resulted in prolonged postoperative swelling despite less bruising. As proficiency increased and technology advanced, vessels were sealed prior to division and little or no char residue was created, resulting in a reduction of both bruising and swelling postoperatively.

## Blepharoplasty

The laser can be utilized for elevating a skin only or a skin-muscle flap (Figure 4-1 A–B). As part of the laser safety precautions, eye shields that cover both the cornea and the sclera are recommended (Figure 4-2). These shields must have a smooth polished surface opposing the globe which should be inspected before each application for possible scratches. In general, patients express less discomfort

**Figure 4-1 A, B**
A) The skin has been incised with the scalpel, and the KTP laser set at 4 watts of power and is used to elevate the skin, leaving the muscle behind with intact vasculature on the superficial surface (black arrow). B) To gain access to the peri-orbital fat, the muscle can be incised or a strip of obicularis can be removed at the caudal edge exposing the septum orbitali. A suction catheter has been attached to the tip of the handpiece and then hooked to the high power evacuation suction.

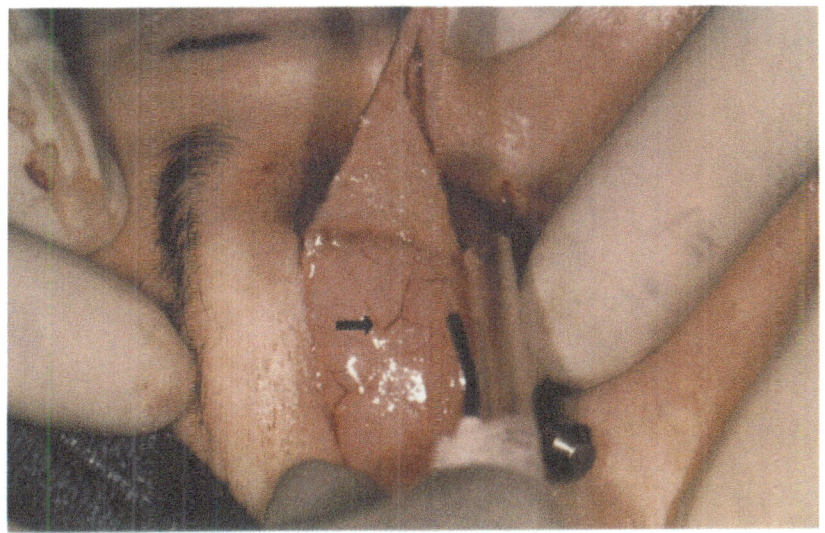

A

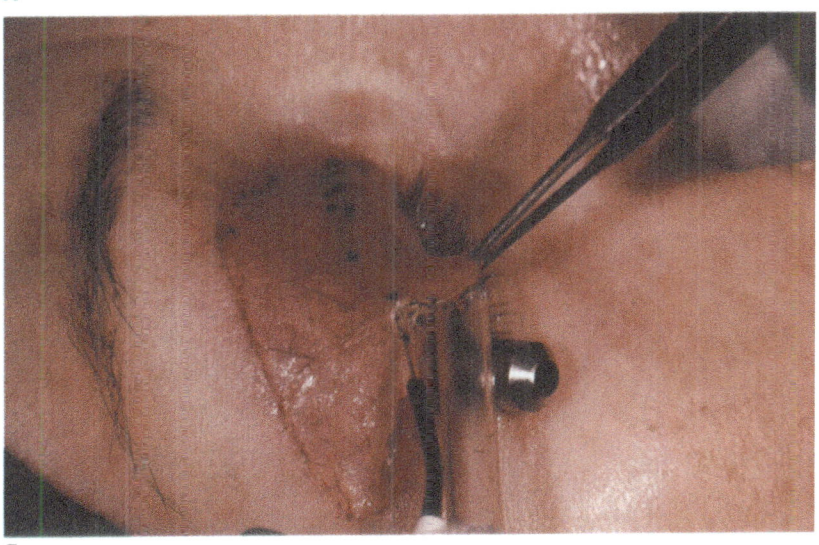

B

**Figure 4-2**
Eye shields have a polished inner surface and a matte outer finish. They are applied with either the suction device shown, or a different manufacturer has a male screw handle that fits into the female opening on the matte surface of the shield. Prior to application, tetracaine is applied to the eye followed by an eye lubricant.

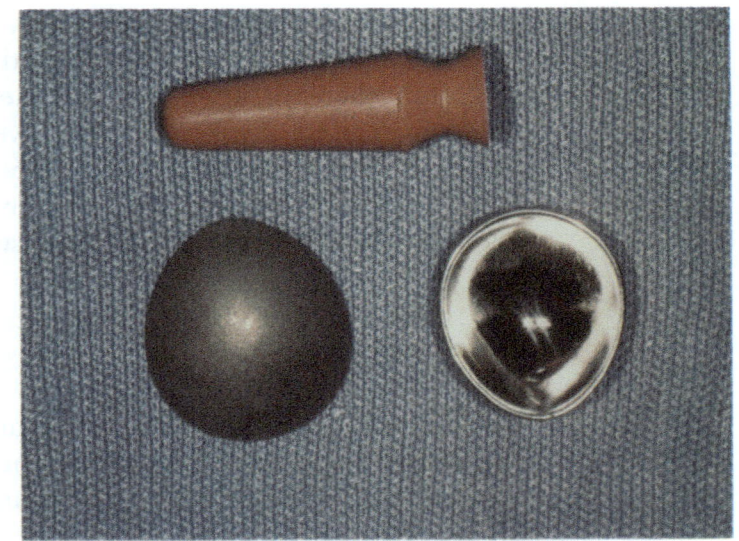

while receiving intravenous sedation during a laser-assisted procedure as compared to conventional surgery using electrocautery for hemostasis (e.g., during the removal of periorbital fat). Local anesthetic is instilled into the fat pockets and similar precautions should be followed regarding over-resection. Proper traction and counter traction is important to assure that vessels are not divided before they are sealed (Figures 4-3 A–B and 4-4 A–H). Whenever possible, vessels should be left intact if division is not essential to the surgical procedure.

## Rhytidectomy

Regardless of your surgical preference as to the level of flap elevation, subcutaneous, composite, or isolation of the submuscular Aponeuritic System layer, the laser can provide a relatively bloodless dissection. Regardless of the level of dissection, it is essential to have proper traction and countertraction to maximize the benefit of the laser. Too little traction requires more laser energy to perform the dissection, resulting in more incidental tissue injury (via heat) and greater postoperative swelling. Too much traction stretches the vessels, making them difficult to identify and thereby increasing the chance of division and retraction prior to sealing. As a result, additional laser energy must be delivered to the site, which is now covered with blood obscuring the vessel, increasing the local trauma and postoperative swelling.

My personal preference is to perform a phytidectomy in which the plane of dissection in the supra-zygomatic region is along the subcutaneous layer, in the mid-face in the sub-SMAS plane, and in the neck along the superficial surface of the platysma muscle. I have performed this type of dissection with both the $CO_2$ and KTP wavelengths obtaining excellent results. The first two zones are connected fol-

**Figure 4-3 A, B**
A) A frequent error is to pull the peri-
orbital fat too much, which results in
transection of the blood vessel prior to
sealing. Gentle traction once the fat is
exposed will allow for vessel sealing.
Unlike the recommendation made regarding the skin incision and the KTP
laser, a hemostatic conjunctival incision can be made with the laser fiber.
B) This figure illustrates the healing at
four days post-transconjunctival blepharoplasty with the KTP laser.

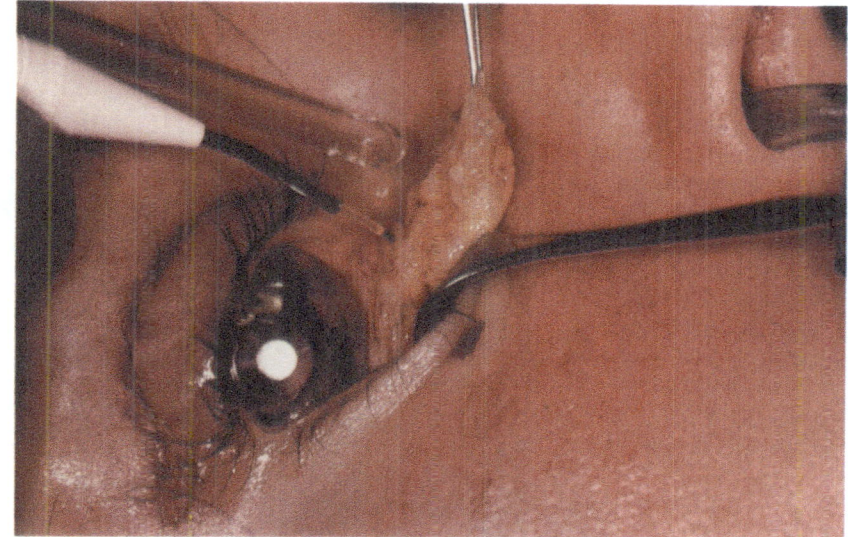

A

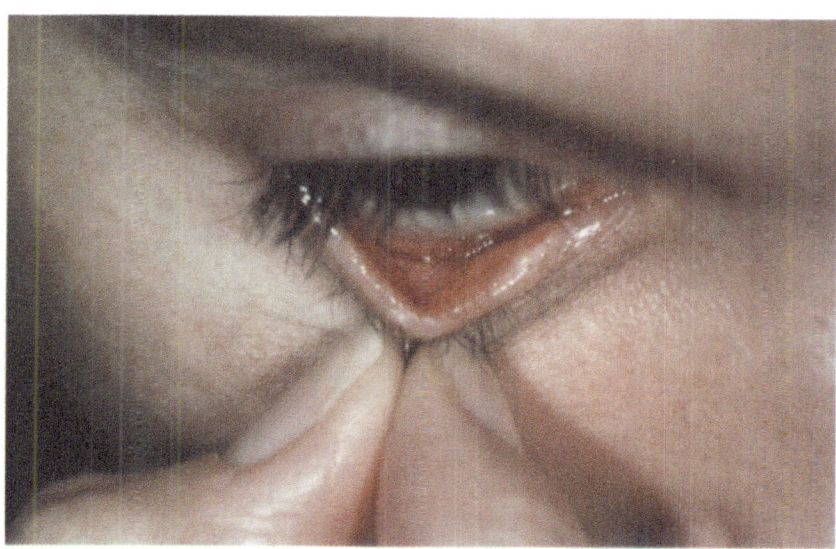

B

lowing the superficial subcutaneous plane into the mid-face, and the
latter planes connected along the superficial surface of the platysma
muscle if necessary for cephalad movement of the flap. Cephalad to
the caudal border of the mandible the platysma and SMAS layer can
be divided at the upper edge and made into a roll to augment the
caudal mandible (4-5N). An alternative would be to dissect along the
subcutaneous layer for the entire dissection.

During flap elevation, dissection must proceed with caution in
certain areas regardless of the laser system used. These are similar to
conventional surgery and include the following:

dissecting in the neck, caudal and posterior to the ear
separating the attachment of the skin over the sternocleidomastiod
muscle
separating the attachment of the obicularis muscle to the skin
dissecting anterior to the parotid gland and along the superficial surface of the zygomaticus muscle

**Figure 4-4 A, B**

A) A blepharoplasty can be performed with the Sharplan laser using either the 125 mm handpiece (Surgipulse setting, 275 millijoules, 7 to 9 watts of power) or the waveguide fiber (450 mm fiber, 275 millijoules, Surgipulse setting, 18 watts power). Both are used in a non-contact mode. The skin is incised (black arrow) with the laser after instillation of local anesthetic. A skin-only resection, as shown, leaving the vasculature on the muscle intact (yellow arrow), or a skin muscle flap can be raised. B) The muscle is incised, septum orbitali divided, and the redundant fat delivered.

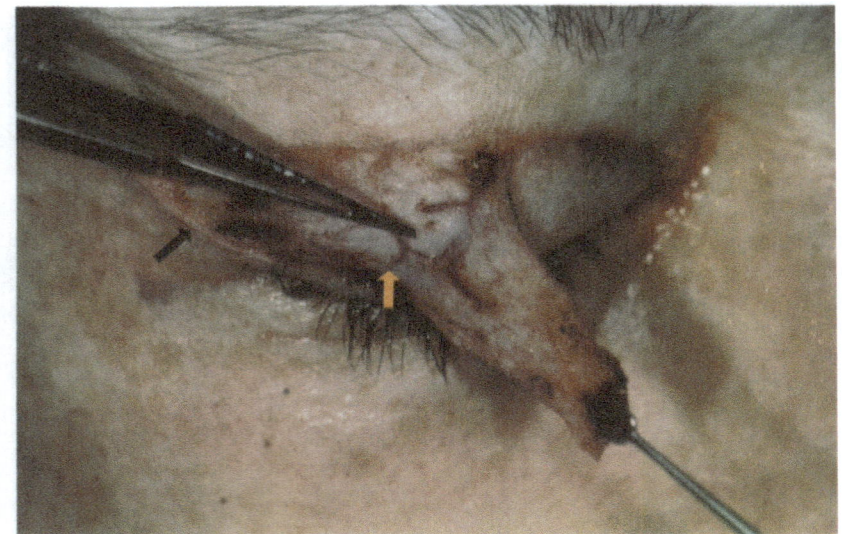

A

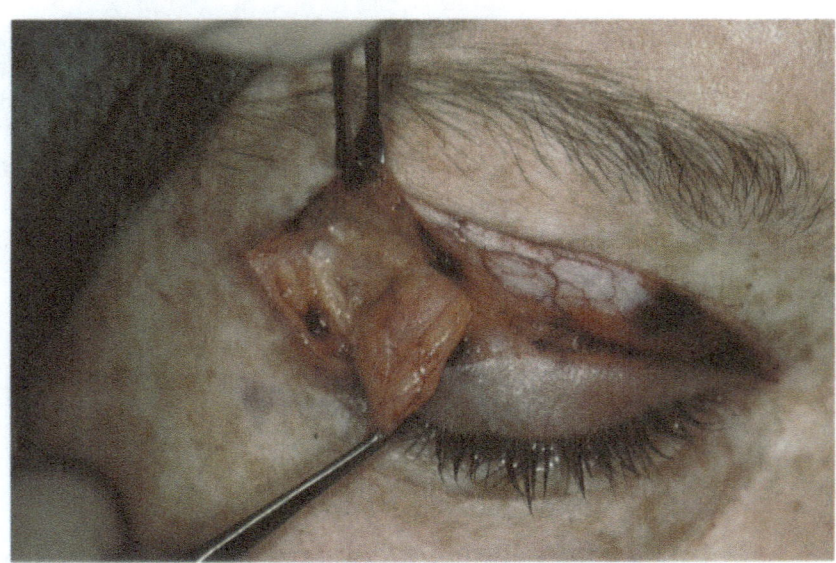

B

**Figure 4-4 C, D**

C) When performing a skin incision along the lower lid, the local anesthetic is injected just beneath the skin and helps protect the pretarsal muscle during the incision. D) A moistened cotton applicator is used to protect and retract the lashes while the skin incision is made. Prior to activating the laser, the handpiece will be lowered so that the tip of the handpiece touches the skin to be incised. White arrow points to the incised skin edge, which is not bleeding. It does not have to be trimmed prior to closure.

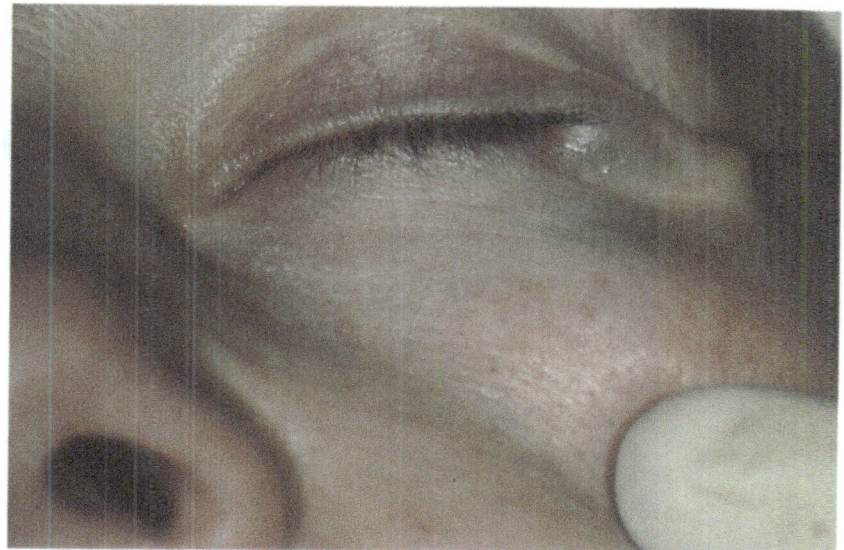

C

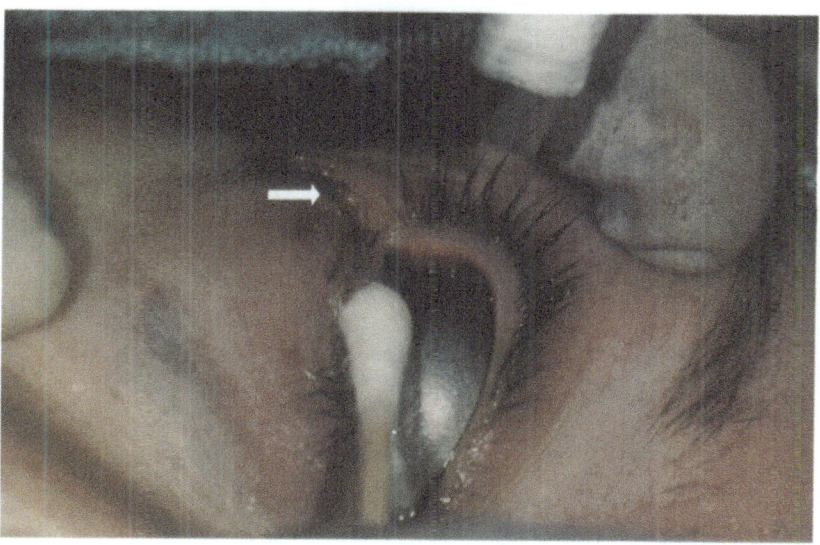

D

**Figure 4-4 E, F**
E) The handpiece is pulled back slightly to cauterize any bleeding points. The junction between the preseptal and pretarsal obicularis muscle is identified. F) The obicularis muscle is divided between the preseptal and pretarsal portions (blue arrow) and the septum orbitali is divided. The laser can be used to divide the lid attachment to the infraorbital rim (yellow arrow).

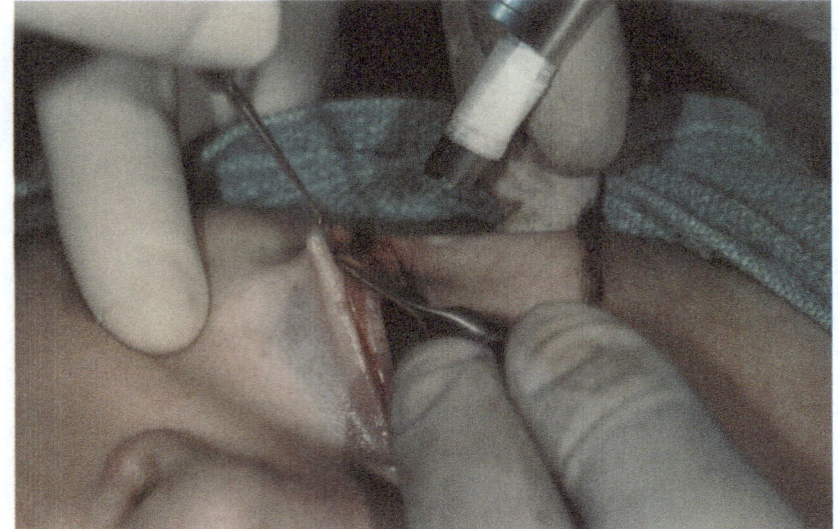

E

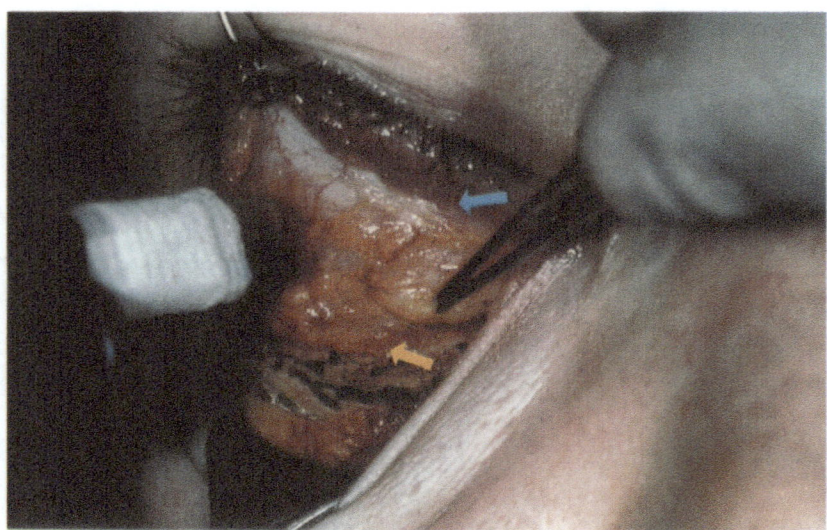

F

**Figure 4-4 G, H**

G) The fat is either removed, melted (vaporized), or relocated across the infraorbital rim (yellow arrow) as determined by preoperative planning. White arrow points to the inferior oblique muscle. H) Skin resection is performed with the laser, protecting underlying structures with a thoroughly moistened tongue blade.

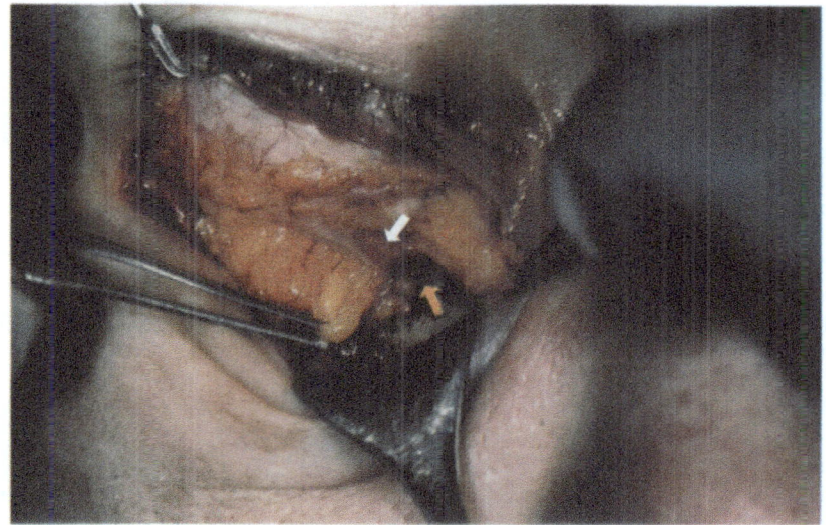

G

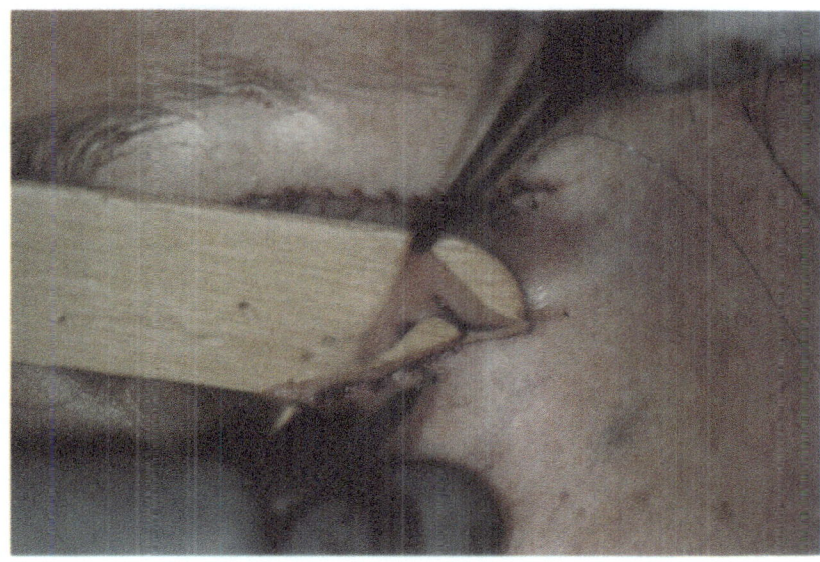

H

dissecting caudal to the angle of the mandible
dissecting in the subcutaneous zone in the superior zygomatic region

Depending on which type of wavelength you are using, various precautions can be taken to minimize the chance of incidental injury. Irrespective of the laser system used, a great deal of the postoperative morbidity is dependent on the type and extent of dissection. These factors may also play a role in the longevity of the procedure. Whenever possible, I try and dissect along natural tissue planes. Figure 4-5 A–W illustrates my standard approach and extent of dissection for most cases.

**Figure 4-5 A, B**

A) Right side. This photo demonstrates
the elevation of the skin flap in the
supra-zygomatic, preauricular region.
The dissection is in the subcutaneous
plane. When using the KTP laser, the
skin incision is made with the scalpel,
which permits bleeding along the skin
edge. The white arrow illustrates the
selective absorption of the KTP laser
energy (green color) by the bleeding
edge of the skin. When using the $CO_2$
laser, the skin incision can be made
with the laser, providing a hemostatic
incision. B) Right side. The dissection
continues anteriorly until the lateral aspect of the obicularis is reached (tip of
the forceps). Black arrow points to a
vessel that is left patent, just below the
subcutaneous plane of laser dissection.

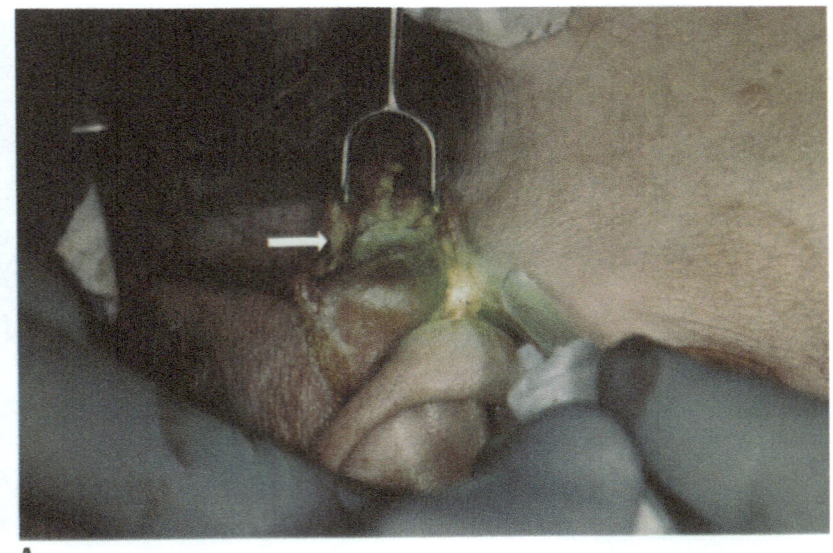

A

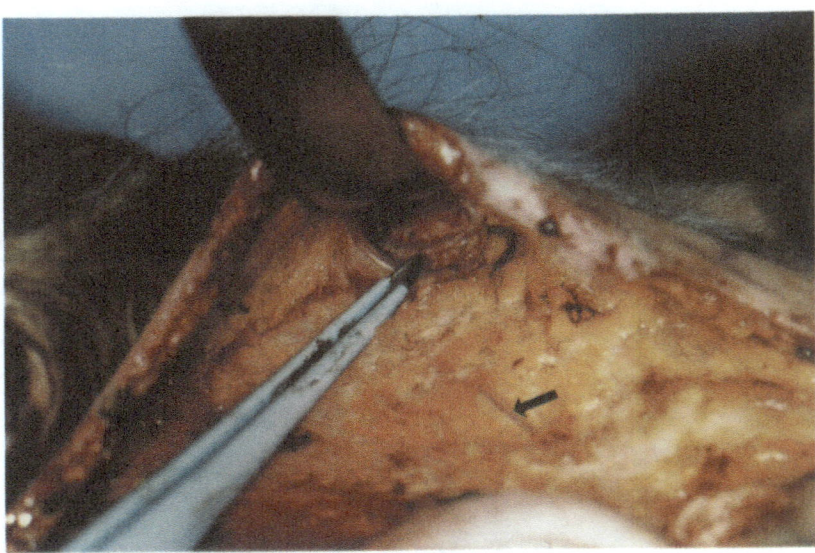

B

**Figure 4-5 C, D**

C) Right side. The dissection is carried caudally in the anterior mid-face along the superficial surface of the zygomaticus muscle. White arrow points to the junction of the zygomaticus and obicularis muscle. Black arrow points to the transition zone between the superficial dissection cephalad to the zygomatic arch and the sub-SMAS dissection in the lower face. D) Right side. At the anterior-caudal aspect of the ear, the dissection starts along the superficial surface of the parotid fascia. Black arrow points to the fascia over the parotid and the white arrow points to the edge of the SMAS.

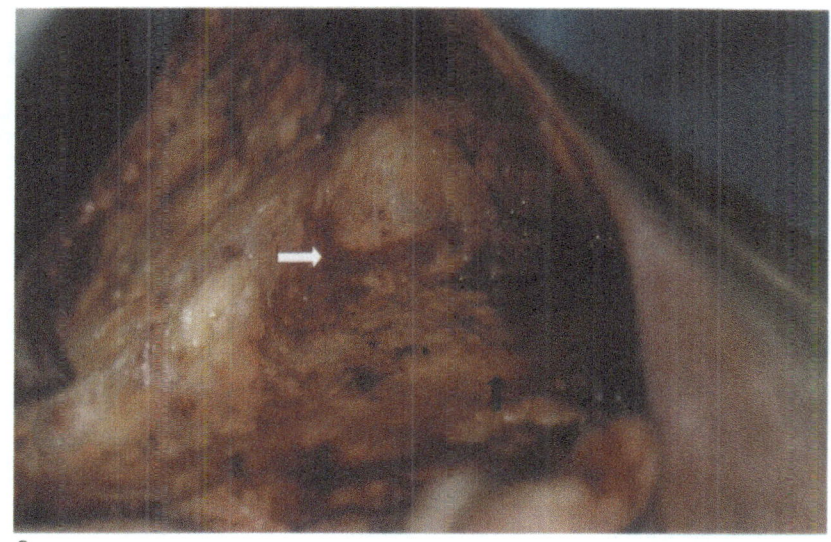

C

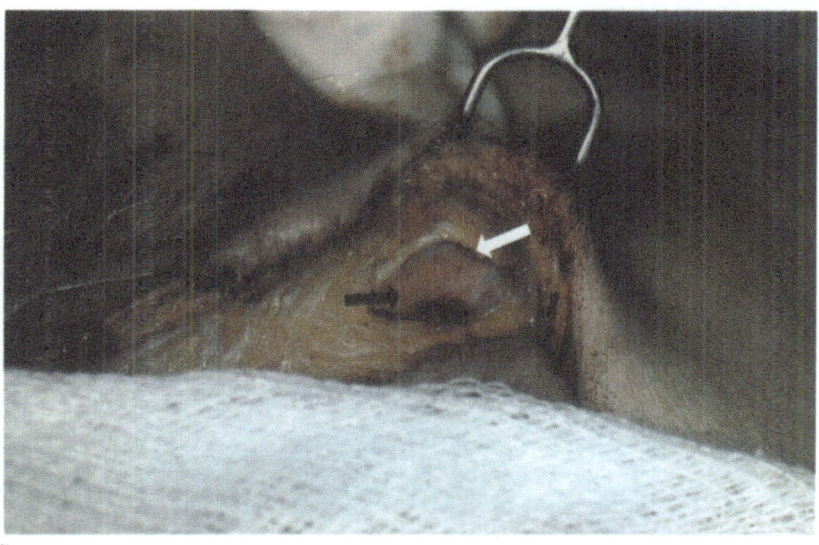

D

**Figure 4-5 E, F**

E) Right side. The white arrow indicates the location of the caudal mandible. The blue arrow points to the zygomaticus muscle. In the anterior face dissection, larger vessels are prevalent. For the purpose of illustration, these vessels are isolated (black arrow). During surgery, optimal handling of such vessels occurs through initial segregation, exposing 2 to 3 mm of vessel length and then activating the laser, directing the energy to the sides of the vessel before transection. F) Right side. The plane of dissection, along the superficial surface of the parotid fascia, is carried anteriorly, along the course of the body of the mandible until anterior to the parotid gland. The plane of dissection then becomes more superficial and is carried further anteriorly, permitting the division of the ligaments caudal and posterior to the commissure of the mouth when necessary. The buccal fat pad, held with the forceps, can be relocated when necessary.

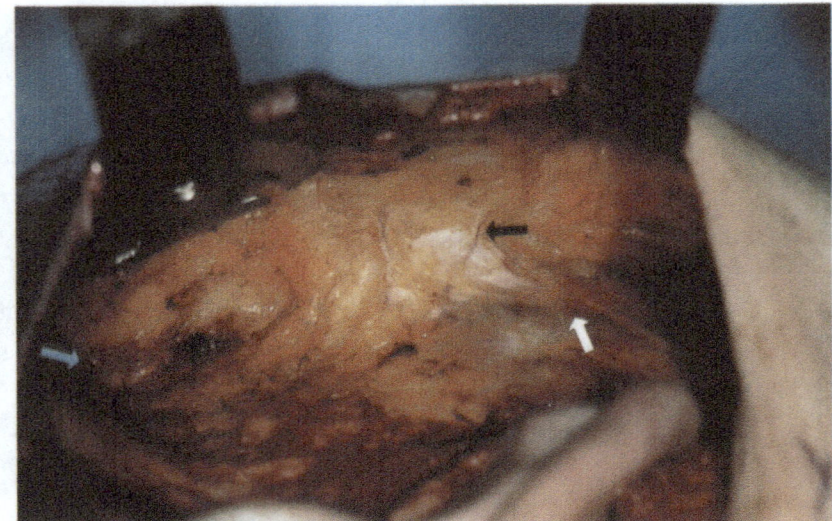

E

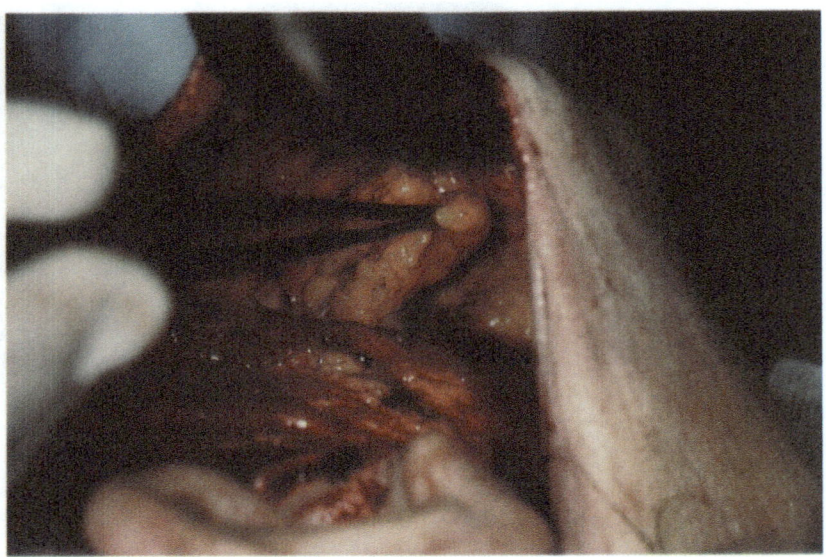

F

**Figure 4-5 G, H**
G) Right side. This patient has more of a fatty consistency in the region of the retaining ligaments of the mid-face. The forceps lie on the superior lateral aspect of the zygomaticus muscle. H) Left side. In contrast, this close-up photograph of a different patient illustrates the fibrous septa in the mid-face and large vessels (black arrow) within this zone.

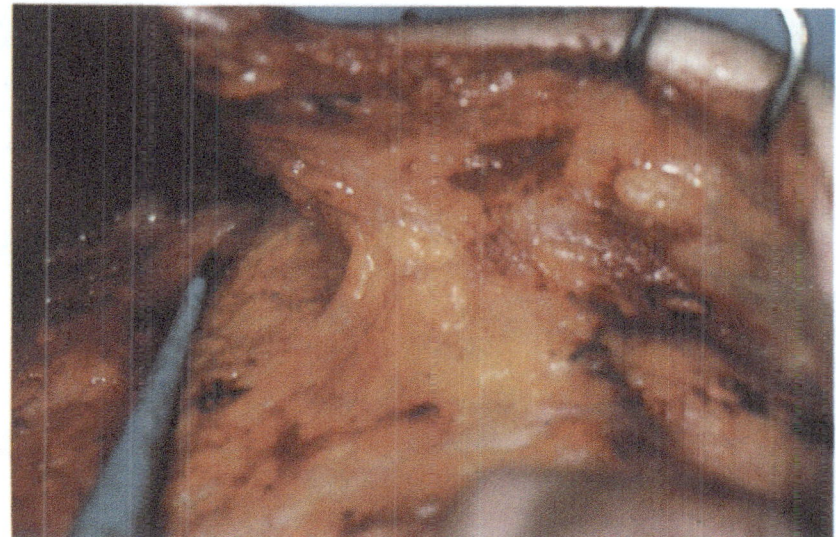

G

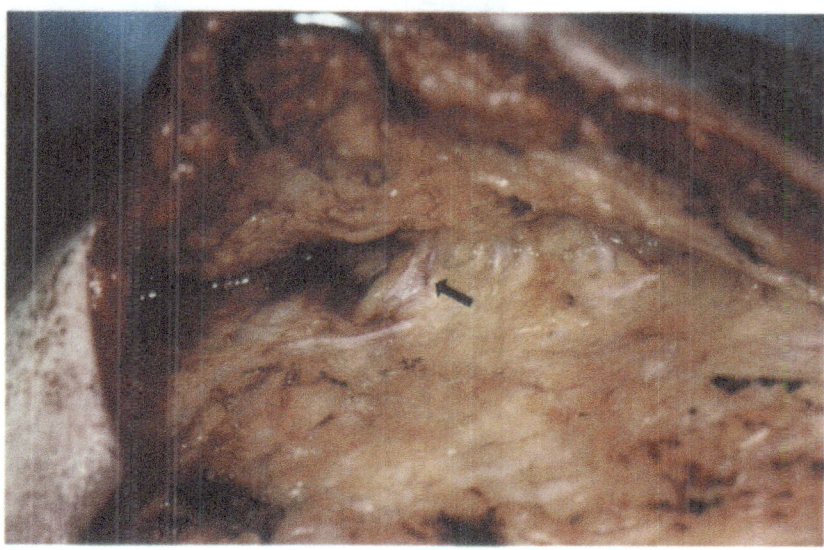

H

## Figure 4-5 I, J

I) Left side. View of the same area as Figure 5. H) From the temporal dissection reveals the relationship of the mid-face suspensory fibers (blue arrow) to the caudal, lateral aspect of the obicularis muscle (black arrow). Traction on the skin flap and mid-face fibers lifts them off the bony support in the mid-face. The white arrow shows the zygomaticus muscle coming into view as the temporal dissection is carried in a caudal, anterior direction. J) Right posterior auricular region. This dissection can be difficult with either the KTP or $CO_2$ laser systems. As with a convention procedure, the goal is to leave the subcutaneous tissue on the flap (white arrow points to a hair blub) but not penetrate the fascia protecting the underlying nerves (black arrow).

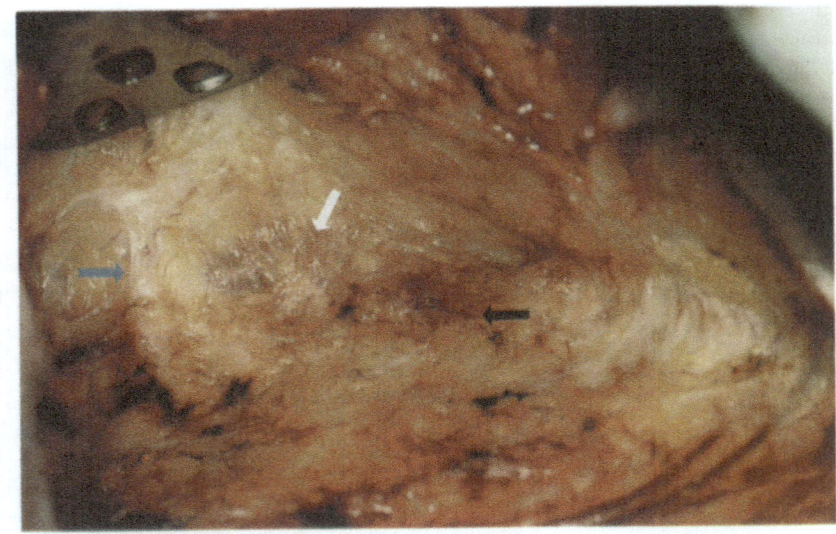

I

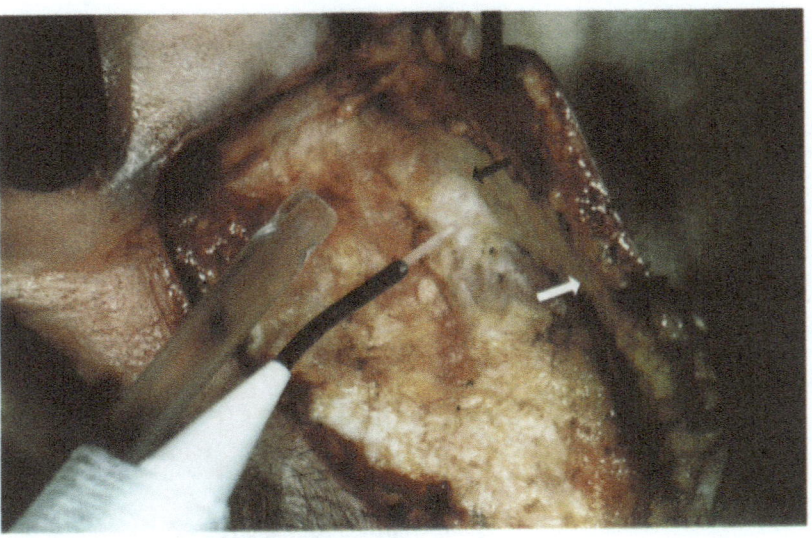

J

**Figure 4-5 K, L**

K) Left posterior neck. In patients with a thin subcutaneous layer, the protecting fascia can be penetrated, exposing the nerves (coursing in the line between the methylene blue lines and the white arrows). In such patients with scant subcutaneous tissue, it may be safer to dissect in this region with conventional methods. When performing this dissection with scissor or knife, expect some bruising in the neck. L) Right side. Even in patients with limited subcutaneous tissue in the neck, once anterior to the sternocleidomastoid muscle (black arrow), the laser can be used to dissect tissue, identifying the posterior border of the platysma muscle (white arrow shows the attachment of the platysma muscle to the subcutaneous tissue).

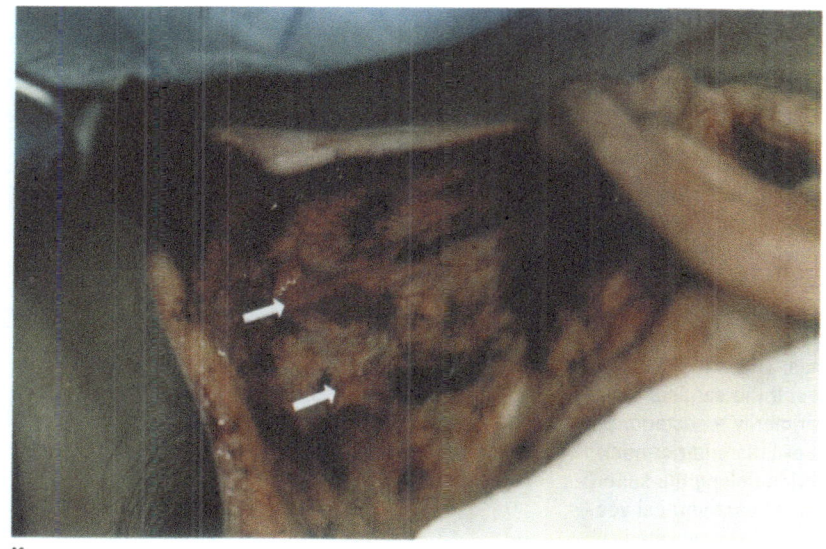

K

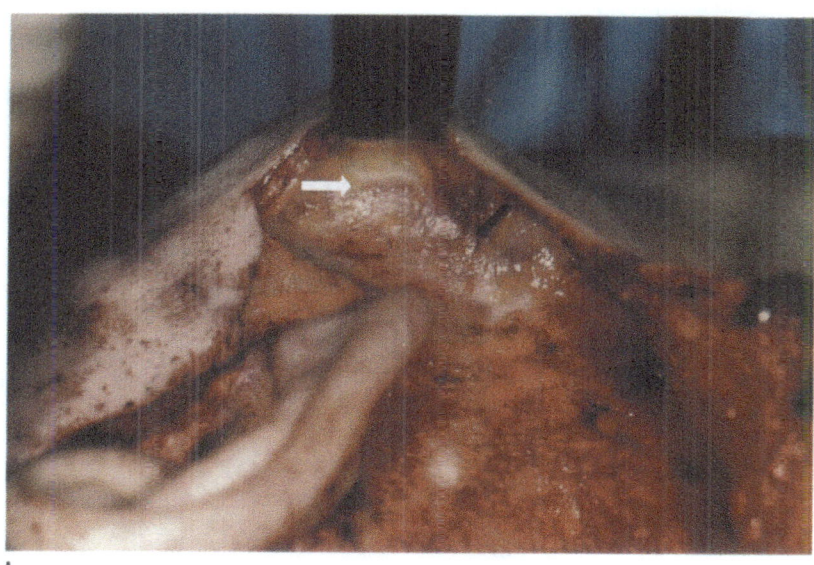

L

**Figure 4-5 M, N**

M) Left side. A fairly constant vessel, 1 to 1.5 mm in width (blue arrow), lies 1 to 2 cm caudal and anterior to the angle of the mandible (tip of white arrow). N) Right side. Illustration of the two planes of dissection in the lower face; subcutaneous in the neck (blue arrow) and deeper over the parotid fascia in the face (white arrow). The yellow arrow indicates the caudal border of the mandible and the junction of these two planes. This bridge of tissue can be left intact if the surgical procedure requires primarily a posterior pull (in cases of no or little anterior neck deformity) or divided along the superficial plane if a significant vertical vector of lift is required. The elevated platysma crossing the caudal mandible with subcutaneous tissue and SMAS attached can be used to augment the caudal mandible if desired (Fig. 4-27).

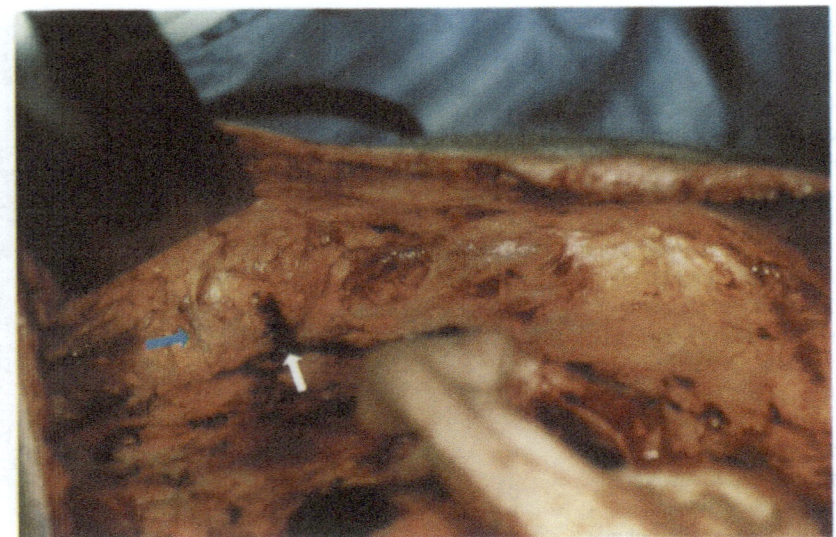

M

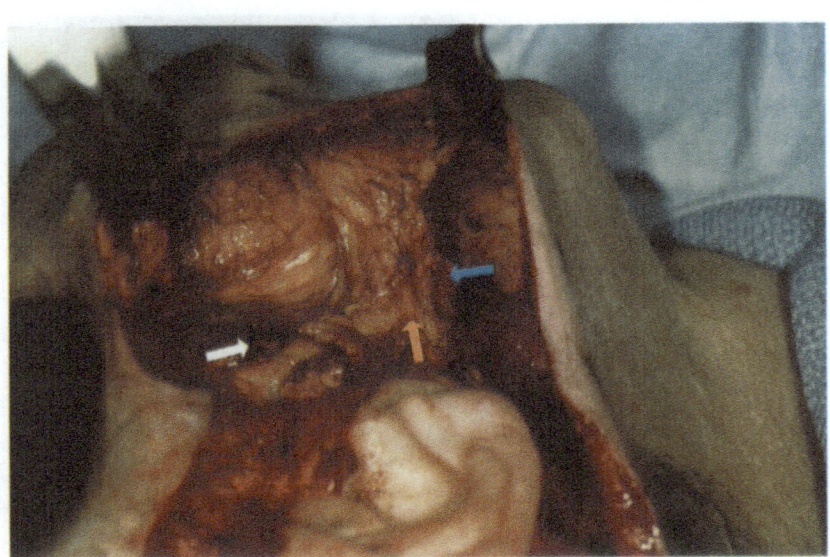

N

## Figure 4-5 O, P

O) Right side, anterior neck. Forceps hold the redundant fat that can be removed off the neck flap as necessary. White arrow points to the methylene blue line placed on the deep surface of the flap. Fat resection remains caudal to this line to provide a more defined jaw line. P) Right side. Yellow arrow indicates the course of the mandible. Whenever possible, vessels are left intact. White arrow points to a fairly consistent vessel which has been preserved and isolated to permit flap mobilization. It is found in the caudal, anterior portion of the neck dissection at the level of the thyroid cartilage.

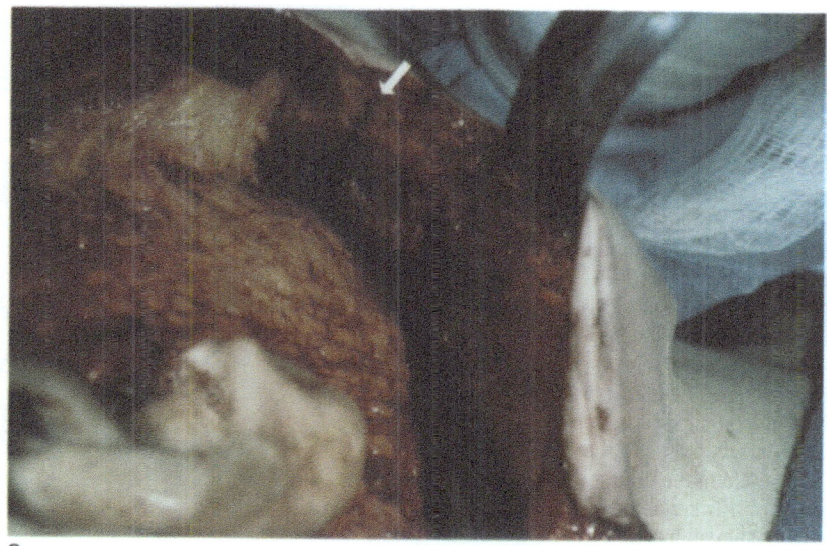

O

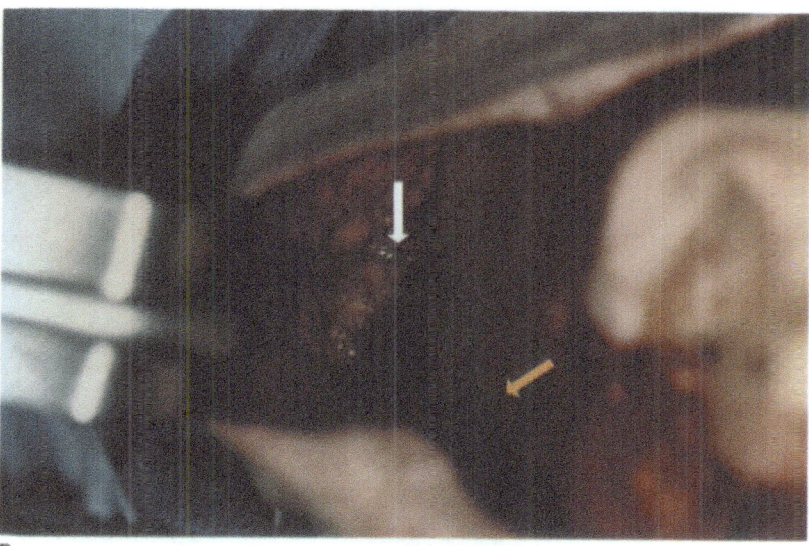

P

**Figure 4-5 Q, R**

Q) Right side. The arrows point to consistent vessels that course in the neck caudal to the corner of the mouth. The black arrow points to a vessel that is approximately 1 cm caudal to the mandible. Division is frequently required. The white arrow points to a vessel that can be isolated and mobilized if necessary for flap advancement. R) Right side. Once the flap dissection had been completed, the deep surface of the flap in the region of the anterior zygomaticus muscle is incised (yellow arrow) and fixation sutures are placed. The white arrow points to the methylene blue line along the course of the zygomatic arch. The blue arrow points to the zygomaticus muscle.

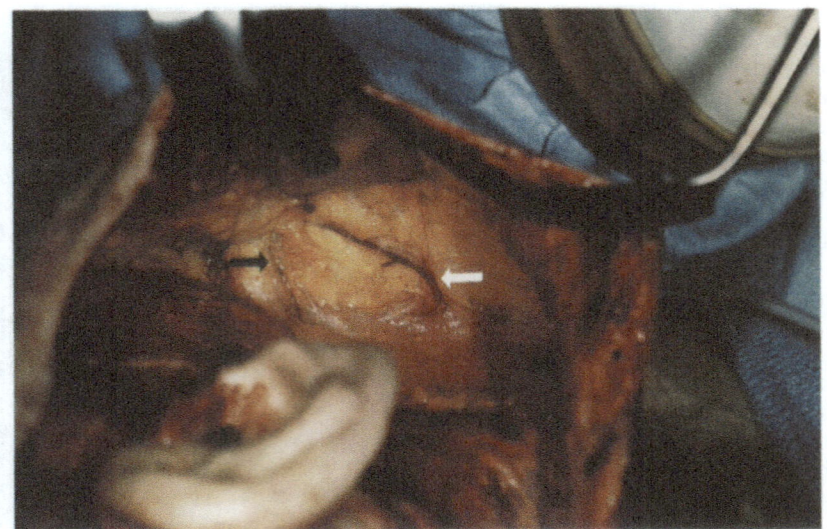

Q

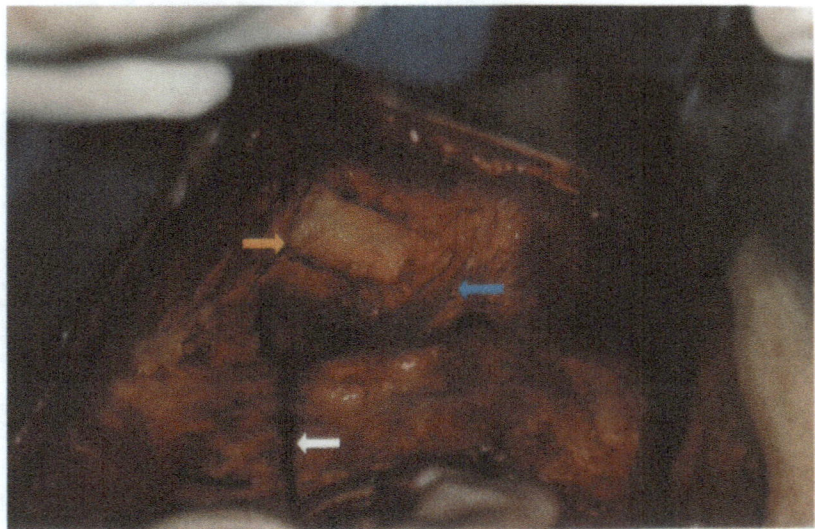

R

**Figure 4-5 S, T**
S) Right face. Yellow arrow points to the methylene blue line along the caudal edge of the obicularis occuli muscle. The double methylene blue lines indicate the course of the zygomatic arch. The forceps hold the fixation suture, extending from the anterior facial dissection (white arrow) to the point of attachment, the anterior zygomatic arch. T) Right side. Reduction in the naso-labial deformity and mid-face support is evidenced by a tethering of the skin flap and elevation (not lateral displacement) of the corner of the mouth.

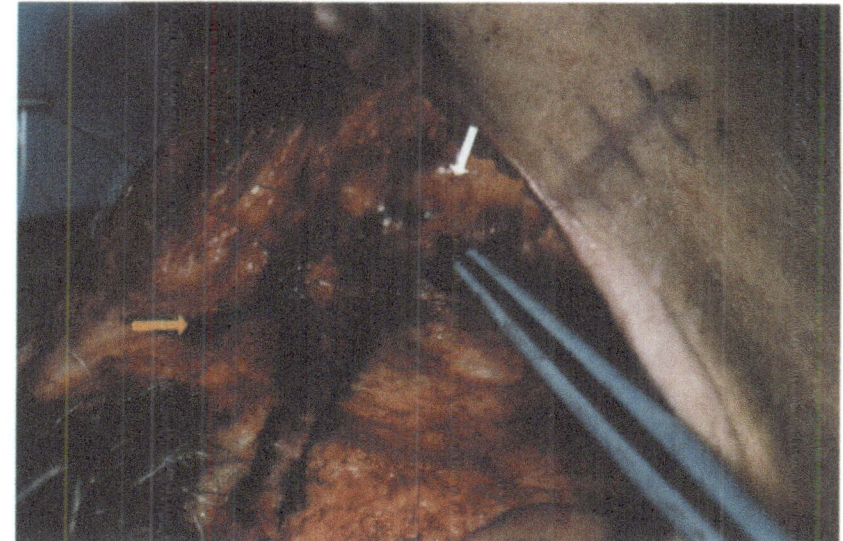

S

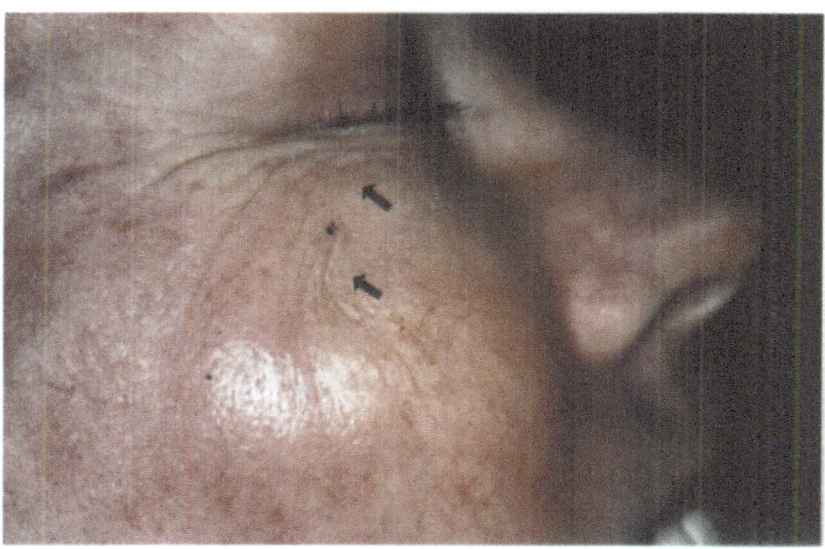

T

**Figure 4-5 U, V**
U) Mouth is elevated in a cephalad direction. V) Left side. A similar procedure is performed on the contralateral side of the face.

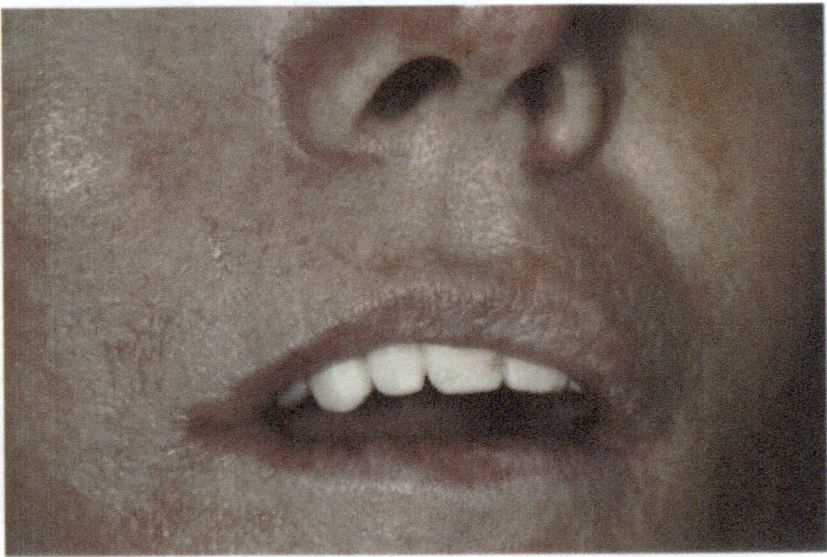

U

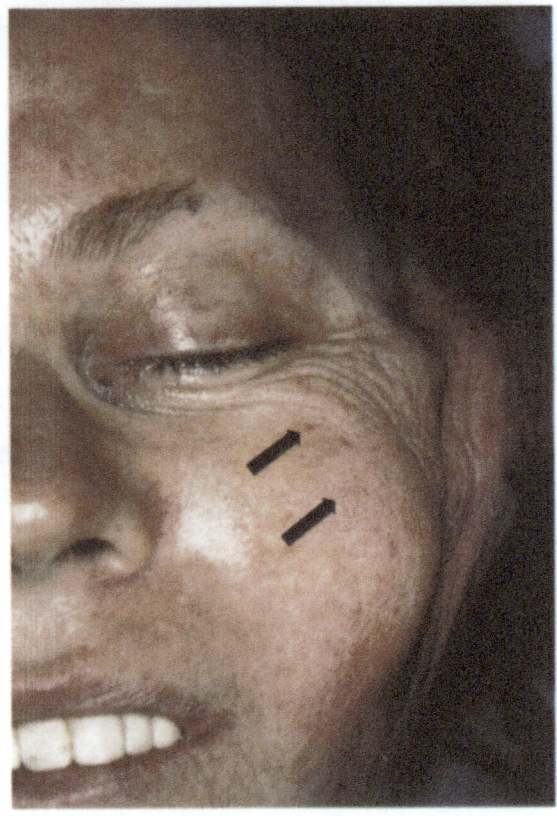

V

Chapter Four   **Aesthetic Laser Surgery**

**Figure 4-5 W**
W) Proper tension is illustrated by symmetrical lip position after both sides are completed.

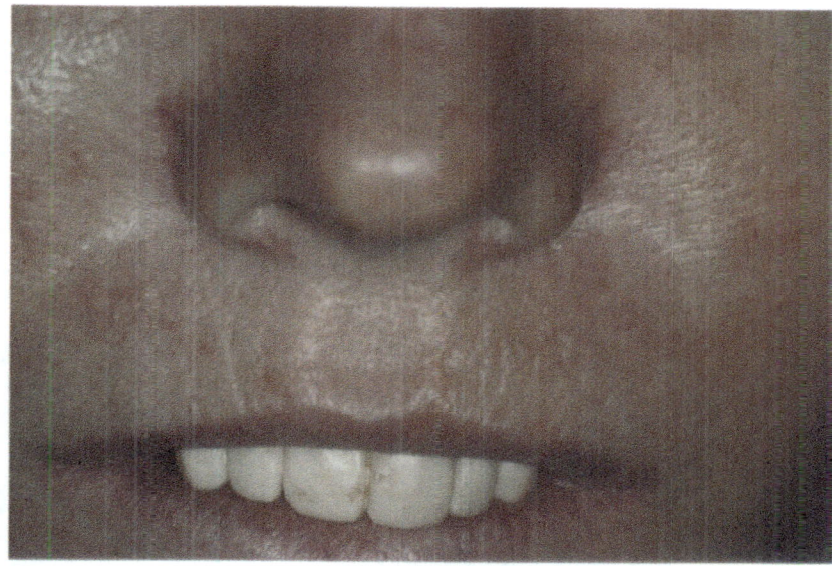

W

## Other Procedures

Once you have gained confidence in your technique and have an understanding of the properties and "feel" of the laser delivery system and wavelength you are using, other laser-assisted aesthetic procedures can be performed, such as the endoscopic brow lift. The principles of proper traction and countertraction, identification of anatomic landmarks, and dissection along tissue planes whenever possible will allow for realization of the potential benefits of laser surgery without additional morbidity. Other nondissecting surgical procedures such as de-epithelialization of the inferior pedicle flap during a breast reduction (Figure 4-6 A–B) are facilitated with the $CO_2$ laser.

## Laserscope Laser: KTP Wavelength

Due to thermal injury, the skin should not be incised with the KTP wavelength and its current delivery system. Once the skin incision is made with the scalpel, skin, skin/muscle, and subcutaneous or composite flaps can be easily dissected off underlying tissue. A setting of four to seven watts of power is all that is required to achieve a hemostatic dissection for either the blepharoplasty or rhytidectomy procedures. The green light (laser energy) can be shown to be selectively absorbed by bleeding tissue (see Figure 4-5 A), which may play a role in the hemostatic effect of this wavelength in addition to the heat at the tip. Local anesthetic instilled into the surgery site will not affect the energy requirements. The delivery device is a sterile, disposable tapered quartz fiber (600 to 300 or 600 to 100 micron tip) which is light and held like a pencil during surgery. Handpieces come in two

**Figure 4-6 A, B**
A) De-epithelialization of breast pedicle using the Sharplan 150 XJ laser, continuous mode, 120 watts, 6 mm handpiece. Average time for de-epithelialization was three minutes. B) The high power histologic section of a random biopsy of the inferior pedicle reveals elimination of the epidermis, upper right-hand corner, with patent, subdermal vessels. (Photographs courtesy of Dr. G. Stevens, Marina del Ray, CA.)

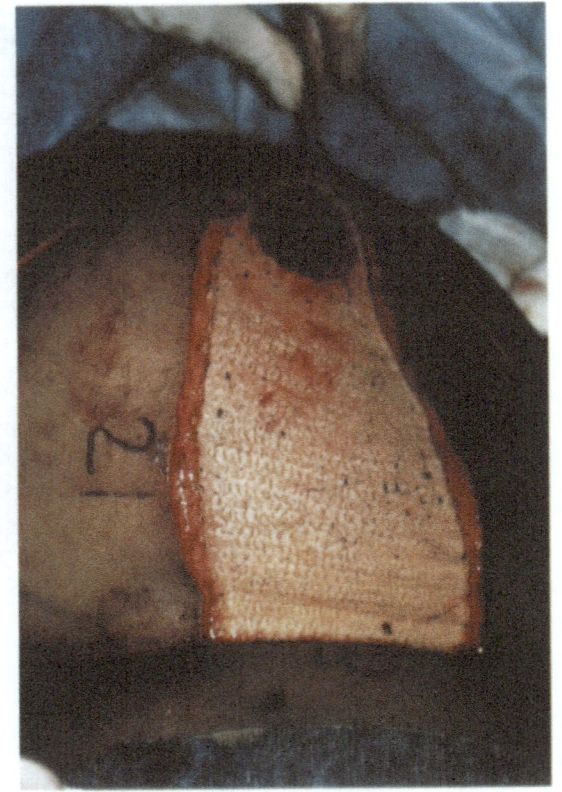

A

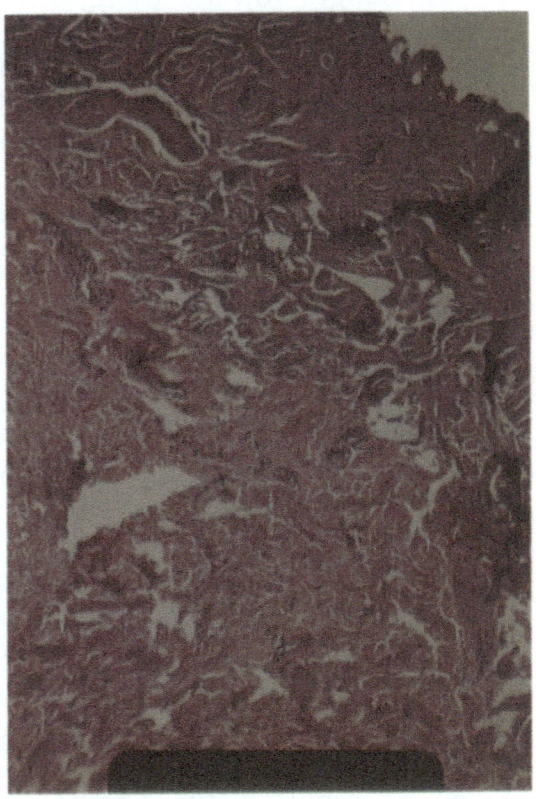

B

lengths: 2.5 and 12.5 cm for near and distant dissection, respectively. A suction catheter can be fixed to the fiber to remove the laser plume (see Figure 4-1). It is advisable to activate the fiber only while it is in contact with tissue to avoid tip overheating with resultant frosting. Once frosted, a greater percentage of the laser energy is transferred to the tissue in the form of heat. Do not use the fiber to separate tissue mechanically, i.e., as a probe, since the clear quartz tip can fracture and may be difficult to recover.

The surgeon should isolate vessels that are 0.5 mm or greater from adjacent tissues for a length of 2 to 3 mm and then expose both sides of these vessels to laser energy in order to seal them prior to transection. This technique should also be used for smaller vessels when the systolic blood pressure is greater than 140–150 mm Hg.

Try to reduce the length of time that you spend in one area with the fiber tip activated to keep the heat transferred to a minimum. Once the fiber tip becomes frosted, due in part to the degradation from heat build-up from length of use or activation when not in contact with tissue, the fiber becomes more and more of a "hot knife" versus light and heat energy transfer. This event can be minimized with the Fiber Life feature of the laser. Another characteristic of the KTP wavelength is that the laser light is visible, which helps to illuminate the surgical field (Figure 4-7). When hemostasis is achieved using the KTP laser, incidental nerve injury is rarely observed as compared with electrocautery in my experience.

Figures 4-8 A–D, 4-9 A–D, 4-10 A–D, and 4-11 A–C illustrate the typical results one can obtain when performing facial aesthetic surgery with the Laserscope KTP laser system. Variability in outcome is related to the aesthetic deformity, surgical technique, procedure(s) performed, patient state of health, and compliance with postoperative instructions.

**Figure 4-7**
Photograph taken without the protective filter. Protective goggles worn by the surgeon reduce the intensity of the light and modulate the color. While not analogous to standard fiberoptic "white" light, illumination during laser activation does help during dissection, especially deep in the anterior face and neck. Black arrow points to the fascia over the parotid gland.

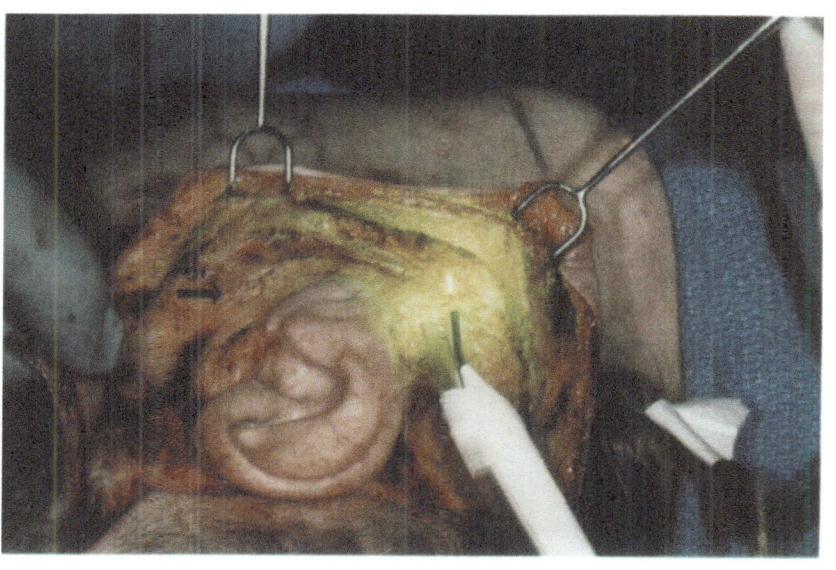

**Figure 4-8 A, B**
A) Preoperative photograph of a 26-year-old female who received an upper lid blepharoplasty with resection of skin and fat and a lower lid transconjunctival blepharoplasty. The surgery was performed utilizing a 600 to 100 micron tapered quartz fiber and 4 watts of power, KTP 800 series laser, Laserscope. B, C.

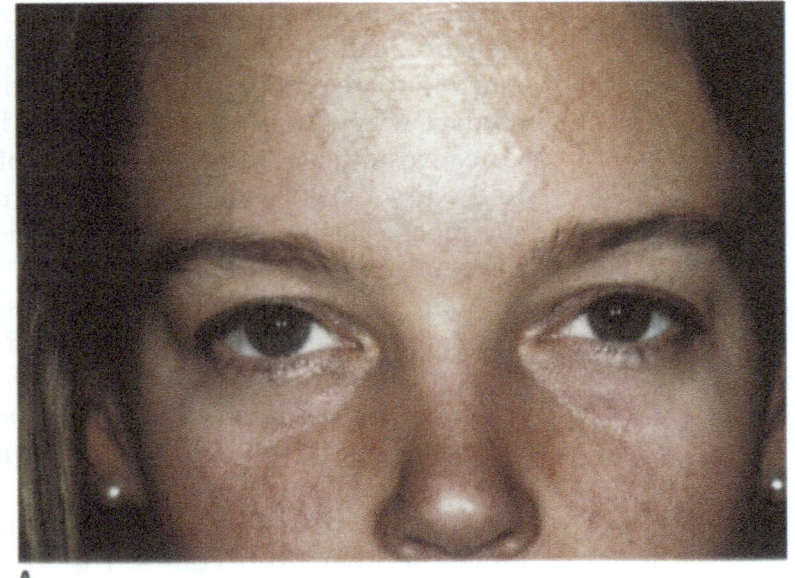

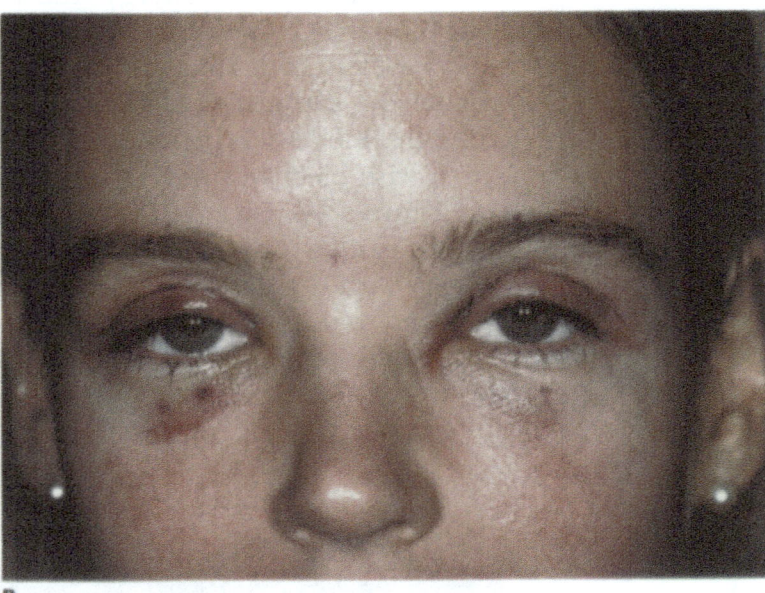

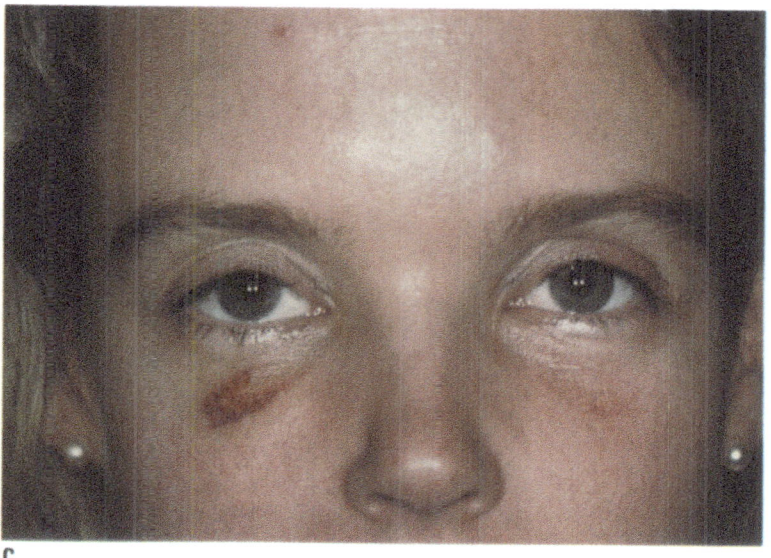

C

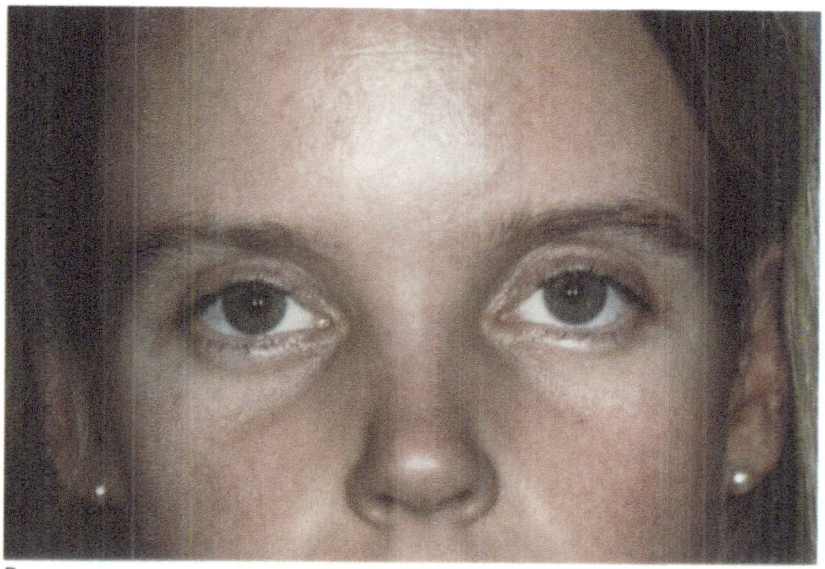

D

**Figure 4-9 A, B**
A) Preoperative view of a 48-year-old female that received an upper and lower lid blepharoplasty with resection of skin, muscle, and fat. The laser and settings were the same as for the patient in Figure 4-8. B) reflect postoperative days 1, 4, and 10, respectively.

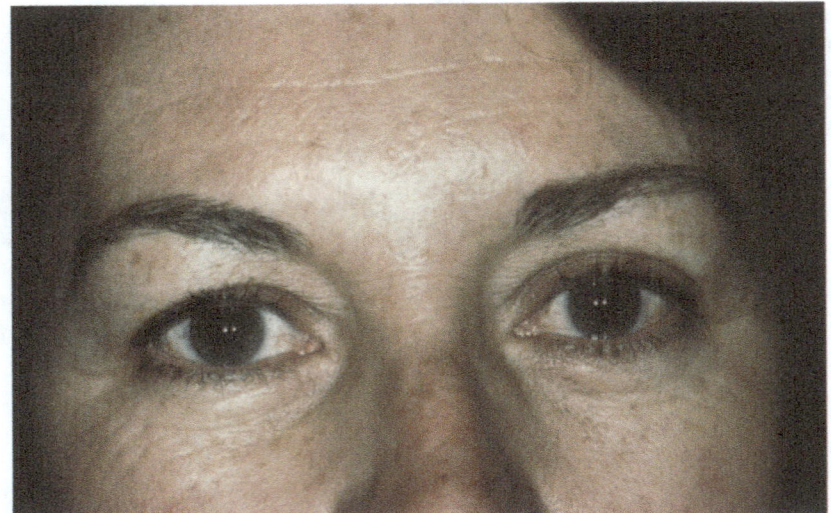

A

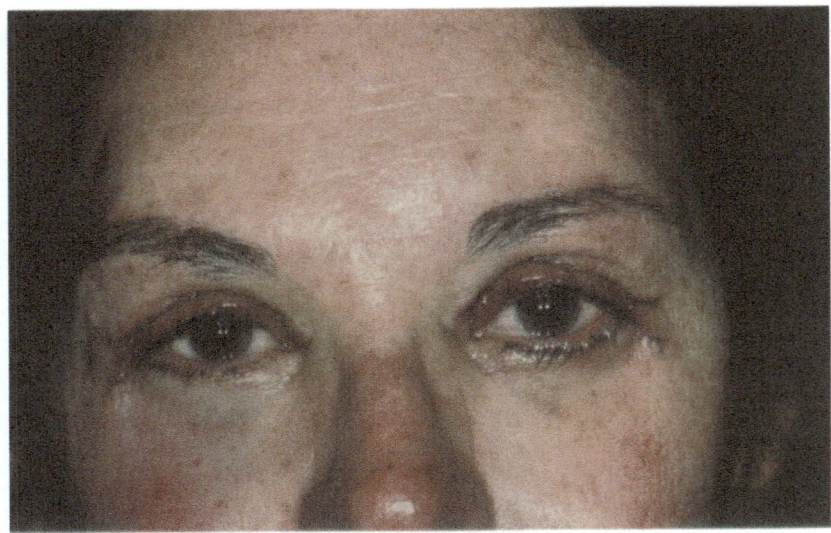

B

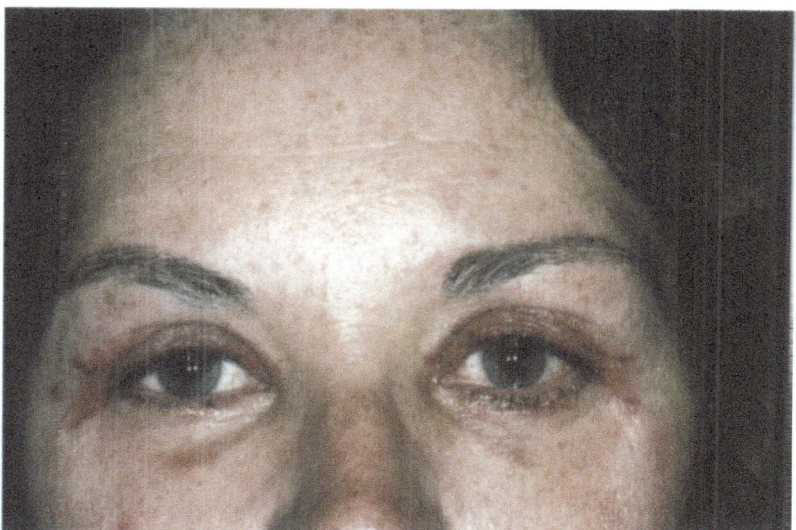

C

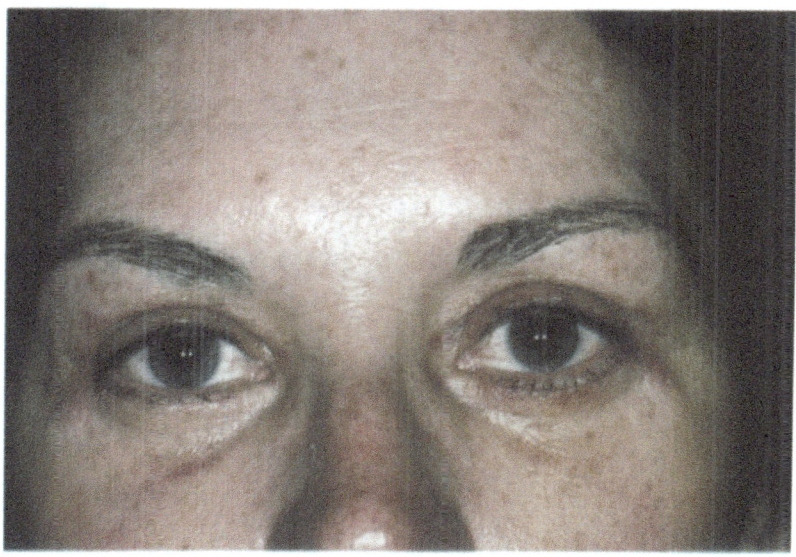

D

**Figure 4-10 A, B**
A) This 66-year-old male would have benefited from a brow lift and upper blepharoplasty as well as the lower lid blepharoplasty and facelift he requested and received. A 600 to 300 micron tapered quartz fiber and 4 watts of power for the eyelid procedure and 7 watts of power for the facial surgery was used with the KTP 800 laser, Laserscope. The photographs illustrate the lateral view preoperatively A), and postoperative days 1 B), 7 C), and 21 D).

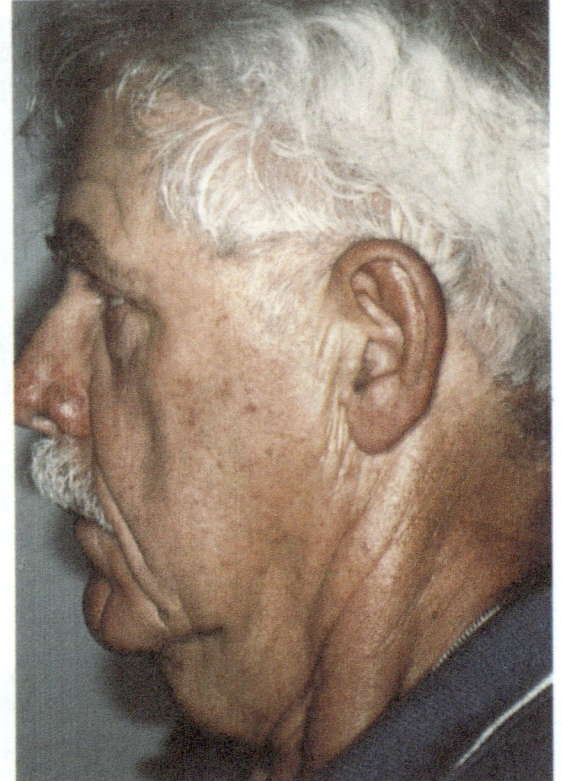

A

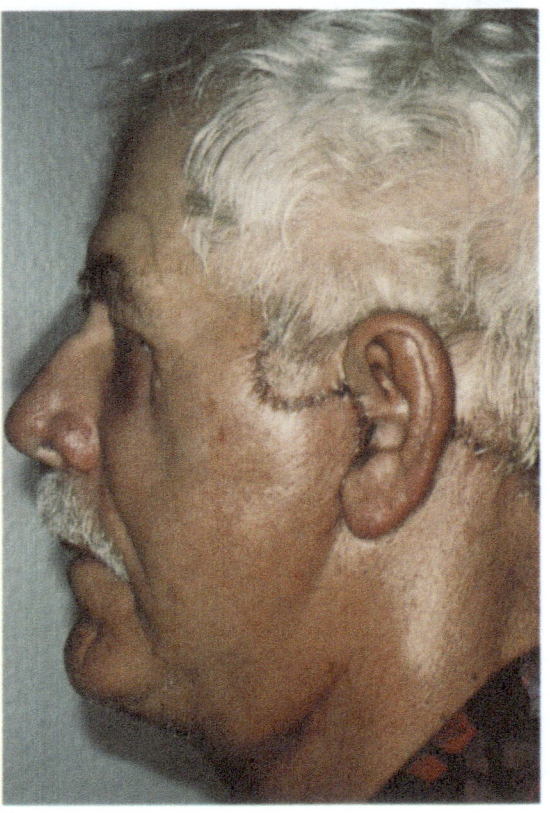

B

**Figure 4-10 C, D**
The photographs illustrate the lateral view preoperatively A), and postoperative days C), and 21 D).

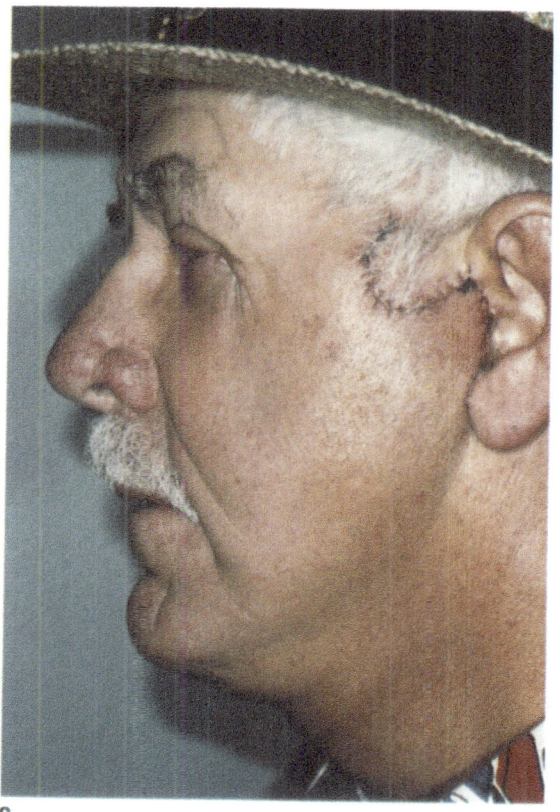

C

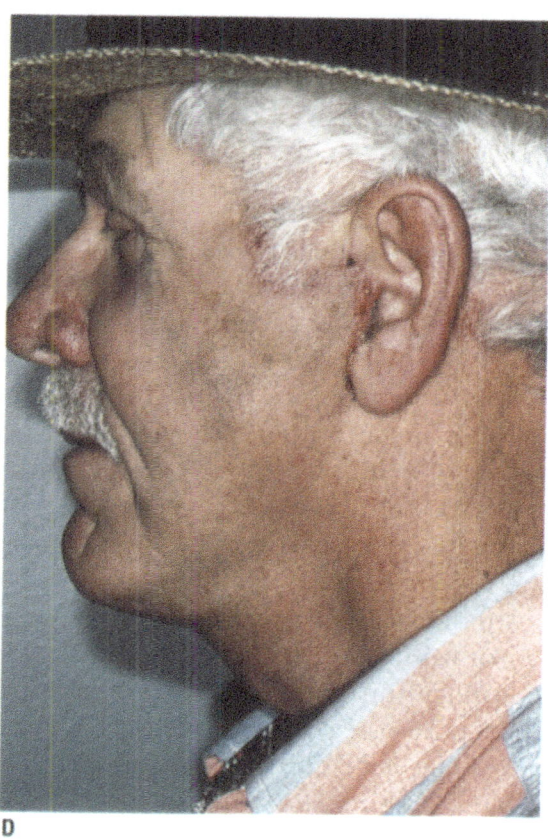

D

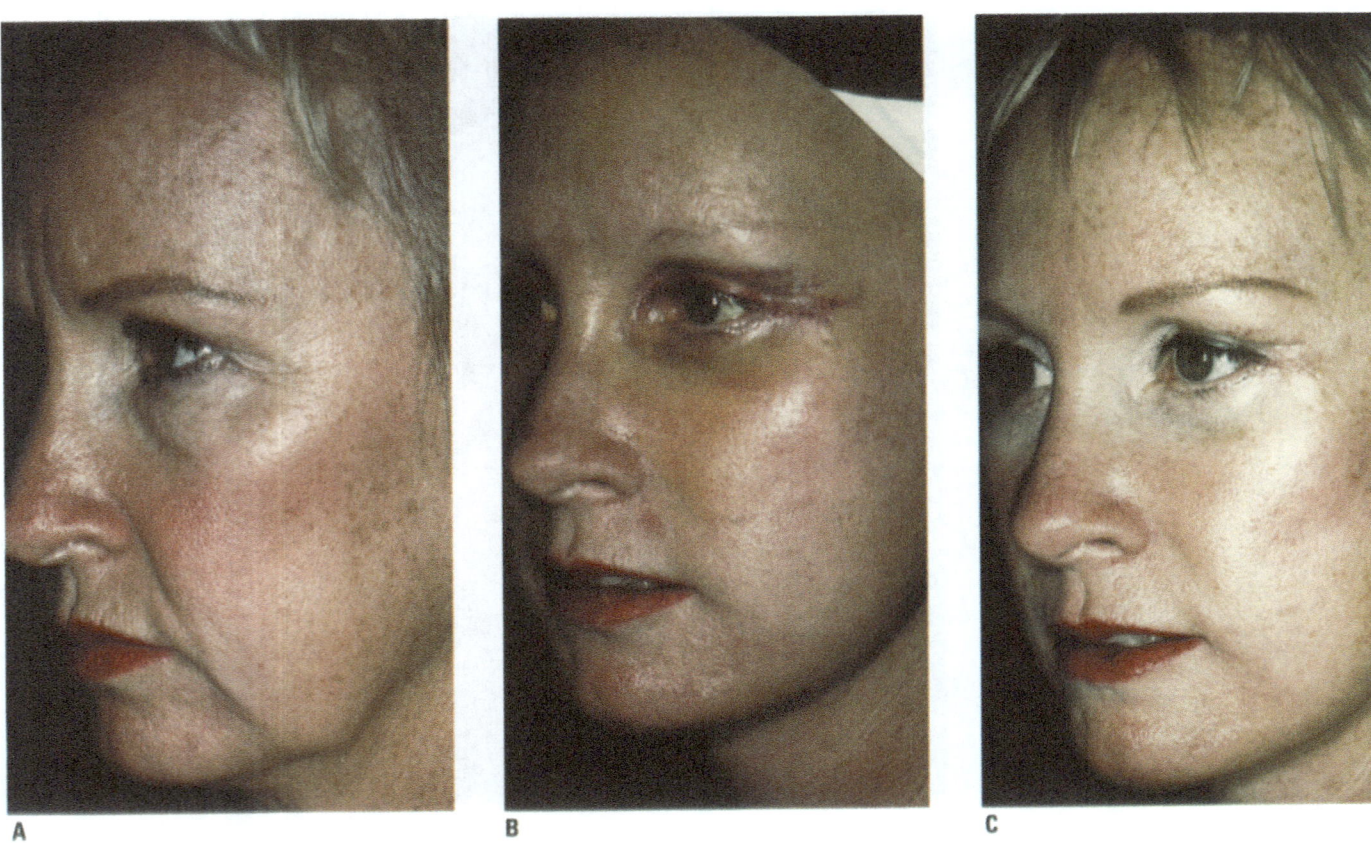

**Figure 4-11 A, B, C**
This 49-year-old female underwent a pretrichal coronal brow lift (subperiostial dissection, release of the lateral orbital ligament and periostial attachments to the supraorbital rim, resection of the attachment of the corrugator and depressor supracilli muscles at the nasion), upper and lower blepharoplasty with resection of skin, muscle, and fat, and facial rhytidectomy as outlined in the text. A) represents the preoperative oblique view of the patient and B) and C) represent postoperative days 4 and 21, respectively.

## Heraeus Laser: YAG Wavelength

### by David Apfelberg, M.D.

The YAG laser (Heraeus Laser Sonics Hercules Model 5040) is utilized with 10 to 15 watts of power transmitted through fiber optics to a frosted sapphire tip of 0.6 to 0.8 mm. Either a continuous wave is used for cutting with coagulation on the face, or lower power (five to eight watts) with 0.01 s pulse and 0.01 s interval for more gentle skin treatment of the eyelids. Skin incision with the laser always produces a narrow zone of thermal necrosis (reported experimentally to be as small as 50 to 200 microns) which is best resected with fine scissors or scalpel prior to closure for prevention of scar formation or wound dehiscence (Figure 4-12). The sapphire tip is carbonized by application to a dry tongue blade to produce a short burning. This prepares the tip for immediate incision when applied to the skin. The YAG laser is "contact" and used as a scalpel, permitting sensory feedback for the surgeon.

Facelift flaps can be undermined easily and almost bloodlessly for a distance of 3 to 5 cm with one exception: transection of large

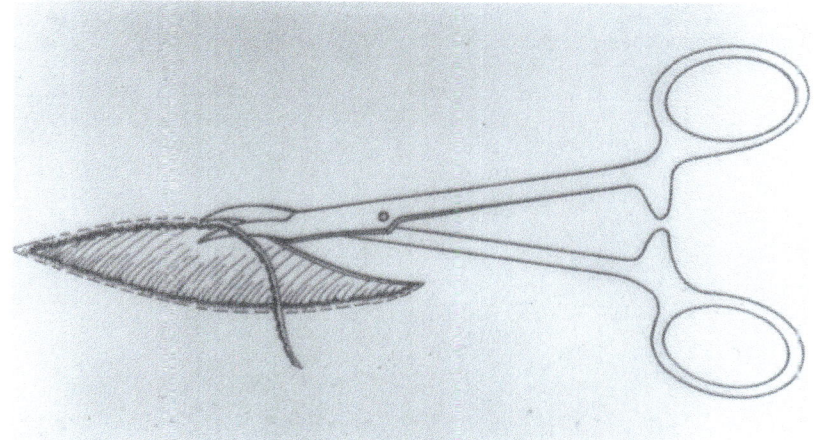

lumen superficial temporal vessels (Figures 4-13, 4-14, and 4-15). Deeper or longer flap undermining is aided by injection and distention of multiple adjacent tunnels with a 14-gauge spatula tip needle and local anesthesia with epinephrine. The tissue between the injected tunnels is then divided with the laser. Care is taken to keep the dissection at the proper level and to avoid "button-holing" the skin. Platysma and SMAS dissection may be performed with the laser, providing a bloodless field for proper observation of important anatomical structures such as facial nerves and muscles. No stimulation of the facial nerve, as seen with electrocautery, results from laser contact. Frequently, no further hemostasis is required after laser dis-

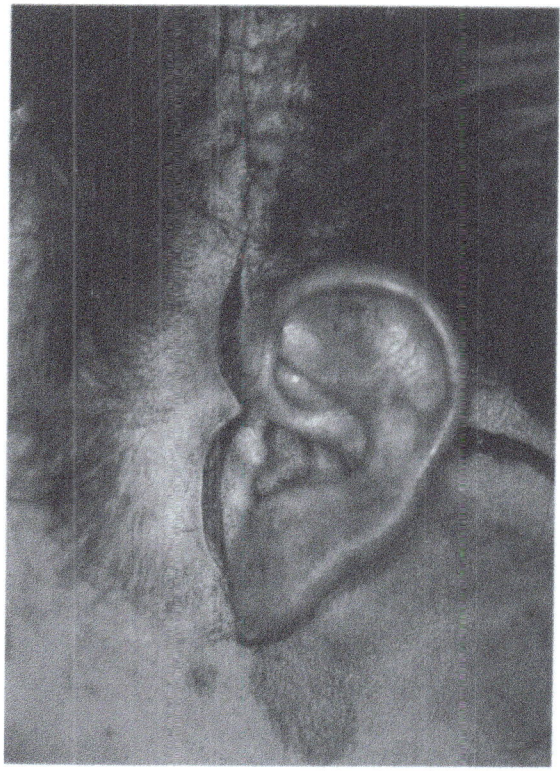

**Figure 4-14**
Contact tip dissecting anterior cheek flap.

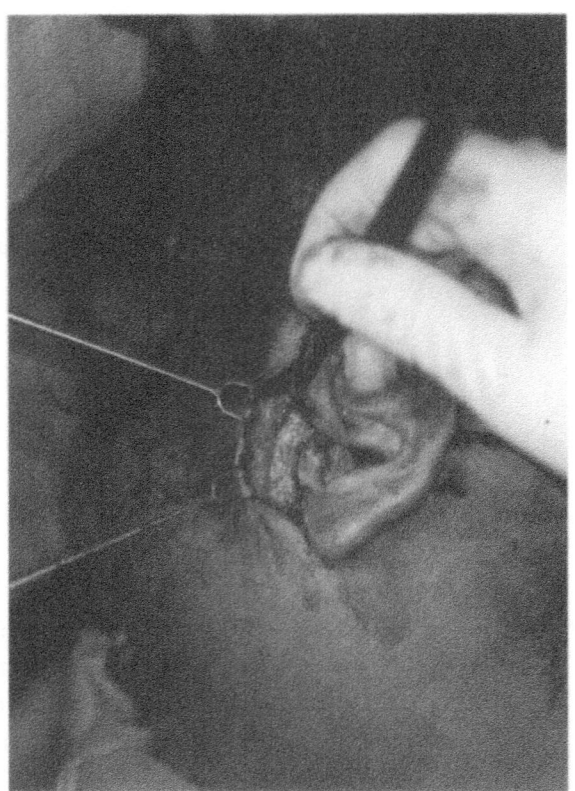

**Figure 4-15**
Contact tip dissecting mastoid skin flap.

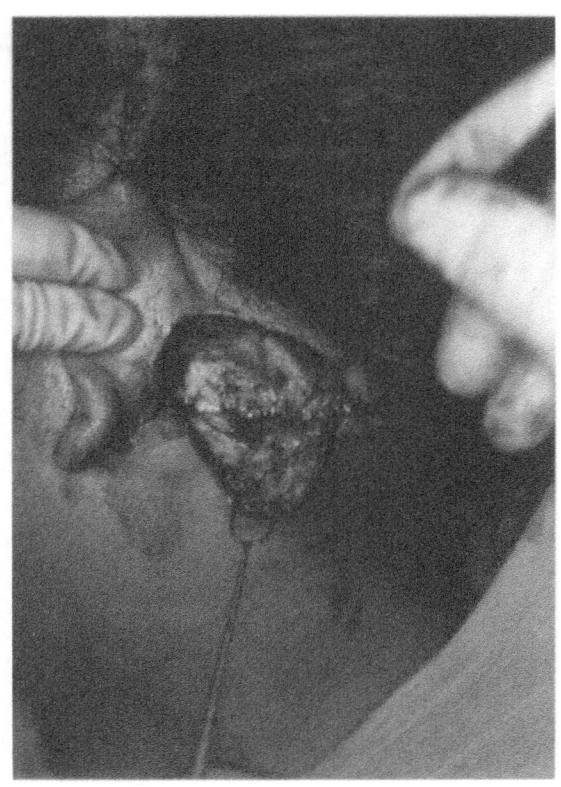

Chapter Four   **Aesthetic Laser Surgery**

**Figure 4-16**
Preoperative patient demonstrating facial laxity and elastosis and moderate blepharochalasia.

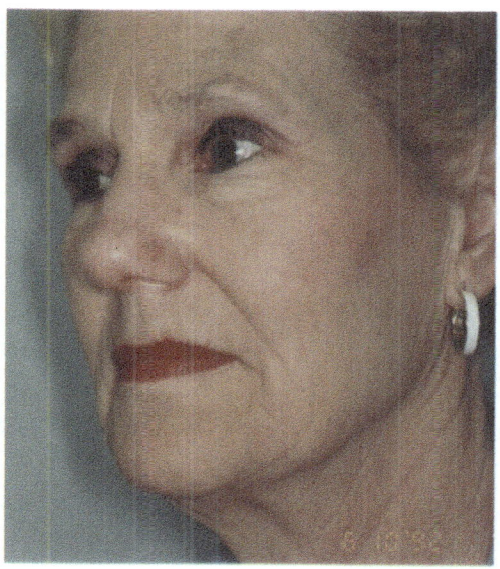

section. Flap advancement and closure is identical to standard facelift techniques. Postoperative course often demonstrates limited ecchymosis and swelling compared to conventional techniques (Figures 4-16, 4-17, and 4-18).

Eyelid surgery is performed in a similar manner with some minor modifications. Protective eye shields are inserted over the globes after application of ophthalmic anesthetic and antibiotic ointments and are removed immediately following the procedure to prevent corneal edema. Skin, muscle, and fat may all be resected with the laser without the necessity for cross-clamping or crushing these structures. Blood loss frequently is reported as 0 to 5 cc for all four lids. Contralateral studies have demonstrated less bruising and swelling on the laser side (Figures 4-19, 4-20, 4-21, and 4-22).

**Figure 4-17**
Four days postoperative photo illustrating very minor bruising and swelling following YAG laser meloplasty and blepharoplasty.

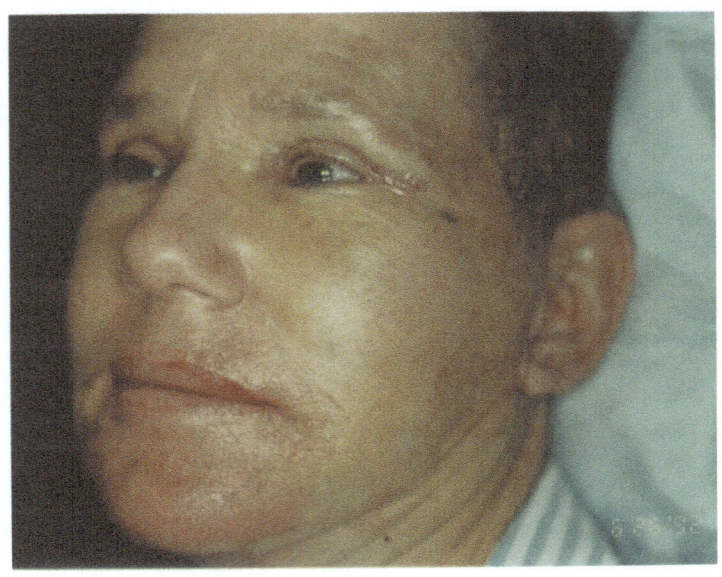

**Figure 4-18**
Final result at three weeks.

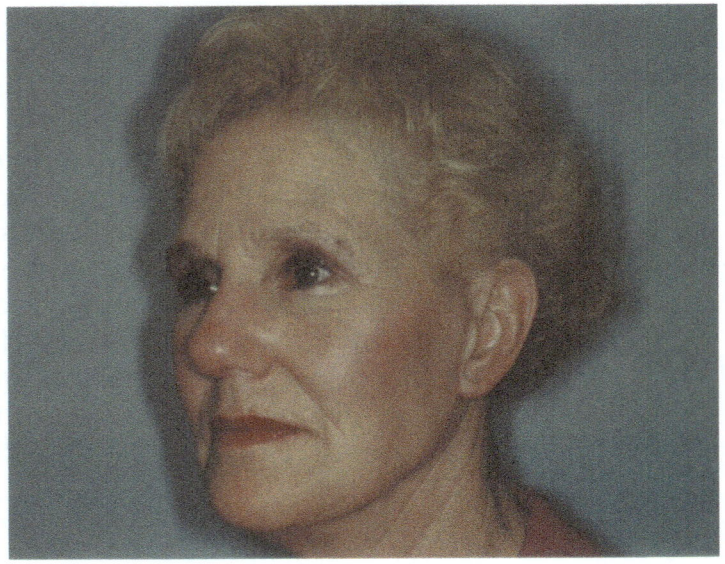

**Figure 4-19**
Preoperative patient with moderate upper eyelid hooding and fat herniations and wrinkled skin in lower lids.

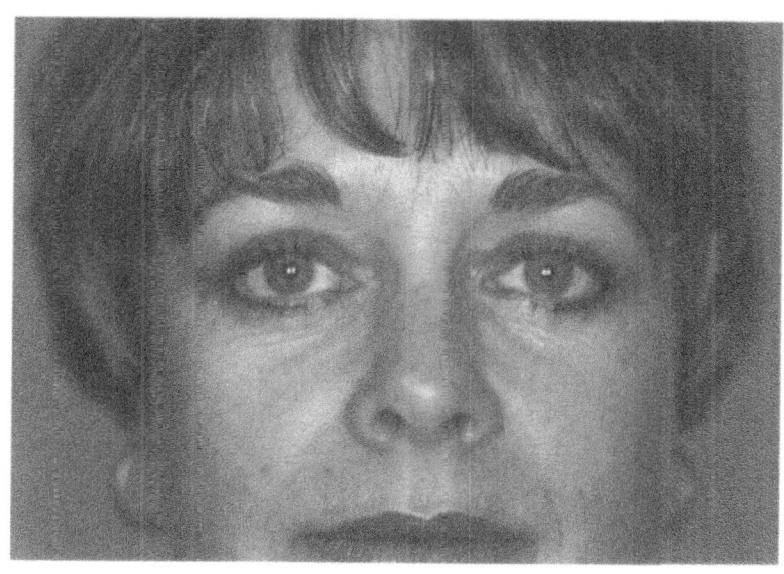

**Figure 4-20**
Patient four days following YAG laser blepharoplasty left eye and conventional scalpel/cautery surgery on right eye. Right eye demonstrates more ecchymosis.

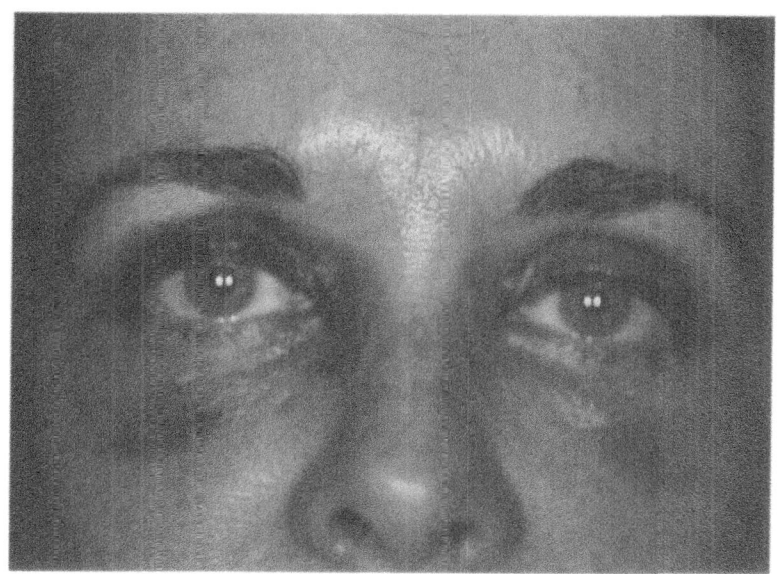

**Figure 4-21**
Nine days post-op, laser eye is completely healed and conventional eye still has bruise, which disappeared by day 14.

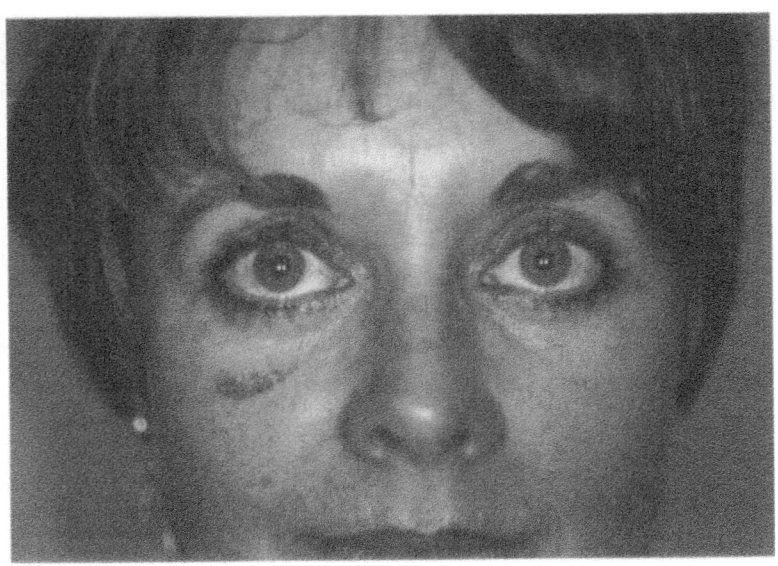

**Figure 4-22**
Final result at three weeks.

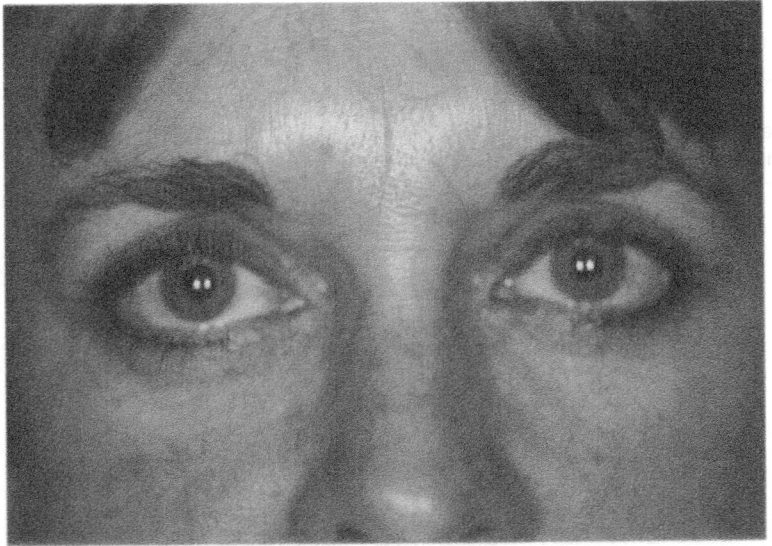

### by Michael I. Kulick, M.D., D.D.S.

Various Sharplan laser models are available, ranging from the 40 watt to the 150 watt XJ machine which I currently use. Using high-pulse energy, the skin can be incised with the CO$_2$ laser. Skin edges do not have to be trimmed prior to skin closure to obtain a fine line scar. The XJ SurgiPulse waveform is a high-energy, short-duration "double pulse" which minimizes adjacent tissue damage and char formation when compared to continuous waveforms. The SurgiPulse "double pulse" allows the tissue to cool and plume to be evacuated in between each pulse delivered to the tissue. The SurgiPulse waveforms are designed never to exceed tissue thermal relaxation time of skin. Less tissue injury and char provides less post-surgical swelling.

For surgical procedures, the two most common devices I use are the 125 mm handpiece and the 450 or 1000 mm long flexible tube waveguides. The 125 mm handpiece has a focal spot size of 0.2 mm. A 50 mm handpiece is available that provides a smaller spot size, 0.1 mm. Of these two handpieces, the 125 mm size furnishes me the best balance between a cutting and cautery device. A HeNe red beam indicates the location of laser beam contact with the tissue. With the 150 XJ laser, I normally use a setting of 275 millijoules and seven to nine watts of power in the SurgiPulse mode with the 125 mm handpiece for a blepharoplasty procedure. The handpiece can be sterilized with the lens removed. Once sterile, it is connected to the lens and then attached to the articulated arm of the laser and the CO$_2$ purge tubing. The handpiece and articulated arm are draped with a sterile sleeve, exposing only the distal end of the handpiece (Figure 4-23). A suction catheter can be attached to the end and connected

**Figure 4-23**
The 125 mm handpiece is connected to the articulated arm and penetrates a sterile plastic sleeve normally used for arthroscopic cameras. Through the clear plastic sleeve you can see the black tubing connected to the hand piece required for the CO$_2$ gas purge. This is the same handpiece that is connected to the Sharplan scanning device for skin resurfacing.

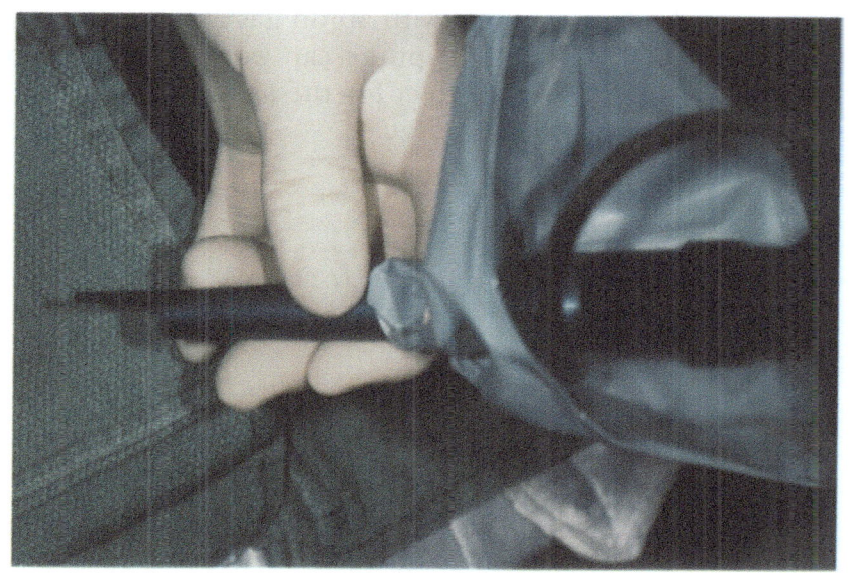

to the high power evacuation machine as an alternative to having the assistant hold a separate suction tubing. Since surgery with the $CO_2$ laser proceeds in a noncontact mode, there is no tactile feedback for the surgeon, which requires an adjustment from standard surgical methods. There is an optimal distance or focal length for cutting, measured from the end of the handpiece to the tissue. A metal extension from the end of the handpiece establishes this distance for the surgeon. Defocusing the handpiece by pulling it away from the tissue will allow for a wider laser beam tissue contact area and permits cauterization. It is the balanced interchange between the focused cutting distance and a defocused cauterization distance that permits a bloodless dissection.

The 125 mm handpiece with the above energy settings can also be used to make the initial skin incisions when performing a rhytidectomy. These settings can be adjusted based on the experience of the surgeon. The amount and location of local anesthetic instilled will also affect the energy settings. The more fluid the laser energy has to penetrate, the more energy required. This can work to the surgeon's advantage when trying to protect the pretarsal muscle when incising the subcilliary skin during a lower eyelid blepharoplasty. The cut is essentially char free and will permit healing with a fine line scar (Figure 4-24 A–D).

The Sharplan Fiberlase waveguides are sterile, disposable hollow tubes that come in three lengths: 300 mm, 450 mm, and 1000 mm. They can be held as stand alone fibers or inserted into a handpiece with integral suction port for dissection under flaps. In the SurgiPulse mode, I set the laser at 275 to 300 millijoules and 15 to 20 watts of power, depending on the waveguide used and the tissue type. These tubes have highly polished inner surfaces that act like mirrors to transmit the $CO_2$ energy. Like the 125 mm handpiece, the waveguide transmits a HeNe guide beam light to indicate the point of laser beam tissue contact since the $CO_2$ laser energy is invisible. To minimize waveguide energy transmission degradation by smoke, debris, as well as the gas used to purge the waveguide, I purge the flexible waveguide with argon gas at 0.5 to 1.0 liters versus the standard $CO_2$ gas. A $CO_2$ purge can work, although I have found less variability in tissue effect for the same laser settings in long procedures with an argon purge.

**Figure 4-24 A, B**
This 35-year-old female underwent an upper and lower lid blepharoplasty with the Sharplan 150 XJ laser using the 125 mm handpiece with the settings outlined in the text. A portion of the lower eyelid fat was removed as well as brought across the infraorbital rim. A lateral muscle suspension suture was placed. The upper eyelids had an initial skin resection, removal of redundant fat, and then a small strip of obicularis muscle excised. A) through D) reflect the patient's appearance preoperatively and on postoperative days 4, 7, and 21, respectively.

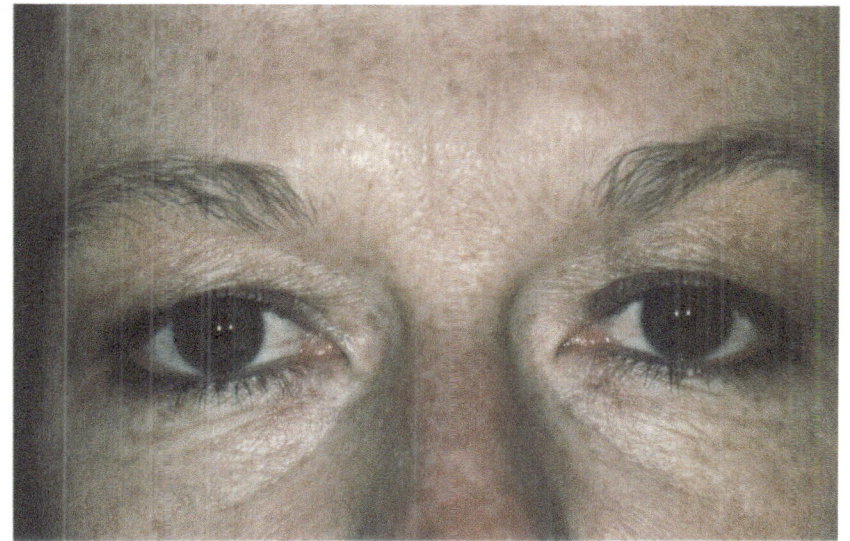

A

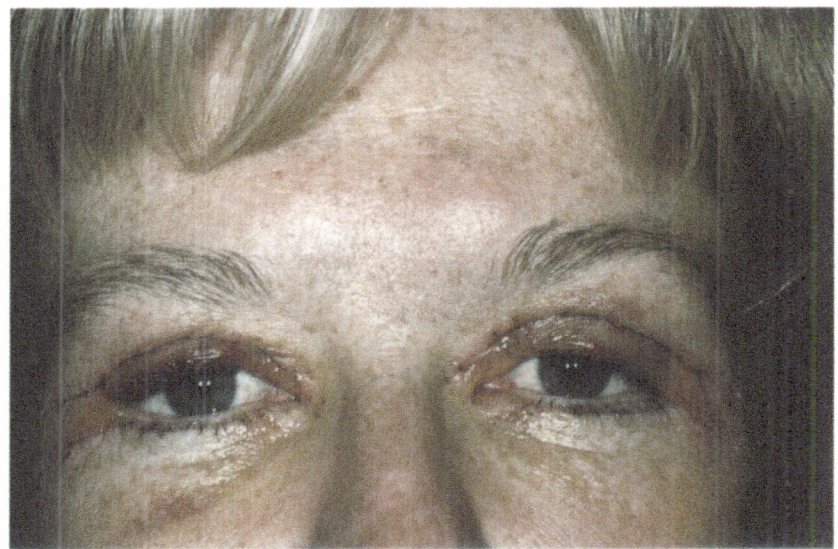

B

Figure 4-24 C, D

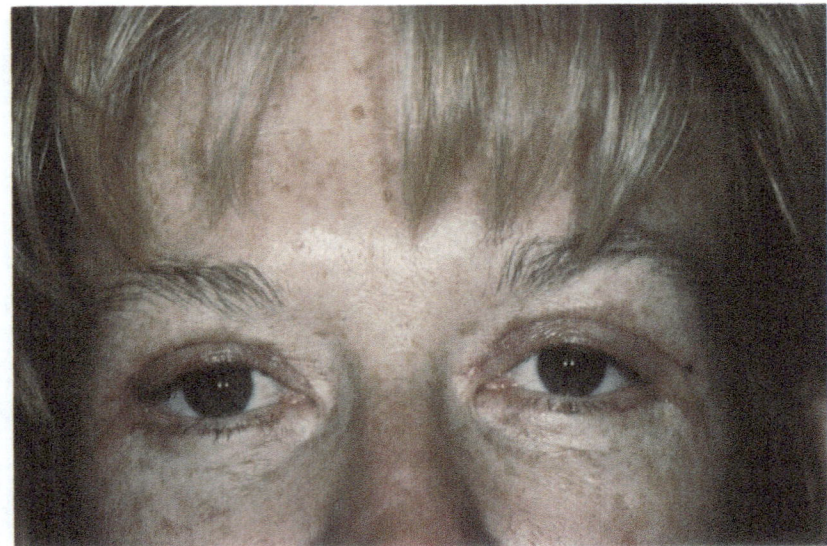

C

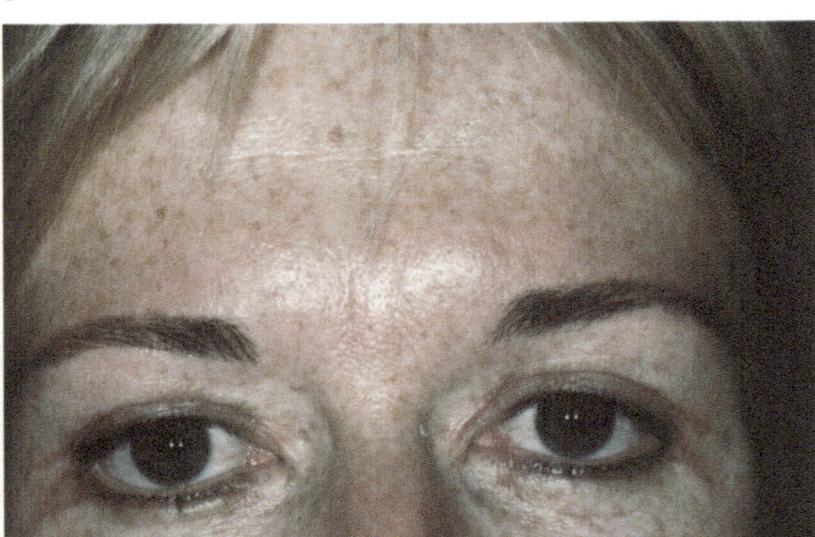

D

The waveguides are flexible, although bending them reduces the efficiency of transmission and the tissue effect for a given energy setting. The spot size ranges from approximately 0.92 mm at 5 mm from the fiber end, to 3.4 mm at a 35 mm distance. This permits both cutting at close range and coagulation when pulling the fiber away from the tissue, similar to the effect obtained with the 125 mm handpiece. To operate properly, the tip of the Fiberlase waveguide must be kept free of debris which can accumulate during a prolonged dissection. The waveguide is ideal for endoscopic procedures and when dissecting under facial flaps anterior in the face and neck. It is attached to the articulating arm of the laser through a coupler device which can be sterilized with the lens removed (Figure 4-25). Once the fiber and the coupling device are attached to the laser, the sterile drape can then be applied to the articulated arm.

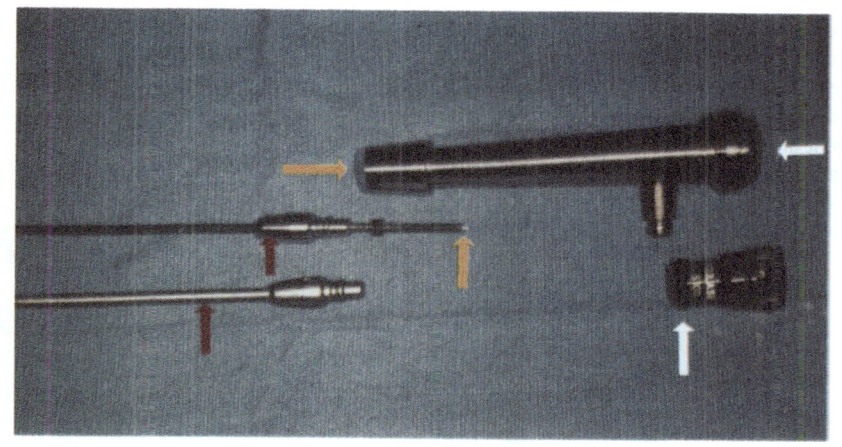

**Figure 4-25**
The waveguide coupler device main body is in the upper right hand corner. The green colored waveguide has been passed through the smaller of the two connector devices (red arrows) that attach the waveguide to the distal end of the coupler device (yellow arrows indicate the end of the waveguide that is inserted into the end of the coupler). The lens is inserted into the other end of the coupler (white arrows), and then this assembly is connected to the articulated arm of the laser.

Regardless of the delivery device or procedure, the surgeon must be aware of the potential pathway of the laser beam beyond the initial point of tissue contact. Inadvertent skin burns or damage to muscle, nerves, etc., can occur when the beam penetrates the tissue being incised and then carries to the next physical barrier. Placement of a wet tongue blade or wet gauze behind the site of surgery, perpendicular to the line of contact of the laser energy and tissue, will help prevent burns behind the immediate surgical site during a blepharoplasty (see Figure 4-4 H). Being aware of the penetration depth will minimize the chance of undesirable tissue injury during brow and facial flap surgery.

When removing adipose tissue, you can either excise the fat with the handpiece in a focused mode for large resections or pull the handpiece back from the optimal focal distance and melt or vaporize the fat, primarily for small resections or removing irregularities. The liquefied fat should be expunged with gauze so that it does not serve as an irritant postoperatively. The defocused technique of energy delivery can be used to smooth any irregularities following surgical resection of fat or muscle. The laser plume must be removed with a separate high power evacuation suction that can be attached to the end of the handpiece or by a suction wand held by the assistant. The $CO_2$ wavelength cuts rapidly through fat and muscle. Thus, the speed of dissection must be adjusted to avoid partial division of blood vessels prior to sealing. The same precautions and method of sealing blood vessels prior to transection exist as outlined for the KTP laser.

Rapid evacuation of the laser plume in confined spaces such as those under facial skin flaps is critical to avoid igniting the non-suctioned plume with laser energy. This phenomena can occur when using the waveguide or handpiece in a defocused mode while defatting an area through vaporization/melting. The plume can build up along the path of the laser beam and ignite if the suction does not evacuate it rapidly due to the volume of plume or a clogged suction port. Inadvertent skin burns or flap penetration can be avoided by periodically palpating flap thickness and dissecting along natural anatomic planes whenever possible.

**Figure 4-26 A, B**
This 71-year-old woman underwent a similar surgical procedure as the patient in Figure 4-24. Photographs represent the patient preoperatively (A) and postoperative days 4 (B), 10 .

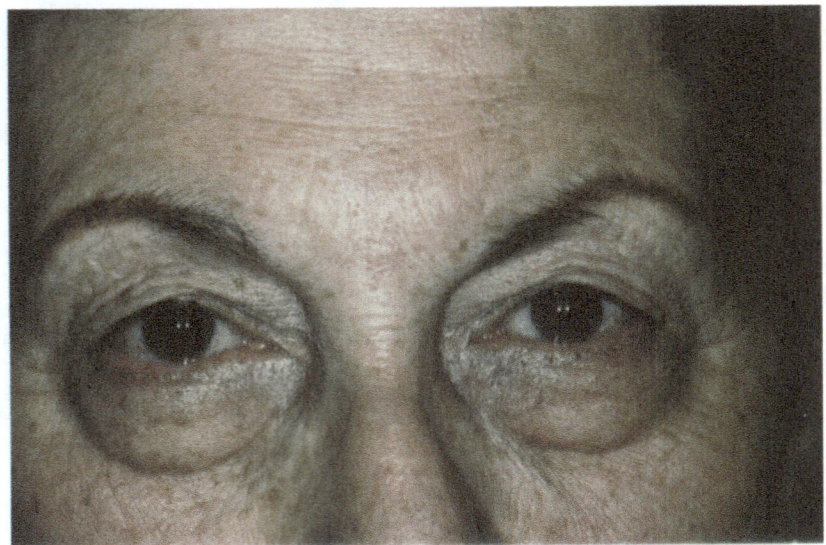

A

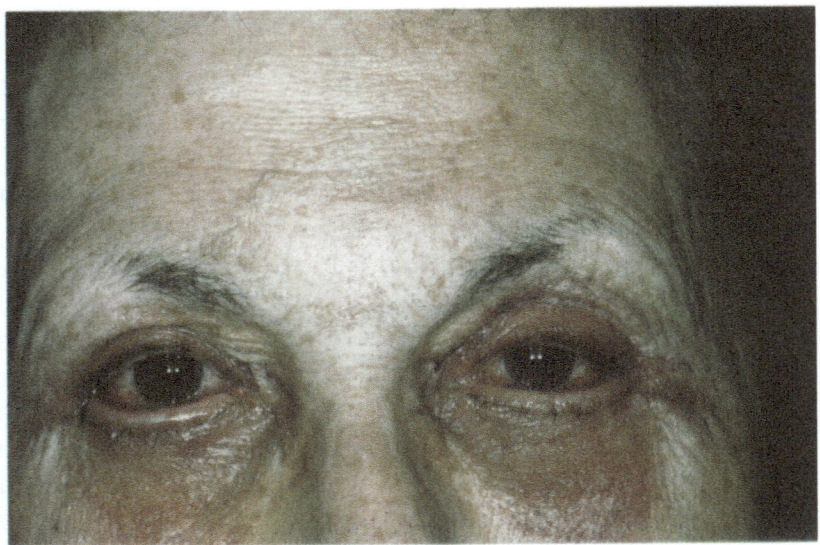

B

The following figures demonstrate the results obtained with the guidelines stated above (see Figure 4-24, and Figures 4-26 A–D, 4-27 A–D, and 4-28 A–D). I have experienced no complications related to the use of this laser (skin burn, ocular or nerve injury, fire, etc.).

**Figure 4-26 C, D**
(C), and 21 (D), respectively.

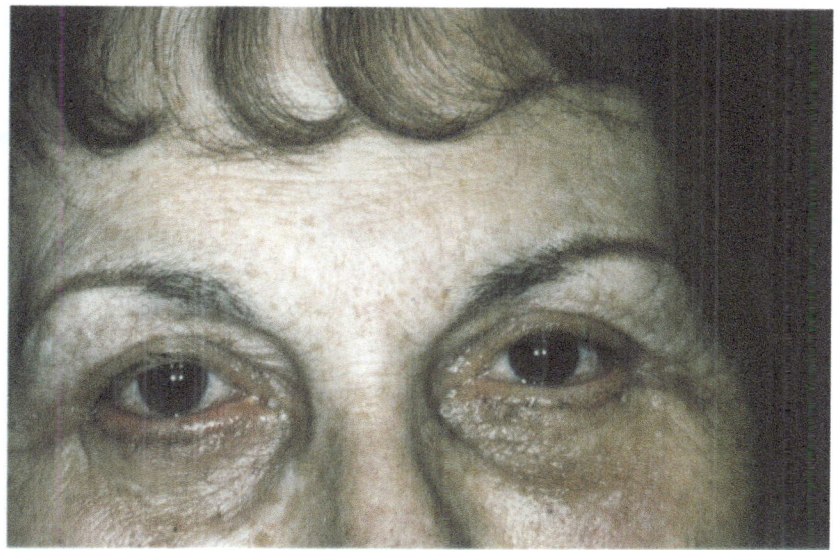

C

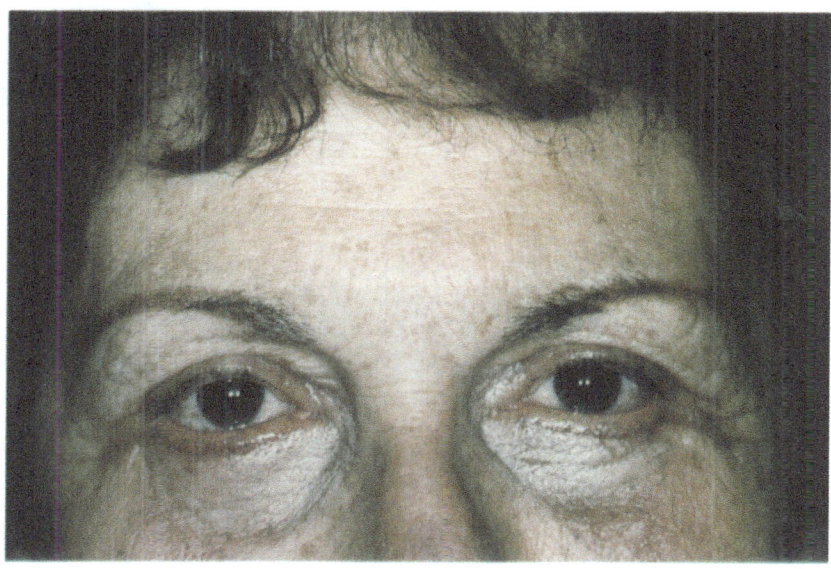

D

**Figure 4-27 A, B**
This 51-year-old woman underwent a coronal brow lift (dissection between the galea and periostium, release at the supraorbital rim, resection of the corrugator and depressor supracilli muscle at the nasion), facial rhytidectomy, and lower eyelid blepharoplasty as outlined in the text. The facial dissection was performed with the 1000 mm waveguide, 150 XJ laser, set at 275 millijoules, 18 watts in the SurgiPulse mode. These figures illustrate the lateral view of the patient preoperatively A) and on postoperative days 1 B), 4 C), and 14 D), respectively.

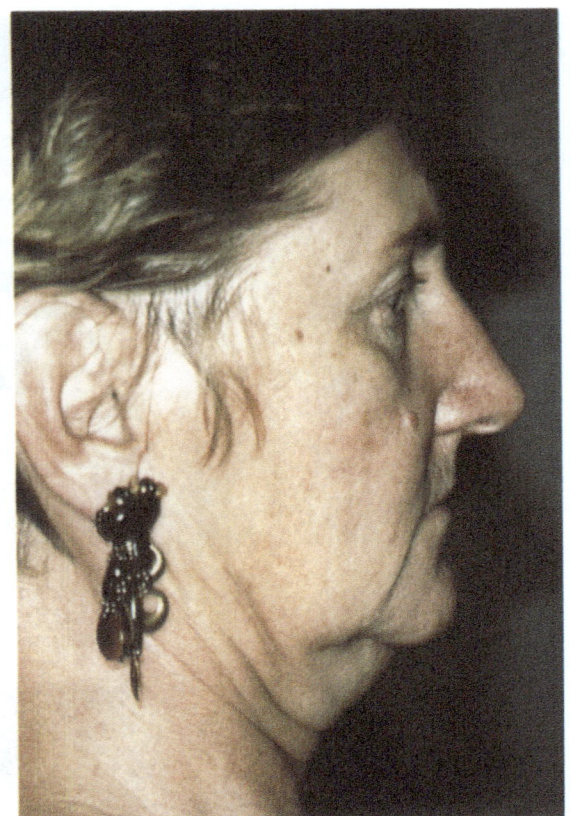

A

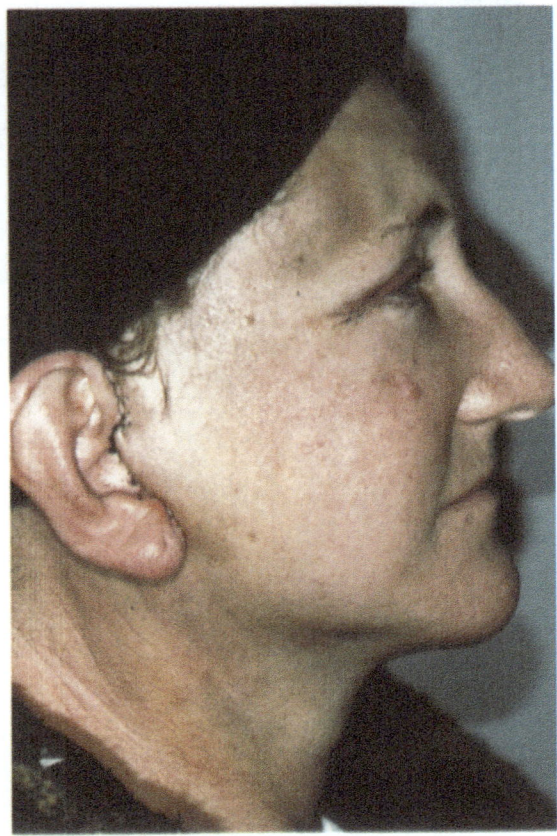

B

Figure 4-27 C, D

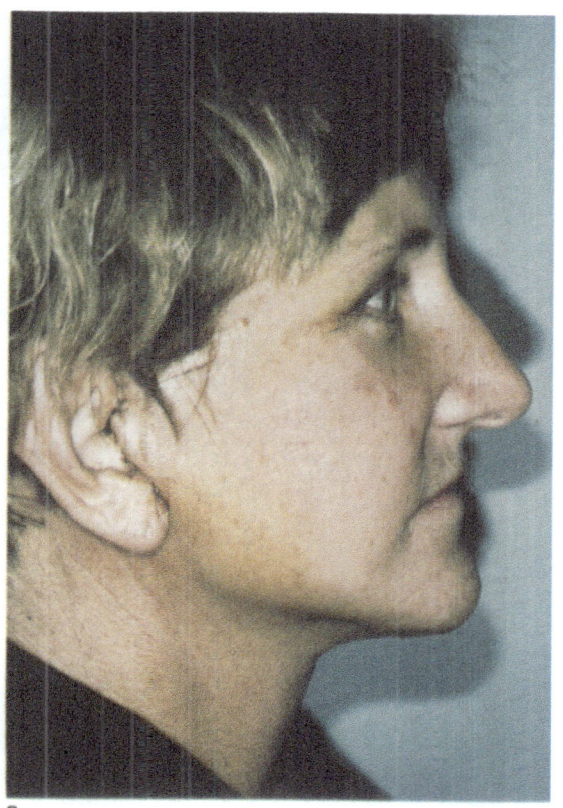

C

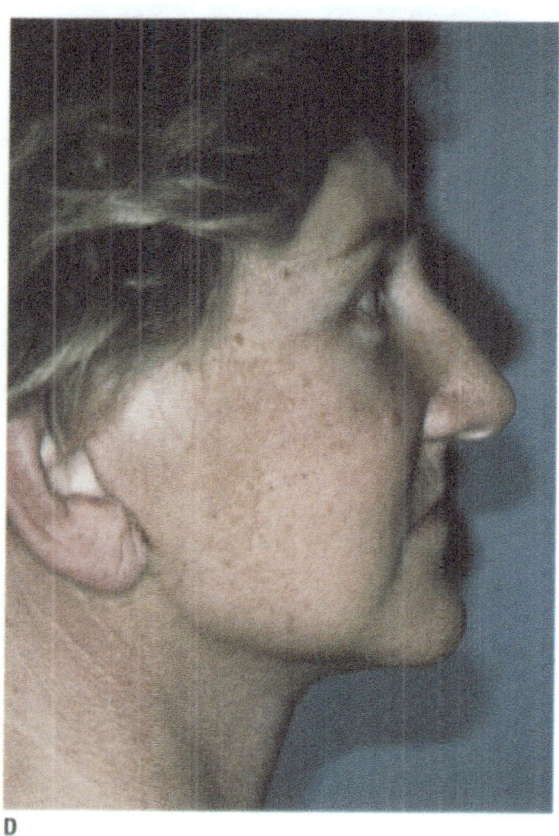

D

**Figure 4-28 A, B**
These figures illustrate the oblique view of the same patient preoperatively A) and postoperatively on days 1 B), 4 C), and 14 D, respectively.

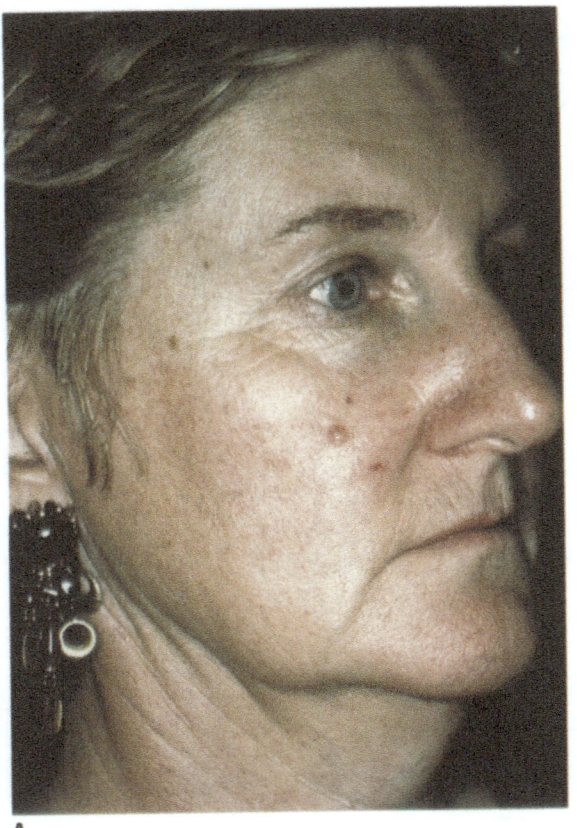

A

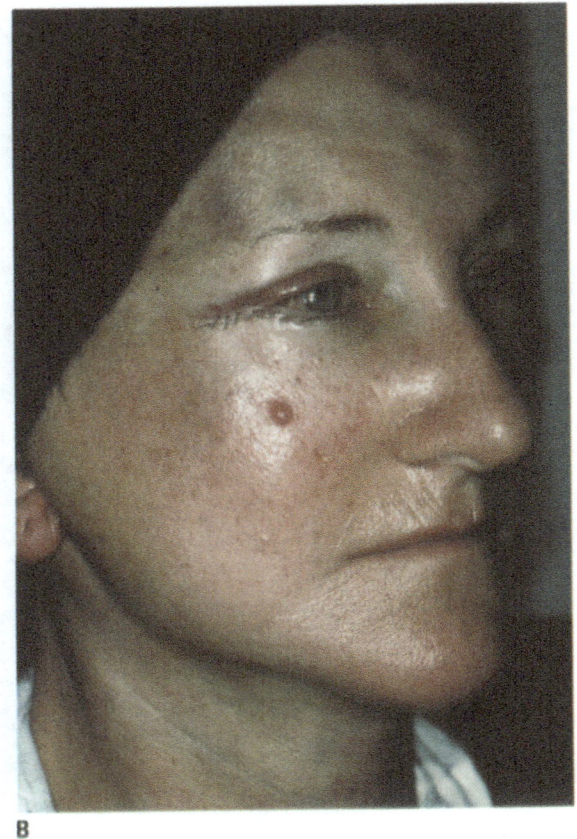

B

Figure 4-28 C, D

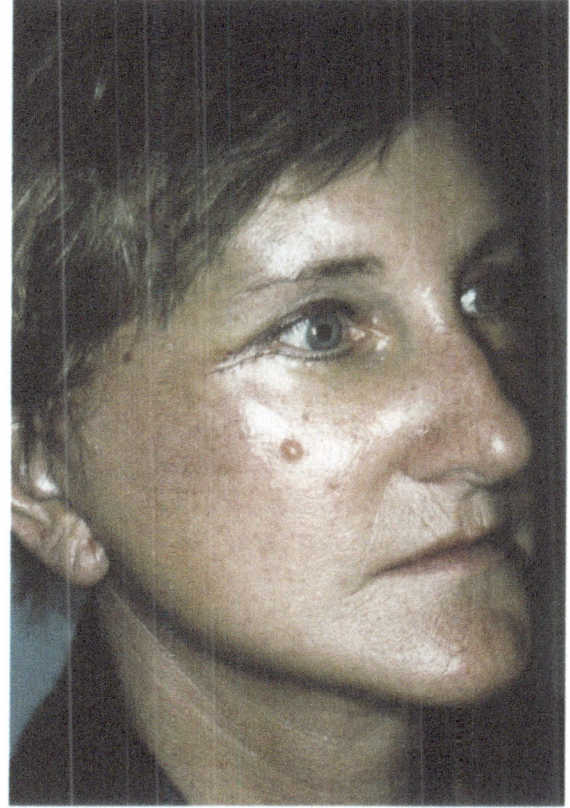

C

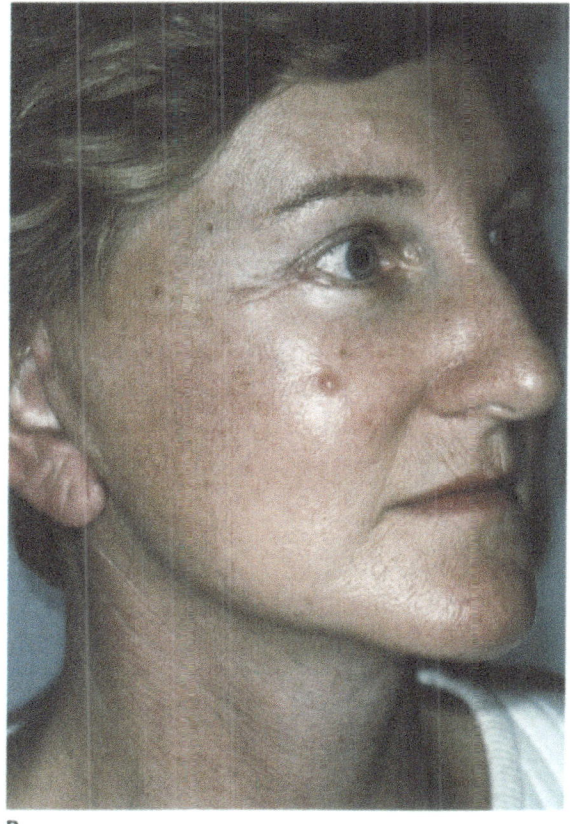

D

**by David Apfelberg, M.D.**

The Coherent Ultrapulse 5000 $CO_2$ laser is used in the "ultrapulse" mode for surgical procedures. To achieve the higher powers than would normally be possible if the laser was operated on a continuous (CW) or superpulsed mode, the laser tube is supercharged with high doses of radio frequency energy for a very short time (pulse). The Ultrapulse can, thus, achieve high power over periods of up to one thousandth of a second. The pulses may be repeated at a certain repetition rate (pulse per second equals hertz). Laser settings that would yield an average power of 5 watts include a repetition rate of 20 hertz, pulse width of about 300 ms, and energy per pulse of 250 millijoules. The clinical result is skin vaporization or incision without char or excessive thermal injury to tissue. The delay between pulses permits the minimal level of heat that has accumulated in surrounding areas to dissipate before the next burst of laser energy is delivered. The result is extremely precise vaporization or cutting with minimal risk of scarring or prolonged healing time from unwanted thermal damage. The Ultrapulse $CO_2$ laser, thus, represents a significant advance over previous continuous wave $CO_2$ laser technology, as it comes close to achieving a "cold incision."

The laser handpiece is held at the focal length and directed toward tissue that is placed on traction for easier separation. Prior to tissue application, the laser is directed toward a moistened tongue blade to check alignment. Utilizing 3 to 5 watts of power, 15 to 25 millijoules, and a 0.2 mm spot size, excellent hemostatic cutting may be achieved. Skin, subcutaneous tissue, fat, and muscle are easily incised. Defocusing the laser beam permits coagulation. Since there is little or no adjacent tissue thermal damage, it is not necessary to cut back wound edges prior to closure.

My surgical procedure is essentially the same as outlined in my section on the YAG wavelength. The skin is incised and flaps can be elevated with the laser beam (Figure 4-29, 4-30, and 4-31). Periorbital structures can be removed with minimal or no use of electrocautery (Figures 4-32 and 4-33). Transconjunctival blepharoplasty may be accomplished safely and bloodlessly as well (Figures 4-34 and 4-35). The laser has no electrical potential, so fat may be draped directly across a small metal retractor and removed without fear of electric transmission and burning of the skin. Moistened applicators should be used as a "backstop" behind tissue that is elevated for removal by the $CO_2$ laser so that the beam will not strike tissue beyond the area to be removed (see Figure 4-33). Excellent results are obtained with the techniques outlined (Figures 4-36, 4-37, 4-38, and 4-39).

**Figure 4-29**
Ultrapulse CO$_2$ laser skin incision.

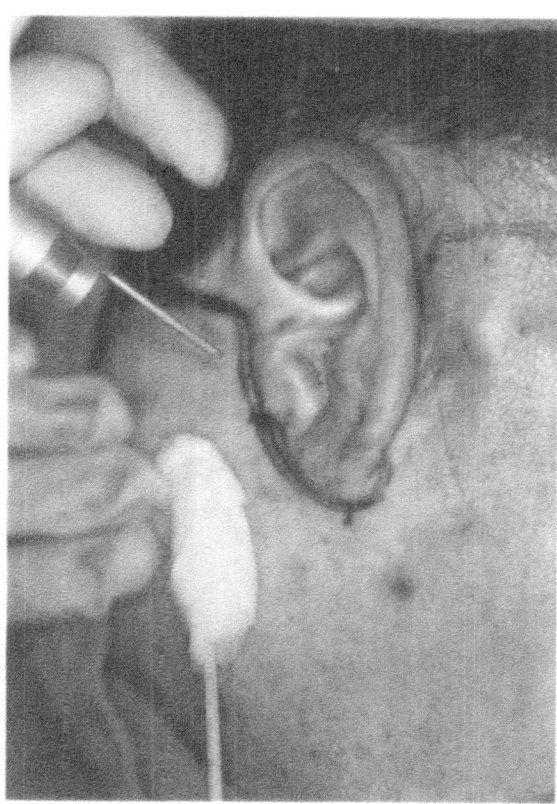

**Figure 4-30**
Dry pocket or elevation of skin flaps using the Ultrapulse CO$_2$ laser.

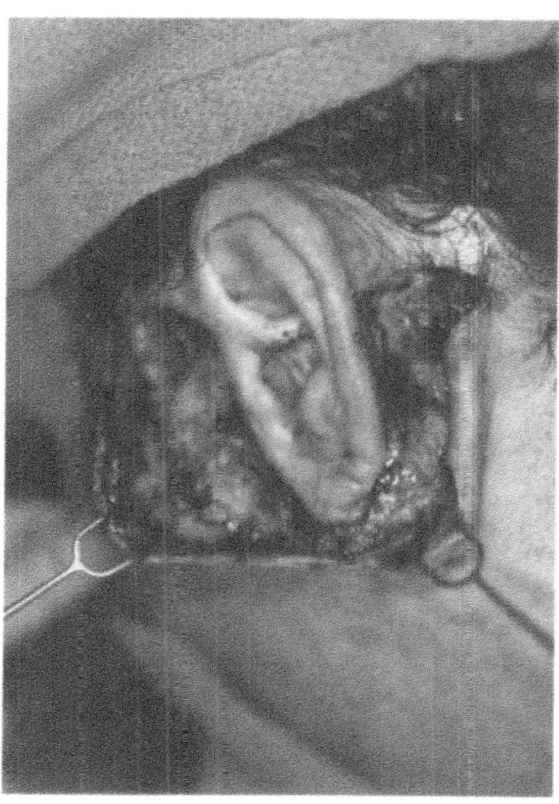

**Figure 4-31**
Ultrapulse $CO_2$ laser development of SMAS flap.

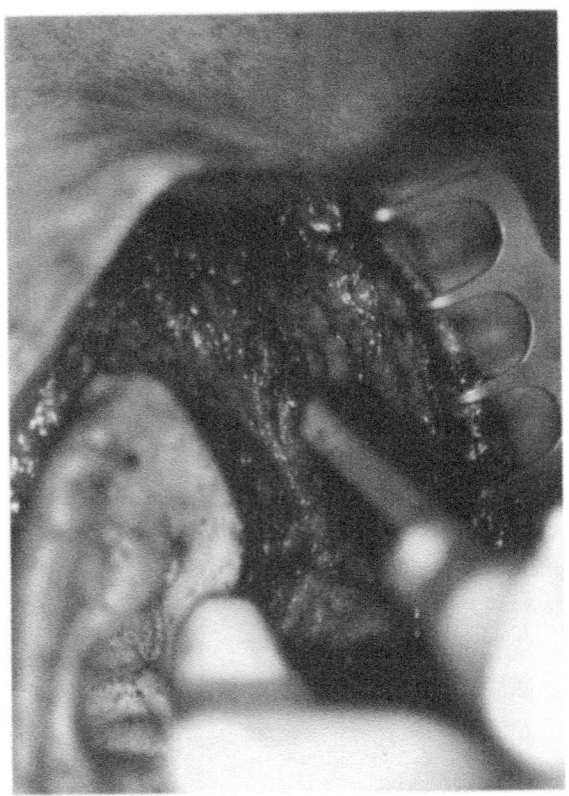

**Figure 4-32**
Schematic diagram of bloodless $CO_2$ laser excision of excess eyelid skin.

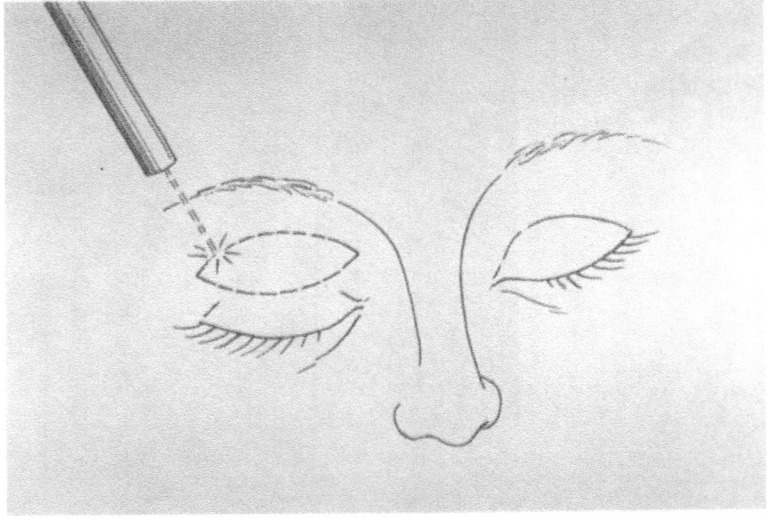

Chapter Four   **Aesthetic Laser Surgery**

**Figure 4-33**
Schematic diagram of removal of skin/muscle flap by $CO_2$ laser. Note moist applicator "backstop" to prevent inadvertent laser burn of nose.

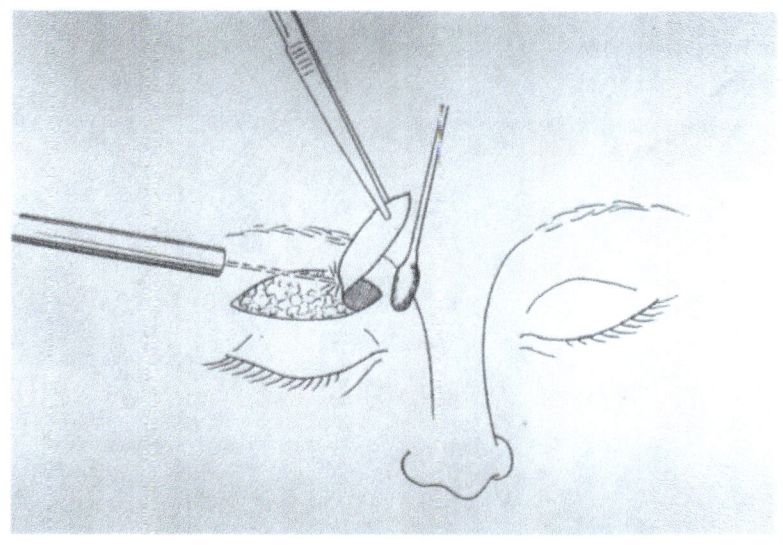

**Figure 4-34**
Schematic diagram of Ultrapulse $CO_2$ laser incision of conjunctiva in transconjunctival lower lid blepharoplasty.

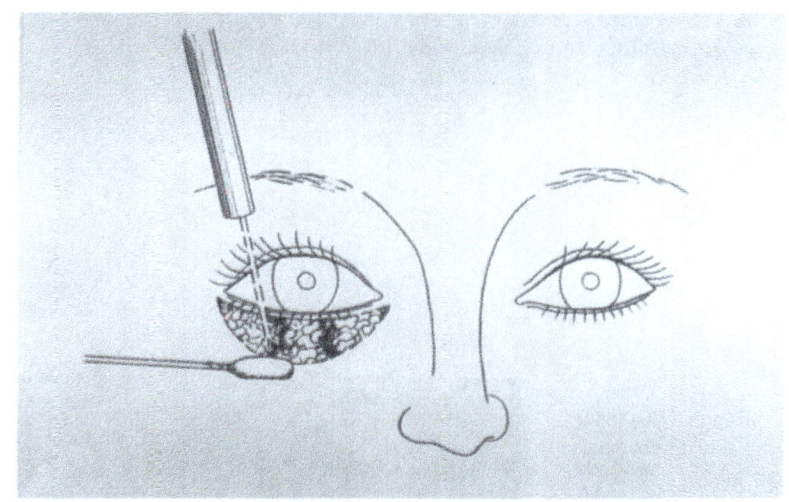

**Figure 4-35**
Schematic diagram of $CO_2$ laser removal of fat herniation with moist applicator "backstop."

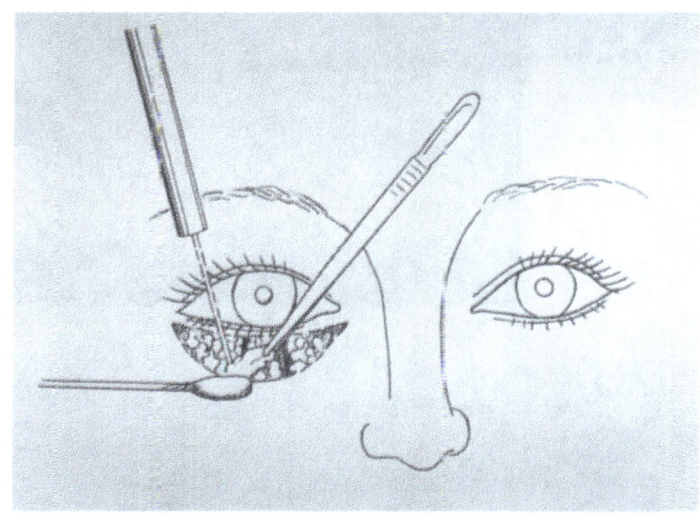

**Figure 4-36**
Preoperative patient with facial elastosis and blepharochalasia.

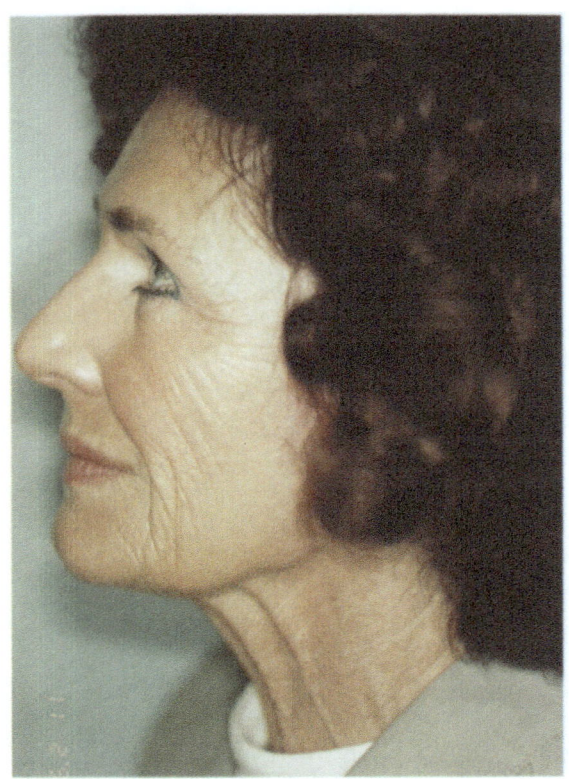

**Figure 4-37**
One day following Ultrapulse $CO_2$ laser
meloplasty/blepharoplasty. Ecchymosis
and swelling are minimal.

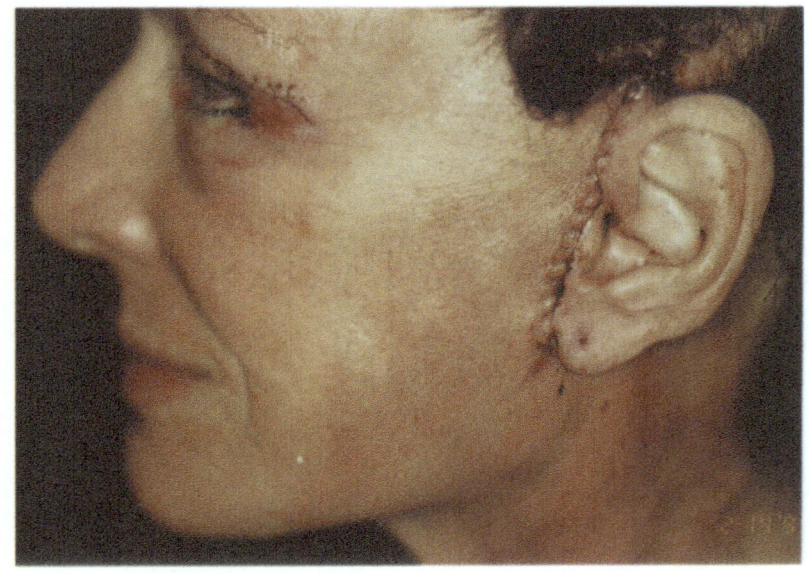

**Figure 4-38**
Postoperative day 4 demonstrating almost complete resolution of bruising and swelling.

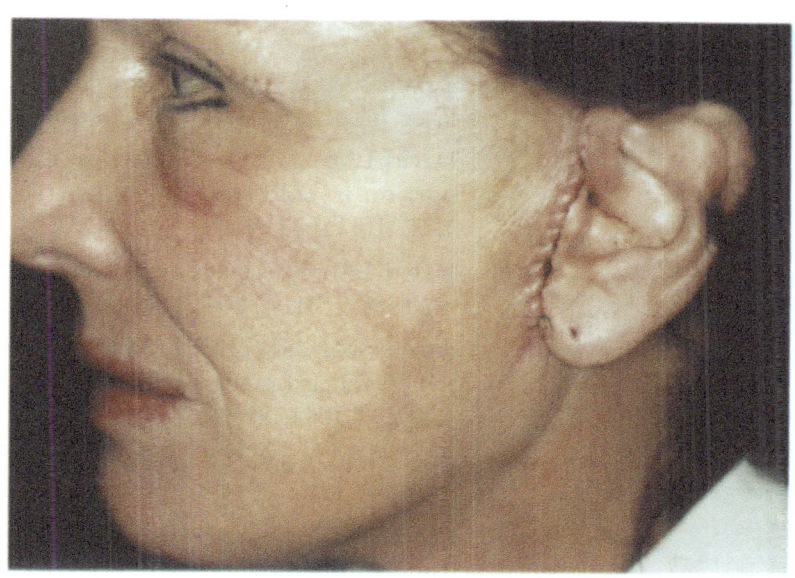

**Figure 4-39**
Final satisfactory cosmetic result at four weeks.

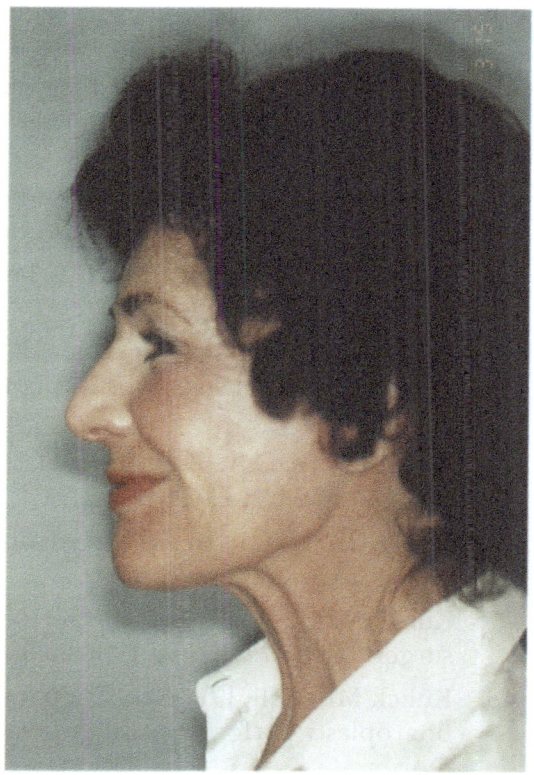

## References

1. Baker SS, Muenzler WS, Small RG, Leonard JE. Carbon dioxide laser blepharoplasty. *Ophthalmology* 1984;91:238–243.

2. David LM, Sanders G. Carbon dioxide laser blepharoplasty: A comparison to cold steel and electro-cautery. *J Dermatol Surg Oncol* 1987;13:110–114.

3. David LM. The laser approach to blepharoplasty. *J Dermatol Surg Oncol* 1988;1:741–746.

4. Trelles MA, Sanchez J, Sala P, Elspas S. Surgical removal of lower eyelid fat using the carbon dioxide laser. *Am J Cosm Surg* 1992;9:149–152.

5. Spadoni D, Cain CL. Laser blepharoplasty. *AORN J* 1988;47:1184–1193.

6. Morrow DM, Morrow LB. Carbon dioxide laser blepharoplasty. *J Dermatol Surg Oncol* 1992;18:307–313.

7. Beeson WM, Kabaker S, Keller GS. Carbon dioxide laser blepharoplasty, a comparison to an electro surgery. *Internat J Aesth Restor Surg* 1994;2:33–36.

8. Mittelman HM, Apfelberg DB. Carbon dioxide laser blepharoplasty—Advantages and disadvantages. *Ann Plast Surg* 1990;24:1–6.

9. Morrow DM, Morrow LB. Carbon dioxide laser assisted lower facelift: A preliminary report. *Am J Cosm Surg* 1992;9:159–168.

10. Apfelberg DB. Ultrapulse carbon dioxide laser resurfacing and facial cosmetic surgery. *Can J Plast Surg* 1995;3:1–4.

11. Apfelberg DB. Laser assisted melopasty and blepharoplasty. In: Alster TS, Apfelberg DB, eds. *Cosmetic Laser Surgery*. New York: Wiley-Liss, 1995: 29–41.

12. Apfelberg DB. The ultrapulse carbon dioxide laser for facial cosmetic surgery and resurfacing. *Ann Plast Surg* 1995 (in press).

13. Putterman AM. Scalpel Nd:YAG laser in oculoplasty surgery. *Am J Ophthal* 1990;109:581–584.

14. Apfelberg DB, Maser MR, Lash H, White DN. Sapphire tip technology for YAG laser excisions in plastic surgery. *Plast Reconstr Surg* 1989;84:273–279.

15. Apfelberg DB. YAG laser meloplasty and blepharoplasty. *Aesth Plast Surg* 1995;19:231–237.

16. Keller GS. Use of the KTP laser in cosmetic surgery. *Am J Cosm Surg* 1992;9:177–180.

17. Kulick MI. Evaluation of the KTP 532 laser in aesthetic facial surgery. *Aesth Plast Surg* 1996;20:53–57.

18. Kulick MI, Mele J, Lee D. Evaluation of complications following blepharoplasty performed with a laser. Submitted Aug. 1996 *Aesth Plast Surg*.

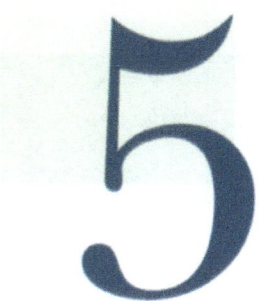

# Laser Skin Resurfacing

Michael I. Kulick, *M.D., D.D.S.*, and
David B. Apfelberg, *M.D.*

Michael I. Kulick, *M.D., D.D.S.*, and
David B. Apfelberg, *M.D.*

## Introduction

The ability to perform a hemostatic dermal injury of varying depths for defects of different size and configurations and produce consistent results is a distinct advantage of laser resurfacing compared to dermabrasion or topical caustic agents. Excellent results are attainable with chemical peels, although depigmentation can be a problem with deep wrinkle ablation (Figure 5-1). While resurfacing was performed with carbon dioxide ($CO_2$) lasers in the 1980s, recent acceptance is due in part to the advanced delivery systems available. These include those made by Coherent, Heraeus, Luxor, Sharplan, and Tissue Technology.

This chapter will deal with two widely utilized $CO_2$ laser systems produced by the Sharplan and Coherent companies. Despite utilizing the same wavelength, the delivery systems of these machines are different, and the surgeon cannot interchange settings between the machines. For instance, increasing the wattage will increase the depth of penetration with the Sharplan system versus increase the speed of delivery with the Coherent system. Due to these differences, Dr. David Apfelberg will discuss the merits of the Coherent system using clinical examples and will outline a review of the literature. I will discuss the efficacy of the Sharplan system and describe my approach to resurfacing. Redundancies or differences are present and allow each contributor to make points he feels are important in the care of his patients.

## Review of the Literature

### by Dr. David Apfelberg, M.D.

Initially described for vaporization of rhinophyma [1–3] and later for actinic cheilitis [4–7], use of the $CO_2$ laser has now been extended to cosmetic skin resurfacing. Laser technology has progressed from continuous wave [8] to superpulse [9–11] to ultrapulse, surgipulse and scanning delivery systems. Reports of regional and full-face laser

**Figure 5-1**
This woman presented to my office with a complaint of the "white lines" across her forehead. Receipt of the operative report revealed that she received a TCA peel to the face with an application of 50% TCA to the transverse forehead rhytids without any attempt to blend these areas into the adjacent, 30% TCA-treated areas. Despite a good reduction in rhytids, she had undesirable hypopigmentation across the forehead. Such an occurrence is possible with laser resurfacing if the surgeon does not "blend" these regions into the adjoining areas.

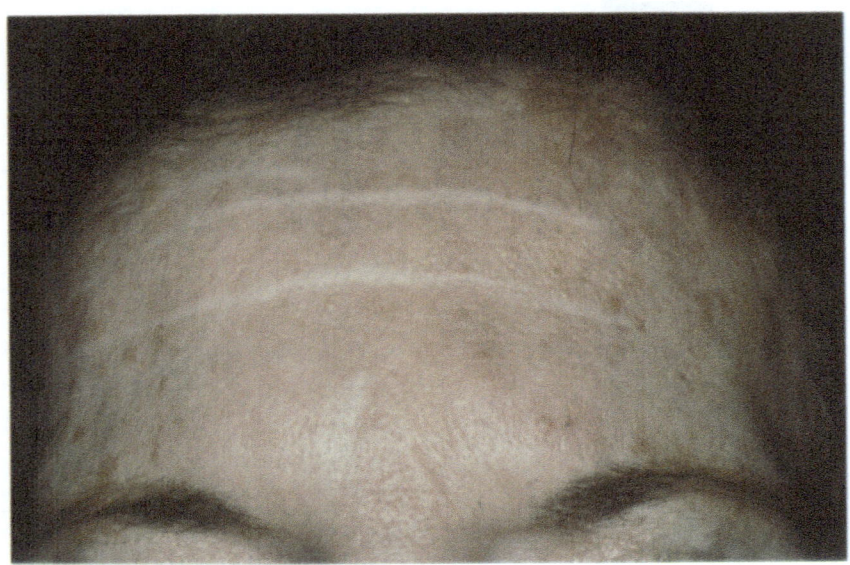

abrasion have defined the procedure. Weinstein [12, 13] and Fitzpatrick [14] have described their techniques for peri-orbital laser abrasion, as have Schoenrock, Chernoff, and Rubach [15]. Apfelberg [16–18] has defined criteria for patient selection, pre- and posttreatment skin care, and sequence of the procedure using the Coherent laser. Optical micrometry studies have demonstrated clinical efficacy with the Sharplan SilkTouch scanner [19]. Comparative studies using the Coherent and Sharplan lasers have demonstrated similar clinical results [20]. Waldorf, Kauvar, and Geronemus [21] have summarized regional laser abrasion using a $CO_2$ laser with a scanning beam. Pigmented patients received 25 to 50% improvement in acne scars and rhytids due to solar elastosis following resurfacing with the Sharplan laser system [22]. Regional and total face rhytids, photoaging, and acne scarring can be improved by $CO_2$ laser resurfacing which has supplanted chemical peel and dermabrasion for many physicians.

## Outline of Personal Technique Utilizing the Sharplan Laser Planning

### by Michael I. Kulick M.D., D.D.S.

When performing skin resurfacing in 1989, there were no time tested protocols or guidelines. The pulse width of the laser was 100 times that which the current laser system utilizes. It was a very "technique sensitive" method. Since that time, a great deal of knowledge has been gained, paralleling the evolution of my resurfacing techniques. Nevertheless, it is the basic comprehension of how the $CO_2$ laser works, experience with pre- and postoperative treatment associated with chemical peels, and an understanding of the management of second-degree burns that provide the basis of treatment associated with laser skin resurfacing.

To standardize the operative experience, it is helpful to outline the defect according to aesthetic facial units, depth of rhytid/scar, and presence or absence of undesirable pigmentation. Patient skin type (oily, dry, atrophic, etc.), general health, and natural skin pigment tone should be recorded as they will factor into the final result. Pigmentation can be standardized using Fitzpatrick's scale [23].

Assessment of wrinkle depth and etiology, skin thickness, and location facilitates customization of treatment. Although inexact, an arbitrary depth assessment (fine, medium, and deep) permits the physician to learn by comparing the results obtained with varying amounts of laser energy delivered to the tissue for a recorded rhytid depth and location (Figure 5-2 A–E). In addition to standardization of results, analysis of deformities within an aesthetic unit helps the surgeon inform the patient as to the potential success of treatment. In my experience, given the same clinical assessment of wrinkle depth, rhytid ablation or amount of reduction differs for the same energy settings, handpiece used, and total fluence delivered depending on the location of the wrinkle. I have found the most predictable rhytid reduction when evaluated six to nine months post treatment occur in treating the periorbital rhytids, followed by forehead/nasion, cheek, and lastly, the peri-oral areas (Figure 5-3 A–D). This may be due to multiple factors: wrinkle etiology due to photo-aging, dynamic muscle attachments, chronologic aging, or a combination of these, as well as skin thickness and hydration.

## Mechanism of Action

The final result of skin resurfacing is primarily the result of two processes: tissue ablation and alteration of the remaining collagen with remodeling. While it is not critical for the clinician to understand fully the scientific equations that form the principles of skin resurfacing, it is helpful when trying to understand the excellent results obtained with the different lasers available.

Clinical observations demonstrate an immediate local shrinkage of treated tissue. This effect may be due to dehydration, alteration of the cross-linking of collagen, a combination of these effects, or another process not yet identified. How much the skin contracts, how long this contraction lasts, and the effect of variables such as patient age, skin thickness, dermal water content, sebaceous gland density, location of resurfacing, and the total fluence delivered to the skin (joules/cm$^2$) have not yet been quantified. Tissue ablation is based on the principle of selective photothermolysis. In this setting, we desire the discriminate destruction of dermis [24]. To achieve this, three requirements must be met: sufficient energy must be delivered (heat the dermis with enough energy to achieve vaporization versus lower energy that would primarily coagulate collagen); a wavelength must be used that is preferentially absorbed by the dermis (we use the high intracellular water content of the epidermis and dermis as the selec-

**Figure 5-2 A, B, C**
A) Illustration of the skin condition prior to treatment with tretinoin. The rhytids lateral to the oral commisure would be classified as deep. The upper lip would be classified as medium, and the chin is scattered with fine wrinkles. B) On the operating table prior to skin cleansing, the medium and deep rhytids are outlined. The skin has a "rosy glow" and a reduction of spotty hyperpigmentation following one month preoperative treatment with tretinoin without hydroquinone. The last two weeks of treatment were with a concentration of 0.1% tretinoin. C) Three months after peri-oral resurfacing and dermal fat augmentation of the upper and lower lip.

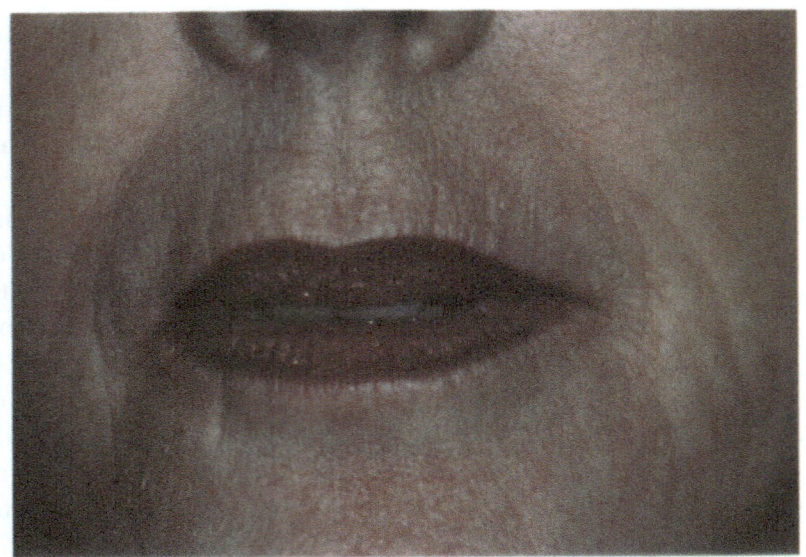

A

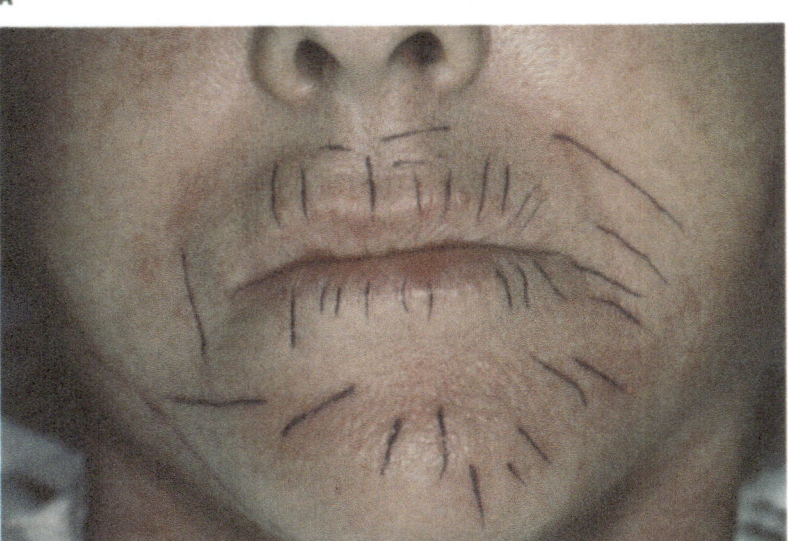

B

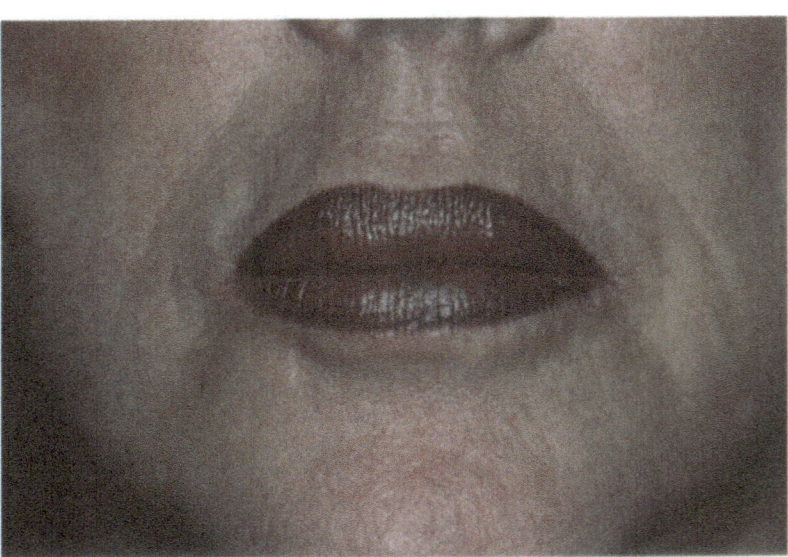

C

Chapter Five   **Laser Skin Resurfacing**

**Figure 5-2 D, E**
D) Right lateral view preoperatively. E)
Three months after peri-oral resurfac-
ing and lip augmentation.

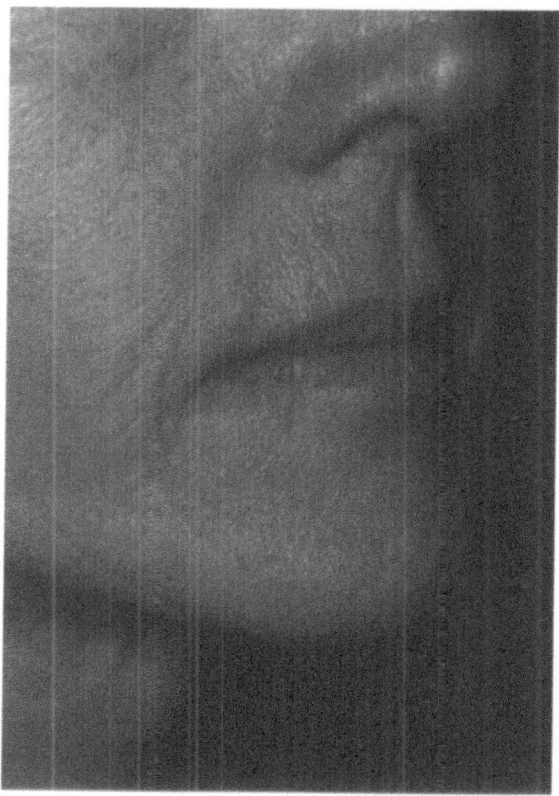

D

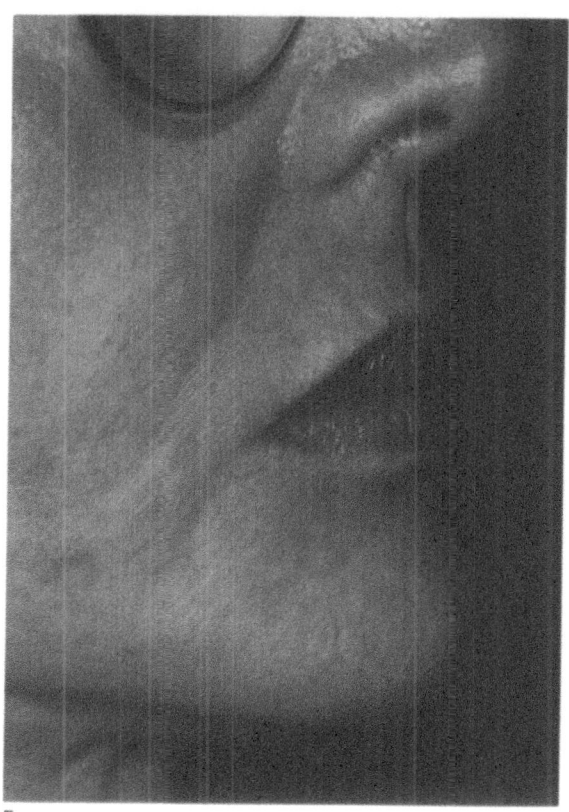

E

**Figure 5-3 A, B**
A) This 48-year-old female had a previous rhytidectomy. She has residual wrinkling along the lower eyelid and peri-oral region, as well as actinic changes of the skin. B) Nine months after a full-face resurfacing, there is excellent reduction of the eyelid rhytids, dark skin pigment of the lower lid region, and actinic skin changes.

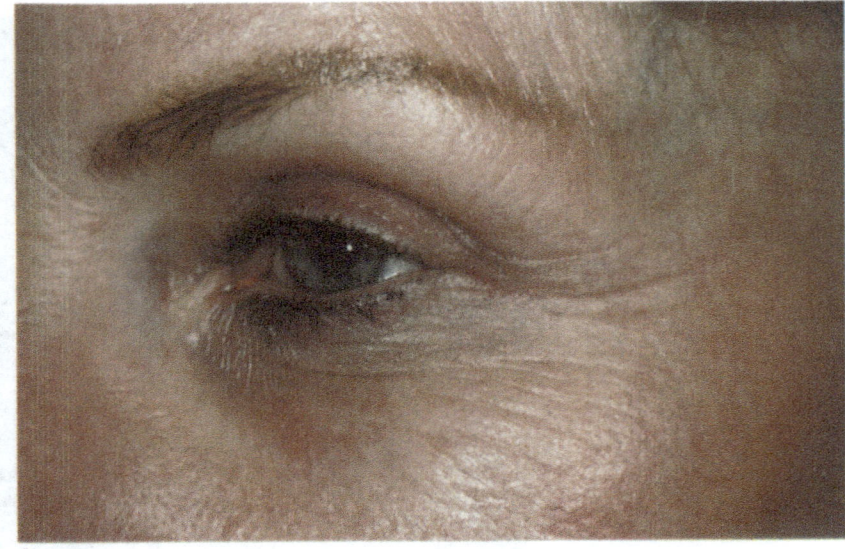

A

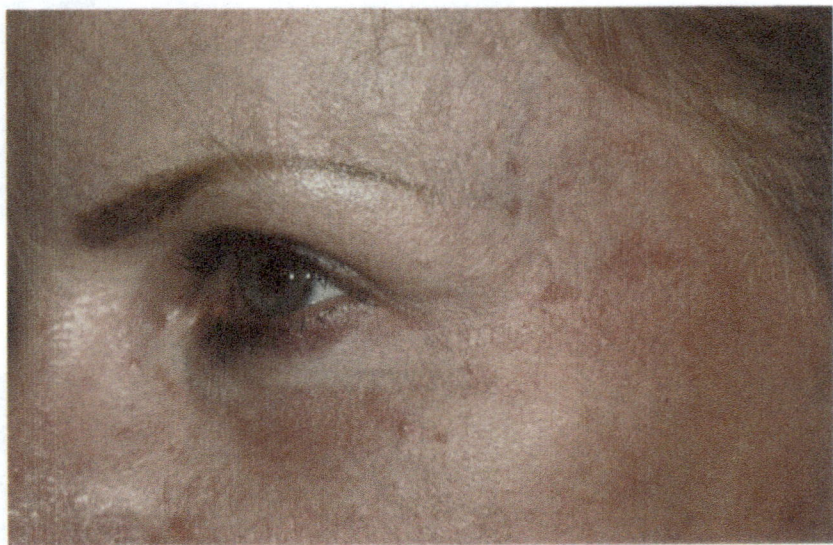

B

**Figure 5-3 C, D**
C) Preoperative view of the peri-oral region with medium rhytids along the patient's right upper lip and fine rhytids on the left. D) Nine months after resurfacing.

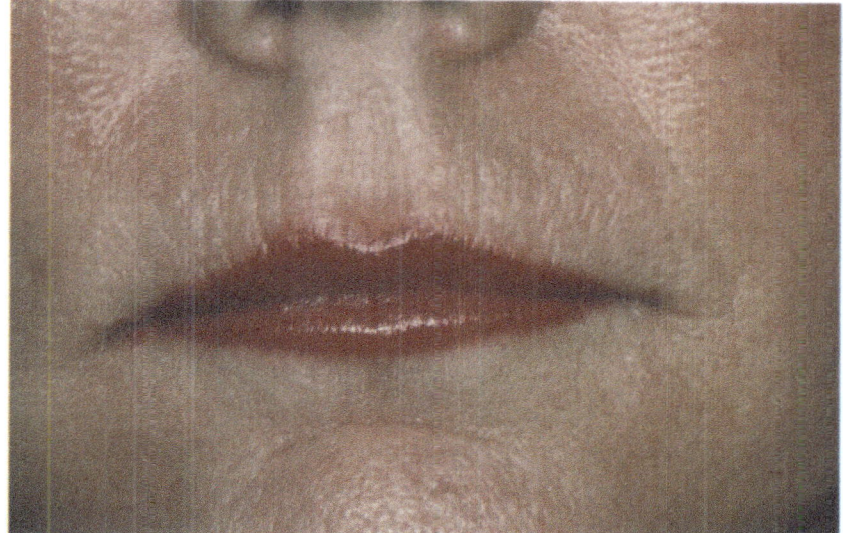

C

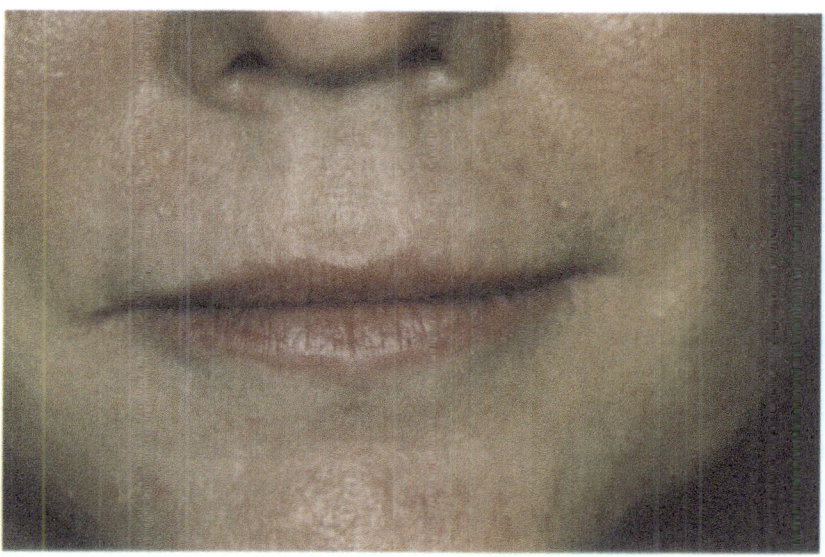

D

tive target for $CO_2$ energy); and the energy to the target skin must be reparted rapidly to minimize incidental heat damage, shorter than the thermal relaxation time (TRT) of the target tissue (time it takes for one-half of the deposited energy to diffuse to the surrounding skin).

Many controlled studies have been performed on animals. Despite the inaccuracy in trying to parallel these findings to human skin, the results have provided a foundation for human studies and clinical applications. At the initial impact of laser energy with the skin during resurfacing, the tissue effect is dependent on the optical penetration of the wavelength, the TRT of skin, pulse width, and the fluence delivered. Using a pulse width of 0.2 ms requires a fluence of approximately 5 joules/$cm^2$ to cause the desired explosive vaporization of dermal tissue [25]. Below this fluence level, the tissue effect is primarily dehydration and or collagen coagulation.

Conceptually, using this information the surgeon would ideally set the fluence on the laser so as to irradicate a rhytid utilizing a single burst of laser energy creating minimal incident thermal injury. The deeper the wrinkle, the greater the fluence. It is accurate that increasing the fluence will increase the tissue ablated, although not in a linear manner. However, in addition to the difficulty in designing a "one pass" rhytid elimination delivery system, there is a limit for each pulse width where increasing the fluence will increase tissue ablation with minimal thermal tissue injury. This is secondary to "plasma" formation above the skin surface. This plasma formation is defined in engineering terms as opposed to our medical understanding of the term plasmas, as intravascular fluid. It represents a high-energy state of electrons which strongly absorbs the $CO_2$ energy and affects the amount of energy imparted to the intracellular dermal water. Clinically, this plasma formation may be evident as a blinding flash. Using a high-energy delivery system and a pulse width of 0.2 ms, plasma formation can occur with a fluence of approximately 13 joules/$cm^2$. Thus, while tissue ablation plays a role in rhytid reduction, the final result for treatment of medium and deep rhytids is also dependent on alteration of collagen at the ablative front with current delivery systems.

It is accepted that the smaller the area of residual damage beyond the ablated surface "debris," the faster the healing and less scaring. Within the dermis beneath the debris, the residual injury is kept to a minimum by having the time the energy is in contact with the skin (pulse width) be less than the TRT of skin. This value differs for each tissue type. The TRT for skin lies somewhere less than 1 ms [26]. This range results from the variables within the skin itself (state of hydration, local blood supply, keratin thickness, etc.), as well as the properties of the energy delivery system. However, the fact that clinically acceptable results are obtainable with delivery systems with a pulse width of 4.0 to 5.0 ms suggests that the clinical results may be more dependent on the heat effect versus tissue ablation.

In addition to altering collagen, some incidental thermal tissue injury is necessary for hemostasis. This energy also raises the temperature of the collagen adjacent to the ablative front above 65°C, which is required for collagen denaturation. There is no "correct" or "acceptable range" of the depth of incidental heat effect to the collagen at the ablative front. In general, the smaller the zone, the less chance of undesirable scaring or pigmentation change. In one investigation, a thermal necrosis zone of 150 microns beyond the ablative front was felt to be acceptable, although the tissue examined was resurfaced, harvested full thickness skin grafts versus skin treated during rhytid reduction [27]. While histologic analysis has been the standard for clinical studies, acceptance of the data must be tempered by understanding the inherent variability due to: sample handling and processing, variations in the actual depth of energy penetration, and variability in effect due to different skin thickness. Theses factors may be significant when reported differences in depth are measured in micron increments.

Tissue histology plays a significant role in the tissue effect of $CO_2$ laser resurfacing due to the different concentrations of water within the various layers of the skin and their thickness. The skin is composed of the stratum corneum (approximately 15 to 20 microns thick, 30% water content), the underlying epidermis (approximately 100 microns thick, 70% water content), and the dermis (approximately 1000 to 2000 microns thick, 70% water content) [28, 29]. The water content is important because the $CO_2$ energy is preferentially absorbed by water. When discussing skin "thickness," reference is made to the thickness of the epidermis (thin skin ranging from 75 to 150 microns and thick skin, 400 to 500 microns). Dermal thickness also varies, with scalp thickness about 1,500 microns and back dermis about 4,000 microns thick. In addition to the variability of skin thickness, the water content varies with age. Therefore, the tissue effect may vary from patient to patient for the same laser settings, skin thickness, and location of treatment.

Long-term efficacy may be explained by the histologic changes observed in the epidermis and dermis following resurfacing. Undesirable pigmentation that resides in the epidermis is removed. Studies demonstrate that there is a layer of collagen deposited at the treatment areas in the superficial dermis [30]. This layer is similar to the collagen deposited after topical phenol treatment, with the collagen bundles more compact and aligned parallel to the surface with new elastic fibers [31]. The lasting effect of laser resurfacing may relate to the elimination of the subepidermal layer of papillary dermis labeled the Zone of Grenz found in sun-damaged skin (this layer lacks elastic fibers) [32]. There is also an actual tissue shrinkage. However, the claim that resurfacing is a substitute for a rhytidectomy, the purported "no incision facelift," should be viewed more as a marketing slogan rather than reality, given today's delivery systems and patient expectations.

## Multiple Passes versus Multiple Sessions

When performing laser resurfacing, there is an initial respect and caution associated with learning a new technology. Depending on the surgeon, the desire to "maximize" the patient's experience may appear attractive. Indeed, the ability to control and see the rhytid eliminated, due to a combination of tissue removal and local swelling, can lure the surgeon to extend the number of passes or increase the wattage with the Sharplan laser for the deeper rhytids.

The $CO_2$ laser allows for tissue ablation (actual removal), a bloodless field, and intraoperative control. It is tempting to think that the more "passes" (a single $CO_2$ energy discharged to the skin in a given area represents a single pass), the more tissue is actually removed with each pass in a linear, controlled manner. This line of thinking is then applied to the theory that one can "shave" or ablate the skin with consistent 30 to 75 micron increments with each laser pass until the wrinkle or undesirable pigment is eliminated. This is not true in the literal sense. It is only the initial pass with laser parameters that follow the guidelines of selective thermolysis that follows a relatively predictable pattern of tissue ablation and incidental thermal injury. Regardless of the laser system used, repeated passes will dehydrate/coagulate the dermal collagen, which subsequently limits the penetration of laser energy affecting both the ablative effect and incidental thermal injury of each subsequent pass. These additional passes essentially "cook" the collagen, with the major tissue effect being heat induced versus photochemistry. Clinically, this is evident by the difficulty in removing the debris with each pass after the first. The intraoperative color change observed in the treated dermis may reflect the denaturation of the dermal protein more than an indicator of dermal depth of resurfacing. This information is obvious to those that have harvested varied levels of split thickness skin grafts and notice no change in dermal color based on depth harvested. The ideal balance of the cumulative fluence delivered to the tissue to provide the optimal tissue removal, long-term tissue shortening, and minimal recovery and morbidity is currently determined by the surgeon's experience with the technology available. I recommend that it is better to afford your patient the opportunity for additional treatments, perhaps at a reduced cost to them for subsequent sessions, than to perform that "additional pass" at the initial session and develop a complication. While collagen coagulation may prevent laser energy penetration into the subcutaneous tissue during resurfacing, the heat imparted may cause a full thickness burn. To minimize the possibility of hypopigmentation and adverse scaring, I rarely treat an individual rhytid with more than two to three passes. This is more critical for brown, yellow, and olive pigmented skin tones.

## Patient Selection

Choosing a patient that understands the process, has realistic expectations, is cooperative, and has uncomplicated defects and fair skin tone will facilitate the surgeon's education with laser resurfacing. Patient compliance is critical, because a great deal of the final result requires adherence to treatment protocol. Special caution should be extended when considering resurfacing patients with diabetes, adrenal gland dysfunction, diagnosed autoimmune disease, or history of keloid scarring. In addition, patients that have been treated with long-term steroids should be carefully evaluated and energy settings reduced to account for skin atrophy. The appearance of pre-existing telangectasias may appear worse following resurfacing secondary to the elimination of the masking keratin and sun-damaged skin. Skin infection, chronic irritation, or excessive steroid use may increase the number of skin telangectasias.

Whenever there is a safety issue, it is prudent to perform a "test patch" in front of the ear, behind the sideburn before beginning treatment. I do not recommend simultaneous resurfacing of skin that has been undermined in the subcutaneous layer by a simultaneous surgical procedure. Resurfacing of adjacent, non-undermined zones, e.g., the peri-oral region at the time of a rhytidectomy, can be performed, although optimal blending methods over the bordering undermined skin can be compromised.

Patients with rosacea should be informed that laser resurfacing will not cure them of their problem. These patients suffer from flushing, telangectasias, papules and pustules of the midface. Prior to resurfacing, I prefer to treat these patients with topical MetroGel and oral antibiotics to obtain the best possible skin condition. I also recommend that patients refrain from foods, beverages, skin care products, etc., that activate their disease. Be aware of post resurfacing rosacea exacerbations which need to be differentiated from bacterial or herpetic infections.

Patients that have received a recent course of Accutane should not be resurfaced for at least six months after discontinuation of treatment. There are no prospective studies regarding this issue. These recommendations are extrapolated from case reports of scarring problems that arose following dermabrasion and Accutane treatment [33–38]. If patients are still reporting the effects of Accutane treatment (dry mouth, skin, etc.) it may be prudent to wait more than six months until these symptoms resolve.

## Informed Consent

Elements essential to the consent are similar to those obtained for dermabrasion or chemical peels. Issues include the possibility of altered skin pigment, scarring, and need for additional laser or other treatments. As part of the discussion, the patient's anticipated recovery should be covered. This would include the length of time for re-epithelialization, with or without occlusive dressings postoperatively, potential sequela if patients prematurely remove any scabbing that develops, length of time the skin will be red/pink, the hypersensitive nature of the skin following treatment, and the adverse effects of the sun and skin irritants. Patients should be warned of the possibility of skin sensitivity to topical creams the patient was normally using prior to skin resurfacing. This may last for four to six months after treatment. Compliance with pre- and postoperative protocols must be stressed, as well as the possible complications that can occur if recommendations are not followed. The consent should indicate no warranty as to the final result, the possibility of the need for additional treatments, and anesthesia risks.

## Pretreatment

Irrespective of the deformity, solar aging, pigmentation disorders, or rhytids, I have found skin preparation very important. While favorable results can be obtained without pretreatment, my results have been more consistent using a preoperative skin preparation protocol. The goal is to enhance healing by stimulating cellular activity, suppressing pigment formation, and modulation of the keratin content of the skin. Achieving these goals will facilitate consistent results. Another benefit of preoperative skin treatment is determining the level of patient compliance. Patients that do not cooperate or fail to follow through with your preoperative protocol frequently continue with defiance or ambivalence after resurfacing which could lead to undesirable effects. As a great deal of the final result depends on patient cooperation after laser treatment, a warning is extended to the physician who treats a patient that will not follow preoperative instructions.

Patients begin with a low dose tretinoin (0.01 to 0.05%) cream that is combined with 4% hydroquinone applied twice a day. Once tolerated, I increase the tretinoin concentration to 0.1%, usually within one to two weeks. If your pharmacy cannot provide such a formula, the patient can mix equal parts of each cream in their palm and then apply this mixture to their face. It is expected that patients will develop some redness and desquamation for the first seven to ten days after initiating topical treatment. This usually diminishes. If significant irritation occurs, the frequency of application can be reduced until the redness subsides and then the cream reinstituted at a reduced frequency (alternate days, then apply once a day, etc.).

Persistent redness and skin ulceration despite reduced dosing may indicate a hypersensitivity to the medication. In these cases, 5 to 10% glycolic peel treatments followed by topical hydroquinone will also prepare the skin for laser resurfacing. Occasionally, a patient will develop a reaction that does not respond to a reduction in concentration and/or frequency of application. In these cases, topical 1 to 2% hydrocortisone cream for four to seven days is helpful. Re-institution of tretinoin is possible if the reaction was not due to an allergy.

The tretinoin/hydroquinone protocol lasts for four to six weeks. This time frame is based on the study that shows significant reduction in hyperpigmentation from sun exposure versus control populations following treatment with tretinoin 0.1% for one month [39]. For patients with minimal pigmentation problems and fair skin, the preparation time can be reduced to one to two weeks. The pretreatment endpoint is the achievement of a homogeneous skin color with a very faint pink tone and smooth texture (see Figure 5-2).

The exact mechanism of tretinoin is not fully understood. It does improve skin texture and undesirable pigmentation and reduce photodamage [40, 41]. It affects the cell cytoskeleton with a correction of epidermal atrophy and dysplasia. New collagen is formed below the epidermis in conjunction with angiogenesis [42]. Histologically, the epidermis becomes thicker with compaction of the stratum corneum. Fading of the actinic lentigines correlates with a reduction in epidermal melanin, possibly due to the reduction in tyrosinase activity [43]. Its effect on the keratinocyte is to decrease the total content of keratin [44]. In my practice, I have found greater consistency in my final results when patients have been treated with tretinoin preoperatively.

Hydroquinone is one of the most effective inhibitors of melanogenisis *in vivo* and *in vitro*. Like tretinoin, the exact mechanism is not fully understood. Part of the efficacy may be due to its ability to serve as an alternate substrate for tyrosinase. Thus, it is a competitor for tyrosine oxidation in active melanocytes which effectively produce less melanin [45, 46]. Its action appears to be independent of the melanin content of the cell. The absorption through human skin has been classified as slow [47]. Although not scientifically demonstrated, the rate of clinical effectiveness is enhanced when used in conjunction with tretinoin. Use of this compound has reduced both the number of laser passes in an area by the preoperative elimination of undesirable hyperpigmentation and the incidence of post treatment hyperpigmentation in my experience.

Certain patients are hypersensitive to hydroquinone. In these cases 1% kojic acid, a fungal metabolic product, can be used. Its effectiveness is felt to be mediated by its ability to inhibit the catecholase activity of tyrosinase, thus affecting melanin formation [48]. Hypersensitivity to this compound can also occur [49].

During this presurgical treatment, patients must wear sun block to protect the skin from ultraviolet radiation. Sun block with a sun protection factor (SPF) value of 15 or more is recommended. Reapplication every one and one-half to two hours is important, as normal perspiration and physical contact with the skin can diminish the cream's effectiveness. A single application in the morning will not provide the desired effects throughout the day irrespective of the SPF value.

I routinely place my patients on anti-viral medication (Zovirax 200 mg qid or Valtrix 500 mg bid or Famvir 500 mg bid) starting the day before surgery and continuing for 10 days after treatment. I also have them take prophylactic antibiotics starting from the day of surgery until the skin is healed.

## Sharplan Laser System

Sharplan has a line of lasers that will perform $CO_2$ resurfacing, ranging from the 40 to the 150 watt XJ laser. Resurfacing can be performed with either the SilkTouch (ST) or the FeatherTouch (FT) delivery devices. Handpieces available are the 125 mm (spot size 2.5 to 3.7 mm), the 200 mm (spot size 4 to 11 mm), and the 260 mm (spot size 7 to 15 mm). Resurfacing patterns can be round or square. Depending on the total area and defect to be treated, the handpieces can be interchanged for optimal treatment. The corresponding power setting (watts, which affects the depth of penetration), pulse interval (time between pulses, which affects the speed of resurfacing), and on time (the time it takes the computer in the laser to trace out the pattern spot on the skin when activated) can be adjusted as necessary for each handpiece. The newer Sharplan laser models automatically set time-on-time for a desired wattage and spot size. It is the scanners' ability to move the approximately 0.2 mm beam contact with the skin rapidly that keeps the effective "pulse width" less than the TRT of skin. Suggested safe parameters for each of the handpieces using the SilkTouch scanner are listed in Table 5-1. For optimal tissue vaporization and minimal heat injury the wattage should not be reduced below the safe parameters to assure that the tissue is receiving the needed 5 J/cm² required for skin vaporization. This is true whether you are blending, treating an area at a second session, using the ST or FT modes.

**Table 5-1.**
Laser Parameters

| Handpiece | Scan Diameter (mm) | Scan Time (seconds) | Power (watts) |
|---|---|---|---|
| 125 mm | 2.5–3.7 | 0.2 | 5–7 |
| 200 mm | 4–9 | 0.2 for 4–6 mm 0.45 for 7–9 mm | 16–18 |
| 260 mm | 7–12 | 0.2 for 7–9 mm 0.45 for 10–12 mm | 36–40 |

Tissue removal with minimal thermal injury is afforded by a fluence approximately $5\,J/cm^2$ combined with a short pulse width (time the energy is in contact with the tissue). Compared to the Coherent system, the peak power is less but the spot size on the tissue is much smaller permitting the surgeon to obtain the desired fluence during the scanning of the treatment spot. This permits the removal of 50 to 100 microns of tissue with the initial pass. Both the FT and ST pulse widths are approximately 0.4 less than the TRT of skin. However, since the ST scanner is not synchronized to the laser as it is with FT, the scanning pattern is repeated twice per exposure. Most of the clinical studies have been performed with the ST delivery device. The benefit of FT is less residual thermal injury and a more superficial vaporization of tissue. Using either the ST with the 200 mm handpiece, 18 watts of power, and a spot size of 6 mm, or the FT delivery system with the 200 mm handpiece, 32 watts, and any spot size produces approximately 70 microns of tissue ablation. With these settings, however, there is approximately 50 microns of residual injury with the ST versus 20 microns with the FT (personal correspondence, Sharplan Laser). Less thermal injury results in less incident tissue injury. The FT delivery system is ideally suited for the treatment of fine wrinkles, blending during zonal resurfacing and treating patients with superficial pigmentation disorders.

### Sharplan SilkTouch Laser Resurfacing Procedure

On the operating room table, the patient's skin is cleansed with a nonalcohol-based prep solution. The face is draped with moistened towels. Tetracaine is applied to the eyes followed by eye lubricant. During the procedure, these shields can shift requiring repositioning. After determining that the surface is smooth, metal shields are inserted that cover the sclera as well as the cornea. The handpiece is connected to the articulated arm after inspecting the internal lens of the handpiece, which occasionally needs to be cleaned with alcohol.

I prefer to resurface each major rhytid in an aesthetic unit initially. The depth of each rhytid is marked with methylene blue. General or local nerve block anesthesia (xylocaine and marcaine mixture) without epinephrine is administered. Do not infiltrate directly into the dermis in areas to be resurfaced as the fluid can absorb the $CO_2$ energy and affect the depth of laser energy penetration.

For the medium to deep wrinkles, I resurface the peripheral edges of each rhytid (the crest) leaving the center 0.5 to 1.0 mm portion or wrinkle depth untreated until resurfacing the entire aesthetic facial unit with the final pass (Figure 5-4 A–D). To resurface the crest of the rhytid, the 125 mm handpiece is used with a 2.5 to 3.7 mm spot size, and the ST is set at 5 to 7 watts. The lower energy settings are for use on the eyelid skin and higher settings on the forehead and peri-oral areas. For machines that do not have default settings the on time is 0.2 s and pulse interval between 0.2 to 0.45 s, utilizing a shorter time as one gains experience which permits a more rapid

**Figure 5-4 A, B**
A) This 48-year-old woman has fine (blue arrow), medium (yellow arrow), and deep wrinkles (black arrow) in the peri-oral region. B) With the 125 mm handpiece and a setting of 6 watts, 3.5 mm spot size, the rhytids are outlined. Notice that the depths of the rhytids are not treated initially, leaving a raised central portion (black arrow) which, preoperatively, was depressed.

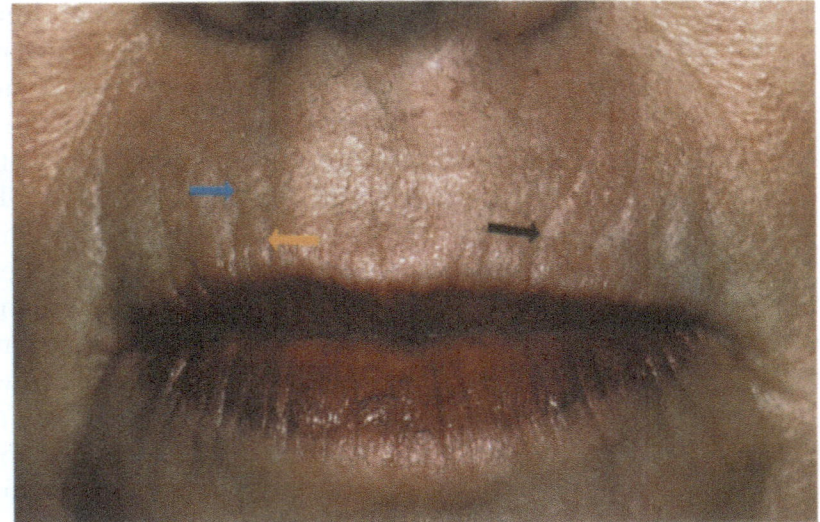

A

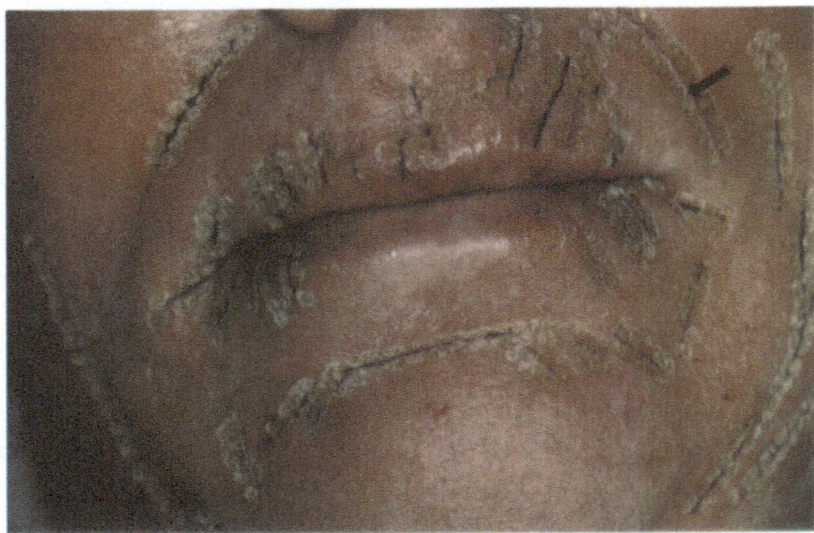

B

**Figure 5-4 C, D**

C) After each medium and deep rhytid and lentigini are individually treated (same color code as above), the entire face is resurfaced with the 200 mm handpiece, 18 watts, 9 mm spot size. This illustrates the appearance after the debris is removed prior to the application of the Vigilon dressing. D) Nine months after resurfacing, only the deep wrinkles remain, although they are less noticeable with excellent retention of natural skin color. The depth of resurfacing has not affected natural hair growth.

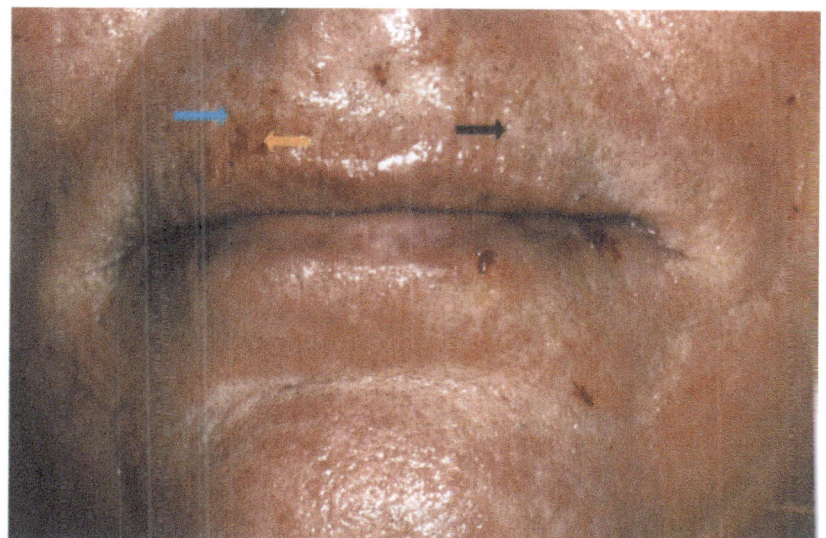

C

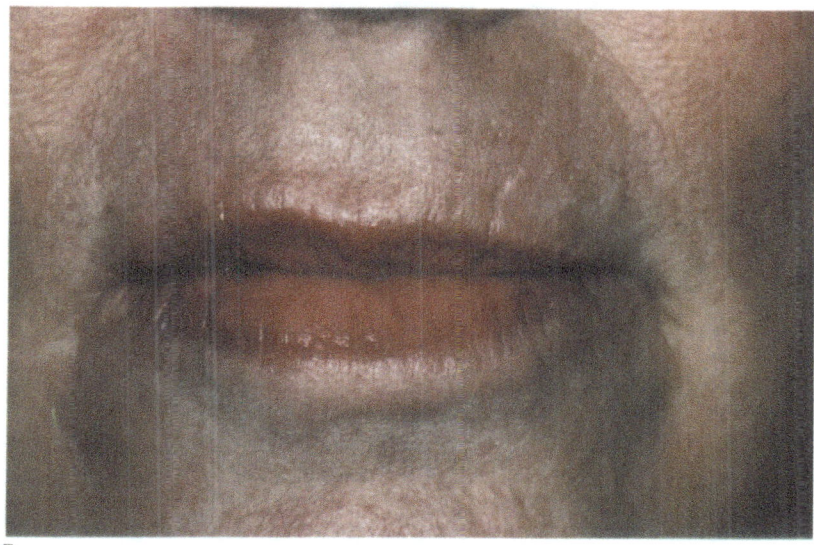

D

procedure. Prior to skin treatment, I test the settings on a wet tongue blade. While treating the skin, the high evacuation suction port is held in close proximity to the treatment area by the assistant or through the integrated port on certain handpieces. In general, one or two passes with the above settings will provide a resurfacing depth into the papillary dermis. Clinically, this depth and temperature effect on the dermal collagen is evident by a very light tan or chamois color (Figure 5-5 A–C). For wrinkles that are within 4 mm of each other or are fine lines (often found on the lower eyelids), I resurface the entire rhytid versus treating the rhytid crest.

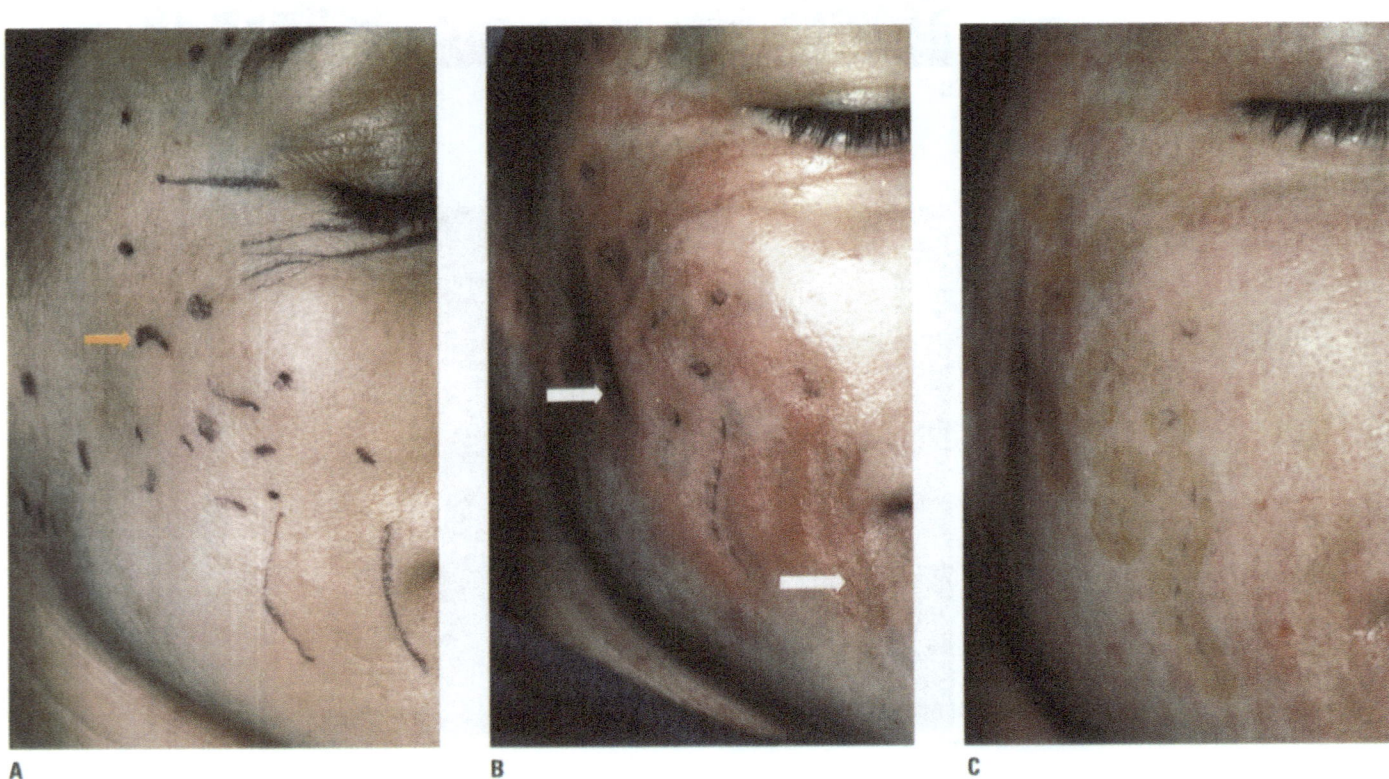

A                           B                           C

**Figure 5-5 A, B, C**
A) In the operating room, the depths of the acne scars and rhytids are outlined. Yellow arrow outlines the irregular acne scarring. B) Following treatment with the 125 mm handpiece, this tangential view allows you to see that the central portion of the rhytids and acne scars (white arrows), initially depressed, are now slightly elevated. The faint tan color is barely visible. At this point, the entire face is resurfaced with the 200 mm handpiece at 18 watts of power, 9 mm spot size. C) The light tan color becomes more prominent after resurfacing the entire face, indicating that maximum safe depth and collagen denaturation have been attained around the depressed regions.

When preparing to use the ST scanner, it is important to keep the handpiece at the proper focal length and keep the beam perpendicular to the skin surface, because the beam is not collimated. This is facilitated by having the end of the handpiece touch the skin (Figure 5-5). This provides optimal tissue destruction and minimal incidental heat transfer. Pulling the handpiece back beyond the optimal focal distance increases the thermal damage. This can result in prolonged redness and undesirable permanent pigment changes. The overlap of the treatment pattern should be kept to a minimum, approximately 1.0 to 3.0 mm, depending on the spot size, to avoid heat build-up and thermal injury in the overlap area. Although not thoroughly investigated, it is felt that the overlapped debris does not transmit laser energy but heats up, causing more thermal injury beneath it. A "quilted" appearance of the skin during the initial recovery period using the laser settings recommended often reflects too much overlap. These patients should be followed closely for possible postinflammatory pigmentation problems and receive treatment with topical steroids and or hydroquinone when necessary (Figure 5-7 A–B).

**Figure 5-6**

The 200 mm handpiece is held perpendicular to the skin and at the correct distance from the skin for optimal ablation and minimal thermal injury. The incomplete pattern ablation (yellow arrow) is caused by not having the foot pedal depressed for the entire pattern. If this area is not treated in a subsequent pass, it can result in residual aged skin, with a color and/or texture mismatch. With the circular pattern, unless there is a slight overlap, there will be diamond-shaped untreated areas (black arrow) between the resurfaced skin. These would have to be treated with individual passes which can be time consuming. Therefore, a slight overlap is necessary and safe using the parameters outlined in the text. Resurfacing is carried into the first line of hair follicles at the brow and forehead. To avoid this, a square pattern can be used for resurfacing.

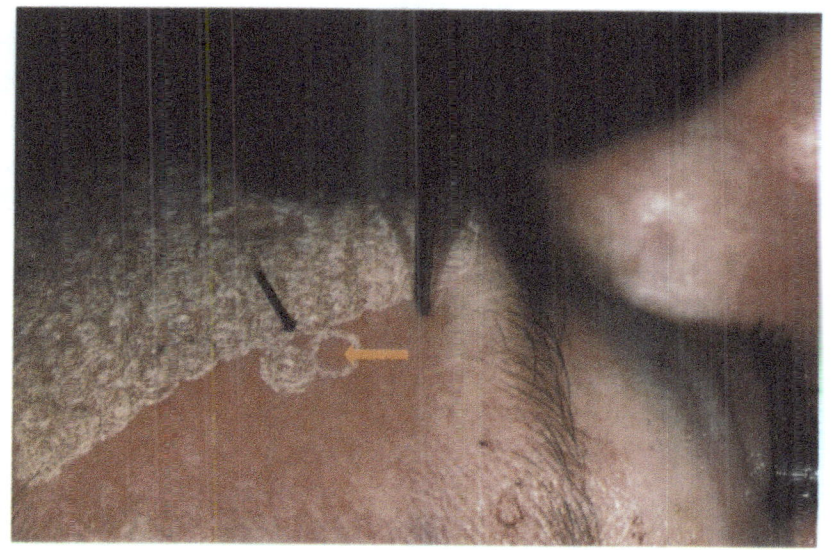

**Figure 5-7 A, B**
A) Too much of a pattern overlap created the "heat sink" in the cheek as reflected by the patches of red hyperemia and edema (black arrow). B) Once the skin re-epithelialized, it was treated with topical steroids with resolution of the redness and a homogenous color without scarring. At this time, the skin was treated with hydroquinone which eliminated the postinflammatory hyperpigmentation after 2 months.

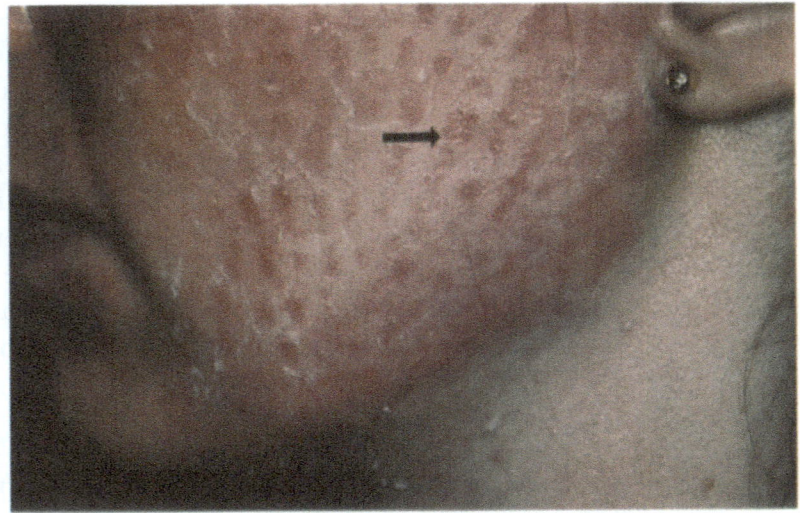

A

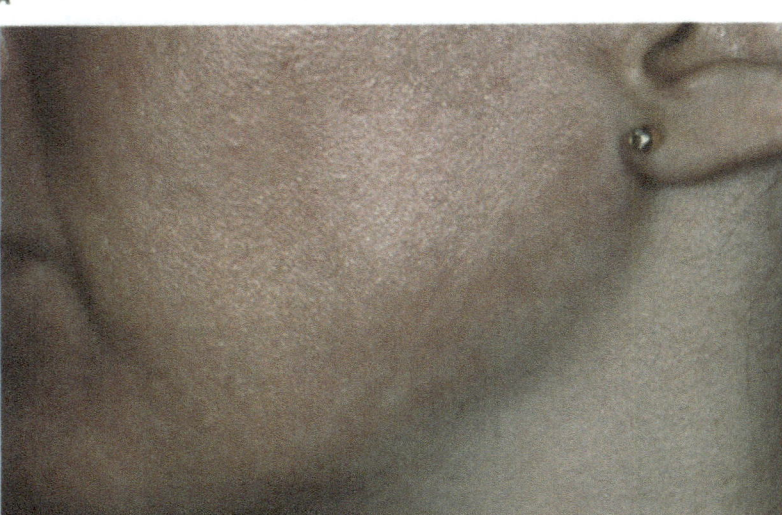

B

Chapter Five    **Laser Skin Resurfacing**

Treatment of medium and deep rhytids within an aesthetic unit must proceed at a rapid pace and continue to the desired end-point (light tan color or wrinkle ablation) to avoid a false appearance of wrinkle elimination due to local swelling. Do not use wrinkle ablation as your endpoint unless it occurs prior to the appearance of the chamois color. Unlike skin peels that use skin turgor as an indicator of depth in injury, the color of the treated skin serves as the indicator of the maximum number of safe passes one can perform during resurfacing. This is true regardless of the skin tone (Figure 5-8).

Once the rhytids within an aesthetic unit are treated, the entire area is resurfaced once with the 200 mm or 260 mm handpiece. Anticipate this final pass when treating individual rhytids so as to not overtreat these areas initially. The light tan or chamois color becomes more prominent in the previously treated areas and the medium, and deep wrinkle center depths, areas not treated previously, are now resurfaced (see Figure 5-5). Only those regions with medium to deep rhytids need to be resurfaced to the light chamois color.

If there are areas of hyperpigmentation in an aesthetic unit not treated as part of individual rhytid reduction, I retreat the hyperpigmented area with a second pass using the 200 or 260 mm handpiece. Never go beyond the chamois color as an endpoint even if some undesirable pigmentation remains. Extending treatment 2 to 4 mm beyond the area of hyperpigmentation in an irregular pattern aids in blending the deeper to the more superficial resurfaced areas.

During treatment, I remove the eschar after each pass in a given aesthetic unit. This is facilitated by a moistened gauze. To standardize your technique, I recommend that you dry the skin before performing another pass. Any fluid left behind will absorb laser energy and complicate the standardization of your technique. During eschar removal, vigorous wiping may cause bleeding. The blood must be removed/stopped before laser energy is imparted again to this area to avoid absorption of the laser energy by blood.

**Figure 5-8**
The chamois color (black arrow) is observed in this hispanic woman who was treated once with the 125 mm handpiece, 7 watts, 3.5 mm spot size over the rhytids, and then with one pass using the 200 mm handpiece at 18 watts, 6 mm spot over the entire area. The yellow arrow reflects the color of the skin after one pass.

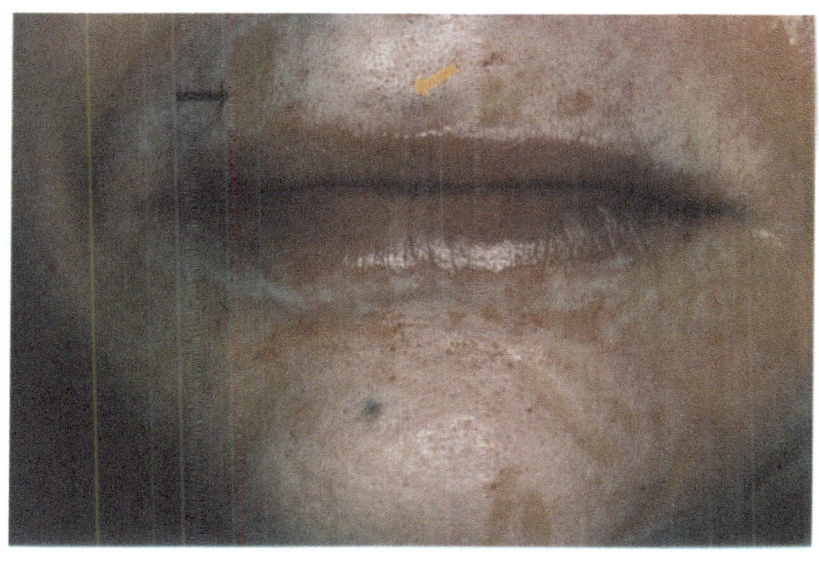

When resurfacing along the hairline or peri-orbital region, the treatment is carried into the first line of hair shafts except along the eyelashes. To avoid a fire hazard, the hair shafts are premoistened. Before resurfacing the eyelids, the eyelashes are protected with a preoperative application of ointment, and then a moistened cotton applicator retracts the lashes during skin treatment. When resurfacing the peri-oral region, the vermilion border is crossed, 1 to 2 mm. Stabilizing the mandible and placing a moist gauze in the labial sulcus covering the teeth will protect the enamel surface from an errant beam.

After resurfacing, I prefer to use an occlusive dressing. The following is my protocol when using Vigilon. The skin is dried and Vigilon dressing applied. A surginet elastic wrap holds the Vigilon in place. This bandage is kept in place until the following day. It is removed and the face gently washed with sterile saline and coarse mesh gauze to remove any debris. A new Vigilon/surginet dressing is applied. This protocol is followed for two to five days, which is sufficient for re-epithelialization in most cases. Others have removed the outer cellophane and allowed the Vigilon to dry, acting like an artificial skin. I have found this effective but could not prevent the occasional collection of debris beneath the dressing in areas of medium and deep resurfaced rhytids. This debris can serve as a nidus for bacteria and resultant infection. Thus, unless a very superficial procedure is performed, I recommend daily dressing changes to minimize the possibility of infection when resurfacing medium and deep rhytids. In addition to Vigilon, other occlusive dressings include xeroform gauze, Silon, Flexzan, and Biobrane.

A postoperative dressing that is used for skin graft fixation and donor site coverage is Mepitel® (SCA Molnlycke). I have applied it to the skin following resurfacing for both zonal and entire face treatment and feel it has ideal properties. Without a chemical adhesive, it adheres to dry skin which facilitates application when treating perioral and periorbital regions. Mepitel is transparent allowing identification and removal of debris on the skin surface without changing the entire dressing. It also has perforations which permits excessive transudate to be withdrawn from the skin surface without lifting the bandage off the skin.

While the occlusive dressings provide greater comfort and may aid in the speed of re-epithelialization, they may increase the chance of infection. When normal skin is occluded with a plastic sheet, the following changes occur in three to five days: an increase in the counts of coagulase-negative staphylocci and coryneform organisms and elevation of the skin pH [50]. Inadvertent contamination with more aggressive bacteria under an occlusive dressing that is not monitored properly and changed when necessary could convert a partial thickness injury into a full thickness wound. Nonocclusive alternative skin coverage includes Crisco®, Catrix®, Vaseline®, and Preparation H® ointment, which are applied daily following skin cleansing. In my experience, patients have less postoperative discomfort and can apply makeup sooner when occlusive dressings are used correctly.

Once re-epithelialization has occurred, the skin is protected with a nonalcohol-based sun block. Creams or powders that use titanium dioxide and or zinc oxide carry the least risk of contact dermatitis. Steroid cream (1% hydrocortisone cream for mild redness, Temovate cream if moderate or severe) can be used twice a day for seven to ten days if redness persists beyond the second week. In general, fair skin color, natural red hair individuals tend to have more redness after resurfacing. If redness persists or does not subside after two weeks of topical steroid use, ask your patient about possible topical treatments they may be applying which may cause a hypersensitivity reaction. Laboratory screening for an undiagnosed collagen vascular condition may also be helpful in assessing a cause for the prolonged redness. While the skin is red/pink, make-up with a green or yellow tint is applied over the sun block. The sun block application is continued for three to six months to avoid undesirable pigmentation changes. If hyperpigmentation occurs, often noticable as the redness fades, it can be treated with 4 to 10% hydroquinone cream applied twice a day. This is continued until the hyperpigmentation resolves. I do not recommend topical tretinoin during the immediate postoperative period due to the irritation it can cause. In patients that are hypersensitive to hydroquinone, an alternative treatment for postinflammatory hyperpigmentation is topical 1% kojic acid, applied twice a day, although I have found it less effective.

Occasionally, antipruritic medication may be necessary during the day. Inadvertent scratching at night can be controlled during the immediate postoperative period by having the patient apply gym socks to both hands prior to going to bed or having their nails trimmed (Figure 5-9).

**Figure 5-9**
Parallel scabbing is consistent with inadvertent scratching, which was occurring at night unbeknownst to the patient despite oral antipruritic medication. The solution the patient preferred was to wear athletic socks over her hands at night versus having her nails trimmed.

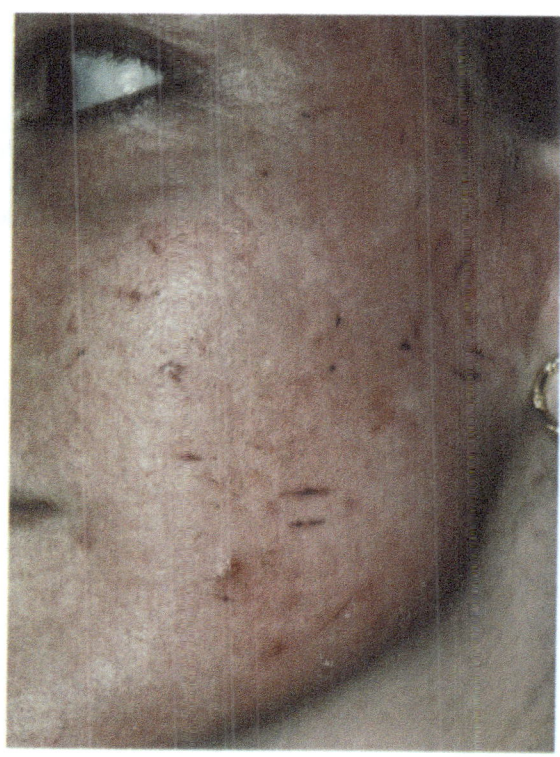

If necessary, retreatment can be performed once the skin color has returned to normal. Treatment while the skin is pink may be complicated with dermal bleeding after the initial pass making it difficult to assess and obtain treatment efficacy. For this second session, I usually reduce the power settings from the initial treatment session by 1 to 2 watts for each handpiece when using the ST or FT mode. However, I make sure to keep the wattage level above the fluence threshold needed for tissue ablation.

### Zone Treatment/Blending

Not all patients request or need their entire face treated. In these cases, treatment of aesthetic units can be performed. In patients with fair skin and even pigmentation, this can be performed following the guidelines above. Once the primary region is treated, a blending or "feathering" to the adjacent nontreated areas can be facilitated in the ST mode by using the 200 mm handpiece, 6 to 10 mm spot size, and reducing the power setting by 1 watt for each adjacent row up until the final treated area is at 15 to 16 watts. Thus, if the primary aesthetic unit was treated at 18 watts, you would have two contiguous treatment areas, one at 17 watts and the last at 16 watts (Figure 5-10

**Figure 5-10 A, B**
A) This is a preoperative photograph of a patient requesting facial resurfacing for acne scarring and skin hyperpigmentation. As the caudal border of the mandible was approached, there was a sequential reduction in wattage. The 200 mm handpiece was used with the 6 mm spot size for the entire procedure. B) After six months, there is a reduction in the preoperative acne scarring and hyperpigmentation and excellent blending with the nontreated neck skin.

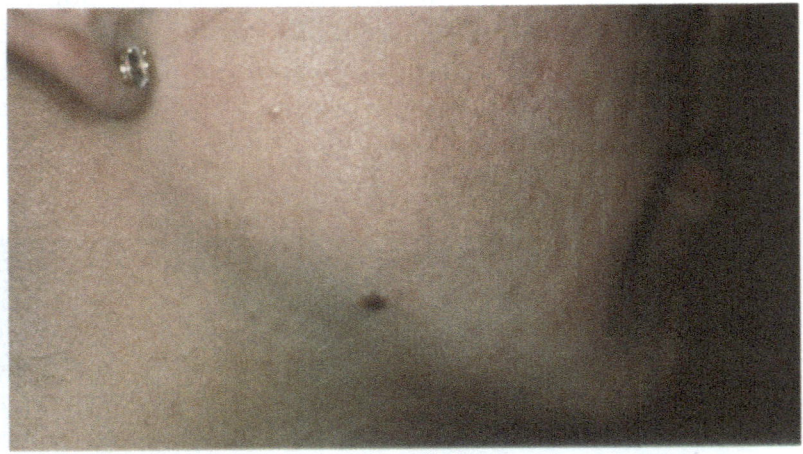

A

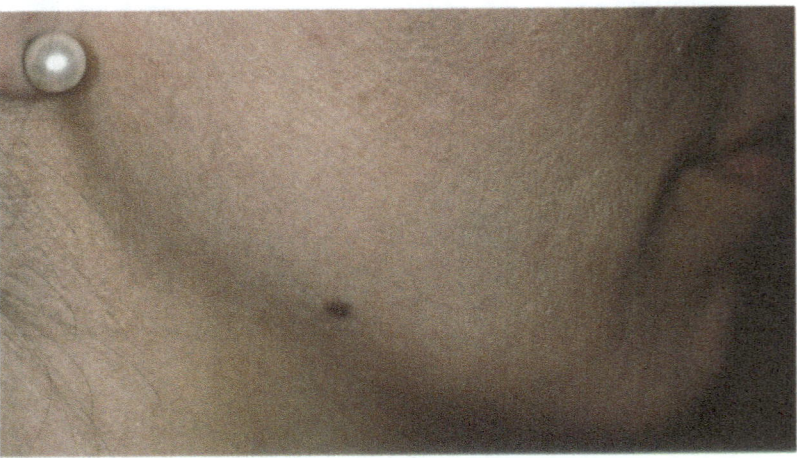

B

A–B). This would provide a transition zone of 12 mm beyond the primary treatment area.

When patients have significant solar damage or a darker complexion, the above treatment may still leave a noticeable line of demarcation. In these cases, an additional blending pass is helpful along the adjacent unresurfaced skin. The 200 mm handpiece, 6 mm spot is moved along the previously unresurfaced skin at a constant speed for one pass with the beam activated (versus the normal usage of holding the handpiece in one location until the entire pattern has been completed) with the wattage set at 16 to 18. This will provide an oval pattern on the skin analogous to the spiral appearance of a stretched, coiled telephone cord. This provides an irregular zone of transition. This blending technique also works when resurfacing the entire face of patients that have a weak or ill-defined caudal mandibular border. Following the same protocol as for zonal treatment, a gradual transition can be obtained (Figures 5-11 A–B, 5-12 A–B). If a distinct line of demarcation remains after healing is complete, re-

**Figure 5-11 A, B**
A) An illustration of the different spot sizes and the coil pattern obtained with constant movement at the optimal focal length during beam activation. B) On the skin, this spiral pattern is faint but noticeable. The numbers on the skin reflect the wattage used with the 200 mm handpiece, 9 mm spot size.

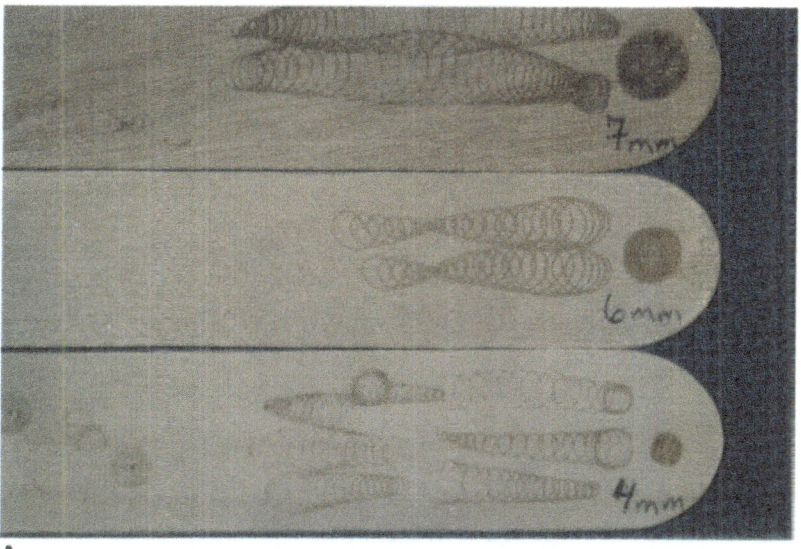

A

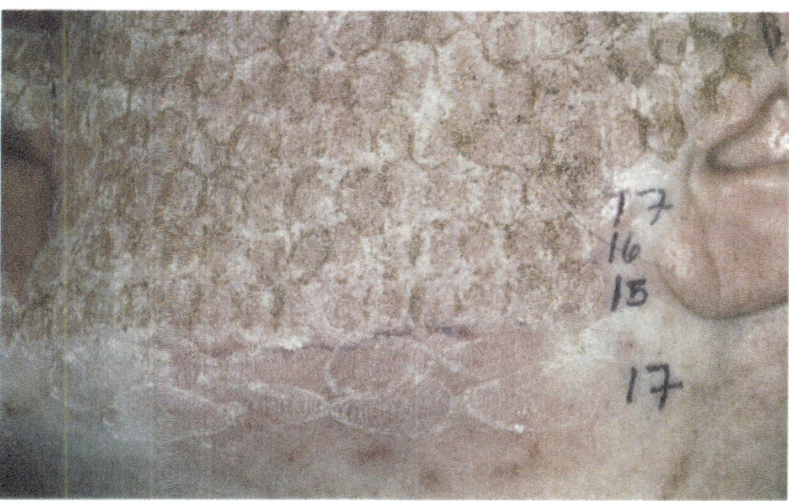

B

**Figure 5-12 A, B**
A) A difficult clinical setting for blending is when a patient has an ill-defined caudal mandibular border and significant hyperpigmentation of the face and neck skin. This preoperative photograph illustrates marked solar changes of the skin. B) Nine months after resurfacing, there is a good reduction of the cheek hyperpigmentation and a gradual transition into the nontreated neck skin using the technique described. Red areas reflect acne flare-ups.

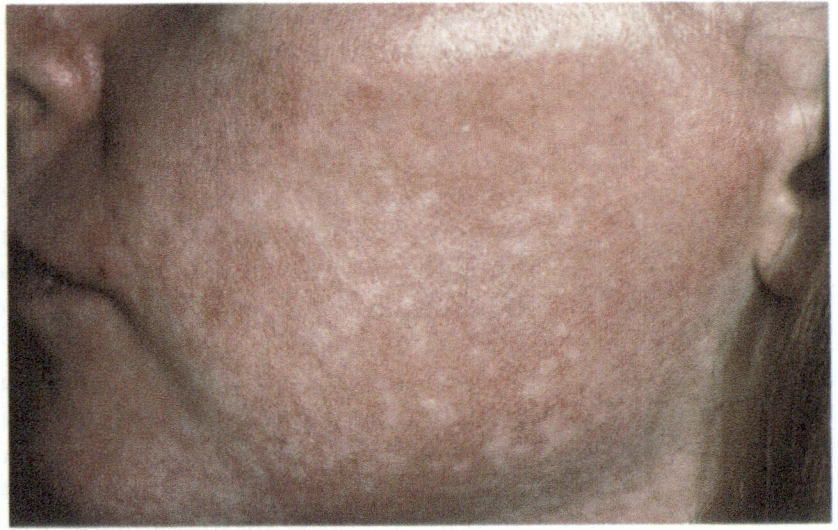

A

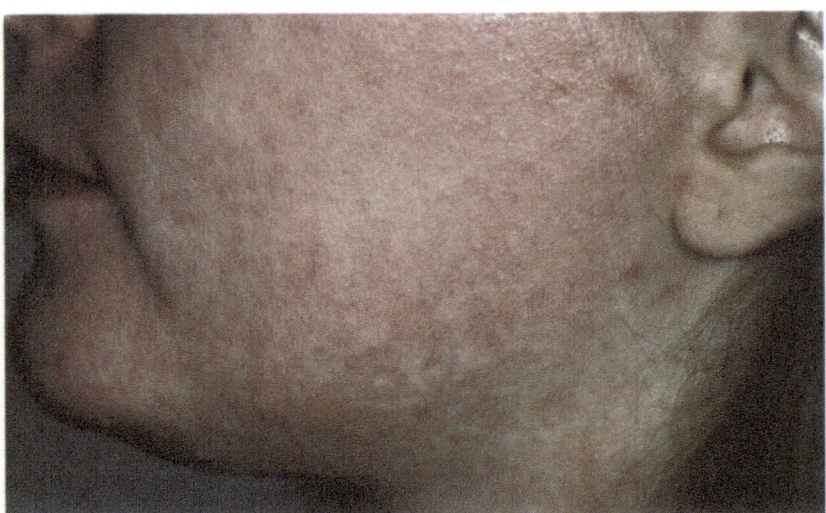

B

treatment or application of 20% trichloroacetic acid (TCA) at the transition zone will help with blending.

Lasers that have FT capability can use this mode to blend treated to nontreated areas. After obtaining the desired end point in the primary treatment area, the laser is put into the FT mode and spot size adjusted so that 2 to 3 contiguous treatment areas of sequentially lower wattage are interposed between the primary treatment area and adjacent untreated skin. If possible, I prefer the last blending pass adjacent to nontreated skin be performed at 33 to 34 watts.

When developing a transition zone, do not try to defocus the handpiece versus reducing the wattage. In my experience, defocusing while resurfacing can lead to more heat transference and prolonged redness and possible pigmentation problems. Also, keep the handpiece perpendicular to the skin. Holding the handpiece at an angle alters the focal length which can create the problems of prolonged hyperemia, hyperpigmentation, and a possible demarcation line (Figure 5-13).

**Figure 5-13**

When sitting at the head of the operating table, there is a natural tendency to allow the handpiece to stray from being perpendicular to the skin. This can result in more thermal injury and hyperpigmentation problems post-operatively.

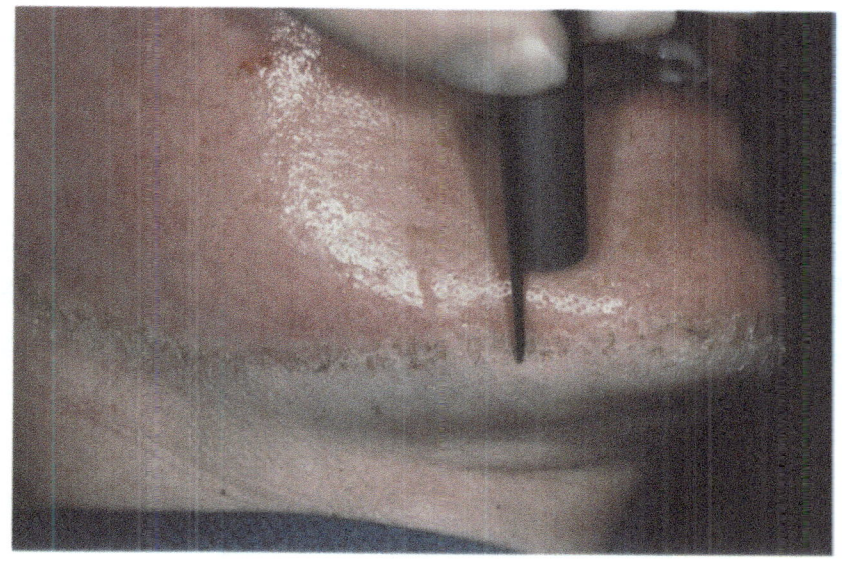

### Resurfacing Darker Skin Tones

Excellent long-term rhytid reduction can be obtained with patients with darker skin tones. Treatment end points are similar to those of fairer skin tone patients, i.e., chamois color. Strict adherence to preoperative skin preparation and the routine use of steroid creams and hydroquinone after the skin has fully re-epithelialized is important. Pretreatment tretinoin and hydroquinone lasts for a minimum of up to 8 weeks in patients with a great deal of heterogeneity in their skin tone. The desired end point is an even, slightly lighter skin tone (Figure 5-22 A–B). The blending techniques outlined above are helpful for the transition areas (Figures 5-14 A–E and 5-15 A–B). When using the FT mode for blending, laser setting of 33 to 35 watts for the outer zone is effective. I have found male patients of dark-skin ethnic groups difficult to manage postoperatively due to their resistance to wearing make-up during the initial phases of healing. When performing "zonal" (regional) treatment, adherence to a proper blending technique is critical. These patients should be prepared to wear make up for three to six months after the skin is healed. If planning on a deeper treatment for reduction of medium and deep wrinkles, it may be prudent to perform a full face versus regional treatment. Transient hyperpigmentation is common and must be treated aggressively with hydroquinone after the initial redness subsides. I often have the pharmacy prepare a 10% hydroquinone cream for these patients.

### Treatment of Scars

Good results are obtained when resurfacing traumatic or acne scars. Prior to laser treatment, optimal surgical results should be achieved. For certain scars, this may necessitate micro-excision and primary closure or elevation of the scar with a punch biopsy knife and release of the feathering fibrous bands. Ideally, the formerly depressed area

**Figure 5-14 A, B, C**
A) This 52-year-old hispanic woman requested facial resurfacing but did not
want her upper eyelids treated. B) In
the operating room, the rhytids are outlined following a six-week preoperative
regimen of topical tretinoin and hydroquinone. C) Two and one half weeks
after resurfacing, the face is red and
Temovate treatment was started.

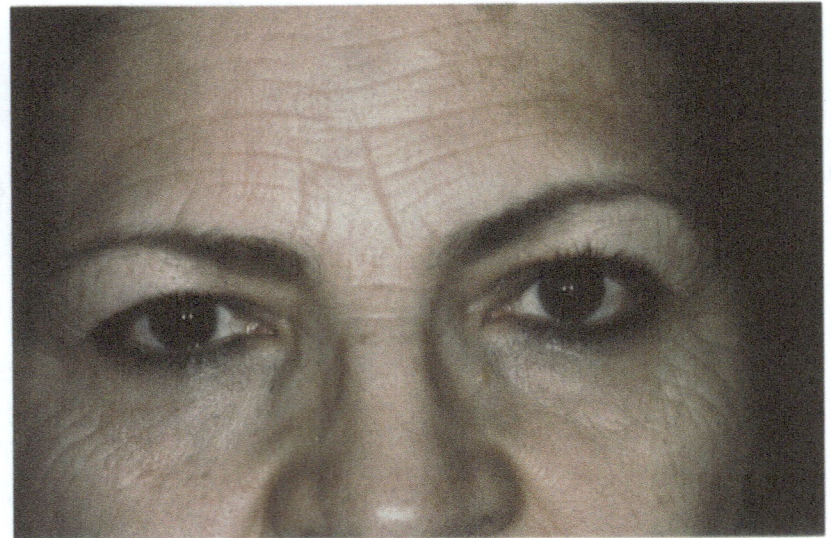

A

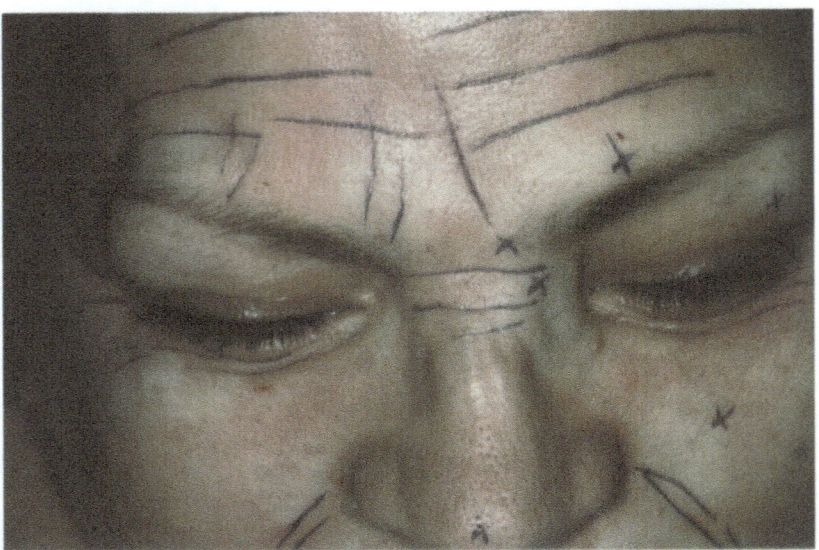

B

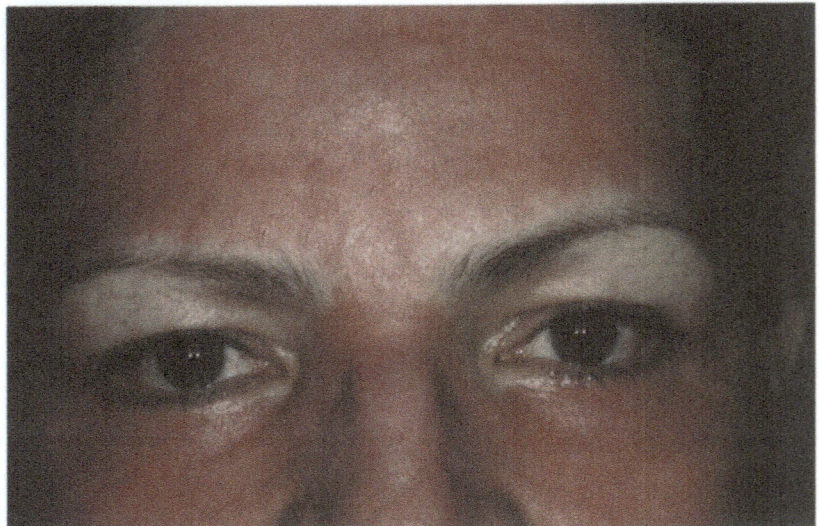

C

**Figure 5-14 D, E**
D) This photograph was also taken two and one half weeks after resurfacing, illustrating that the red color can be covered with make-up that has a green and yellow tint added. E) Six months after resurfacing there is an excellent reduction of rhytids.

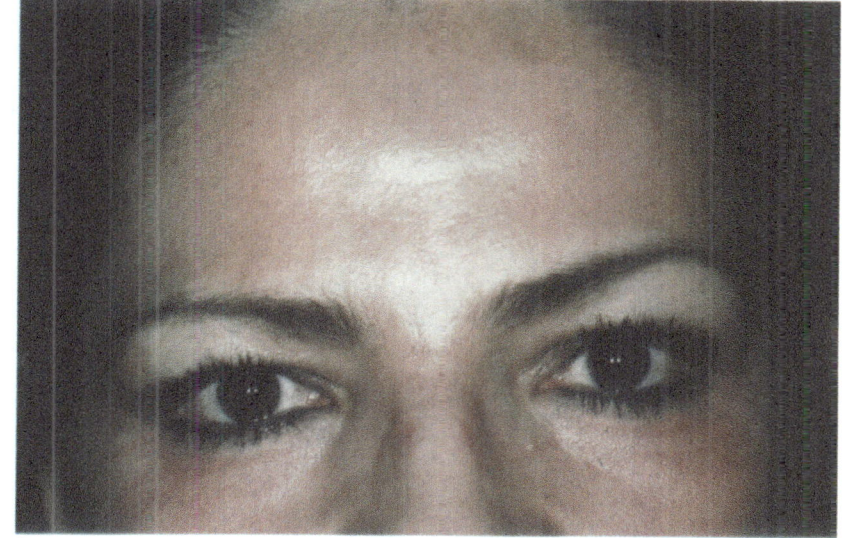

D

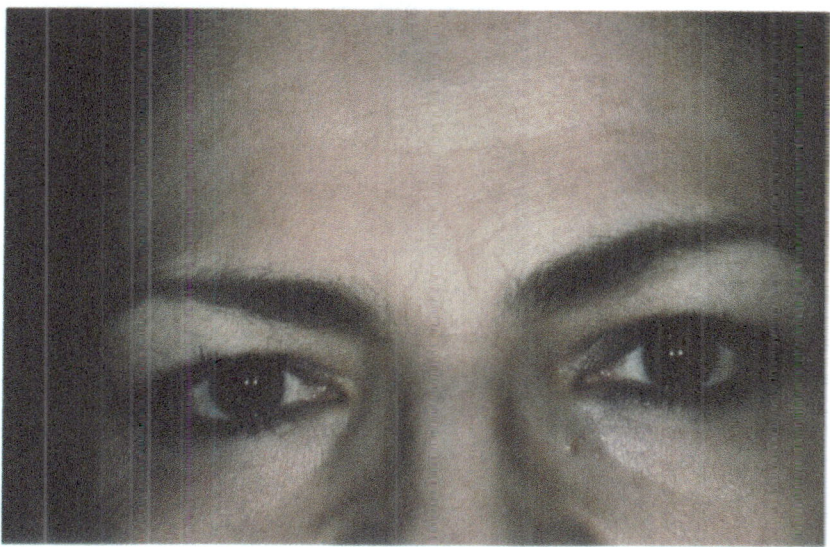

E

**Figure 5-15 A, B**
Pre (A) and six-month post (B) resurfacing photographs showing reduction in forehead lines and retention of normal skin color.

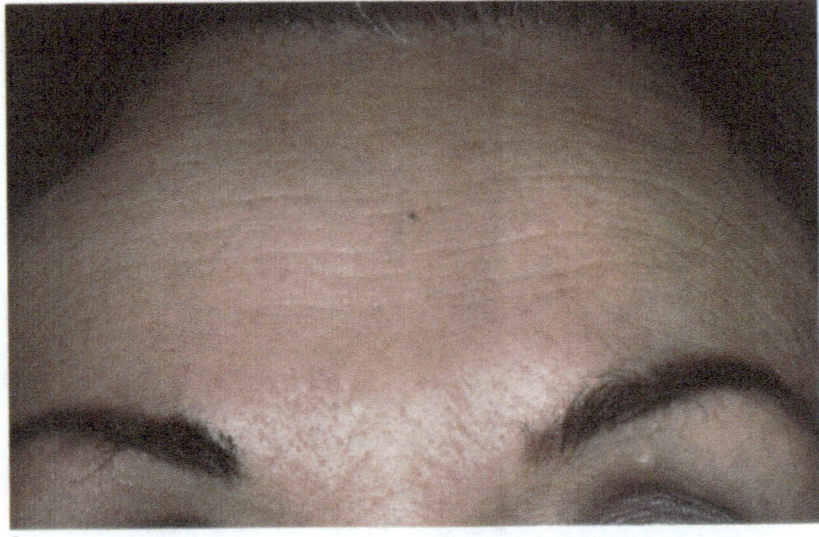

A

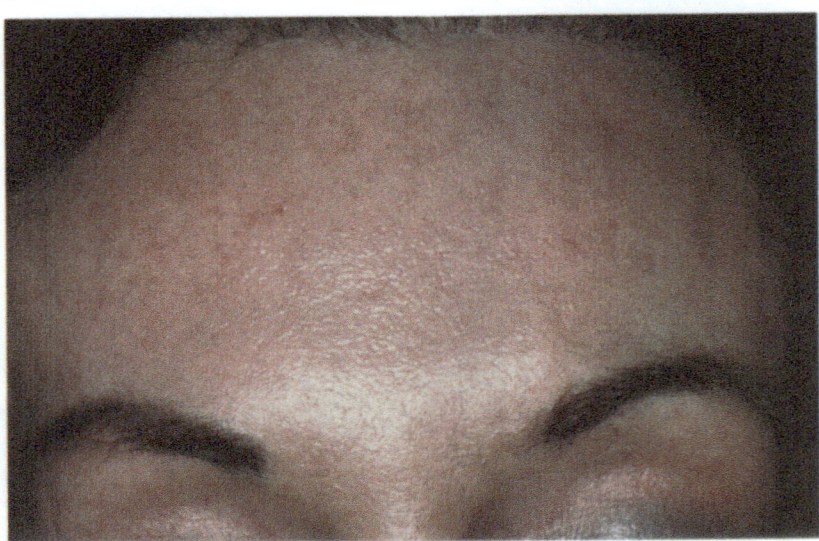

B

should be at or above the plane of the normal skin before resurfacing. Once the revised scar is pink in color, the region can be resurfaced, treating the area immediately adjacent to the scar as one would treat the crest of a deep wrinkle, followed by resurfacing of the entire area, including the revised scar with a larger spot size (Figure 5-16 A-B). In cases where there are isolated facial scars that could be revised, initial resurfacing followed by same day surgical scar revision can be successfully performed. In these cases, I recommend an occlusion bandage that is changed daily. Sutures are removed in five to seven days.

**Figure 5-16 A, B**
A) Photograph of a traumatic scar across the lip in a hispanic woman. B) Postoperative photographs are taken six months after resurfacing (scar revision performed three months prior to resurfacing).

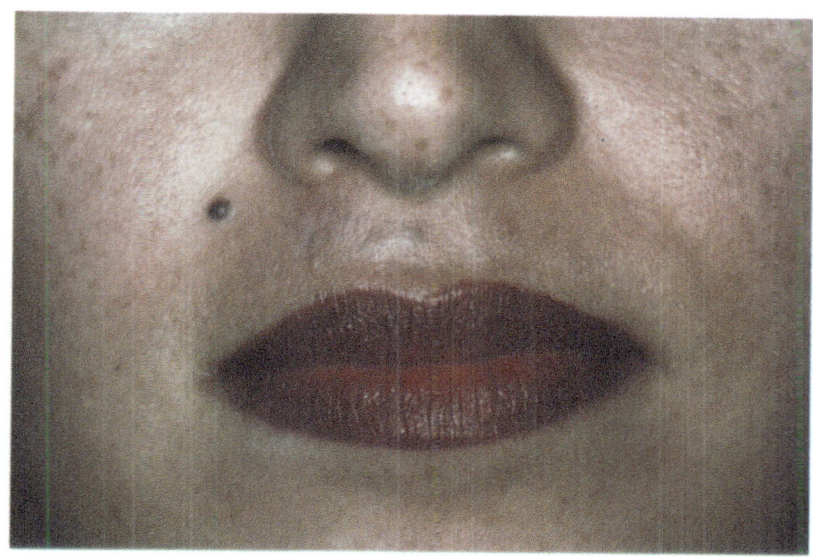

A

B

**Figure 5-17 A, B, C**
A) Preoperative views of a 51-year-old woman who requested a lower lid transconjunctival blepharoplasty and lower eyelid resurfacing. Blending technique described in the text. B) At two weeks post treatment, the skin is red–pink. C) Postoperative photographs taken six months after resurfacing showing good elimination of the rhytids and lower lid hyperpigmentation.

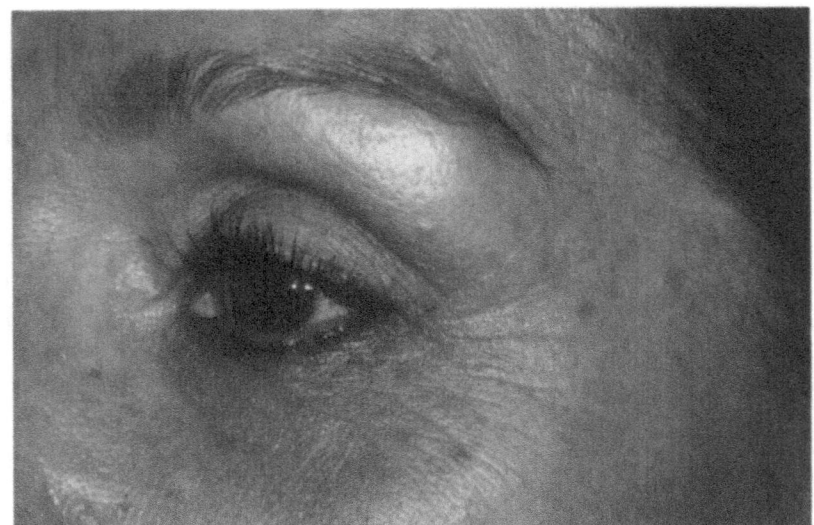

A

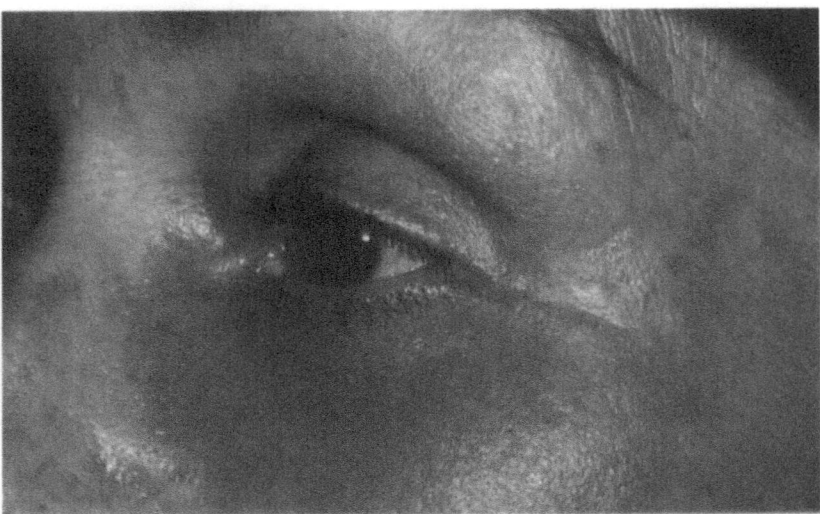

B

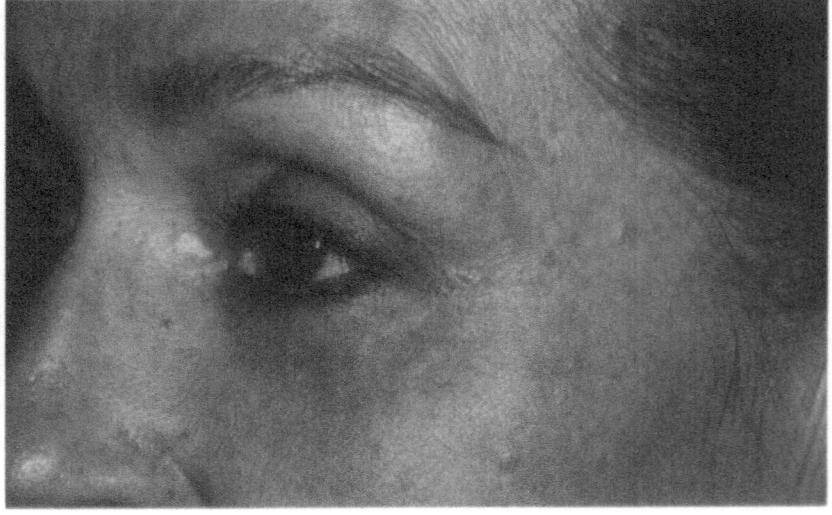

C

**Figure 5-17 D, E**

D) Side view showing preoperative herniation of fat and fine skin rhytids. E) Side view six months after resurfacing demonstrating good contour and excellent blending into the nonresurfaced areas.

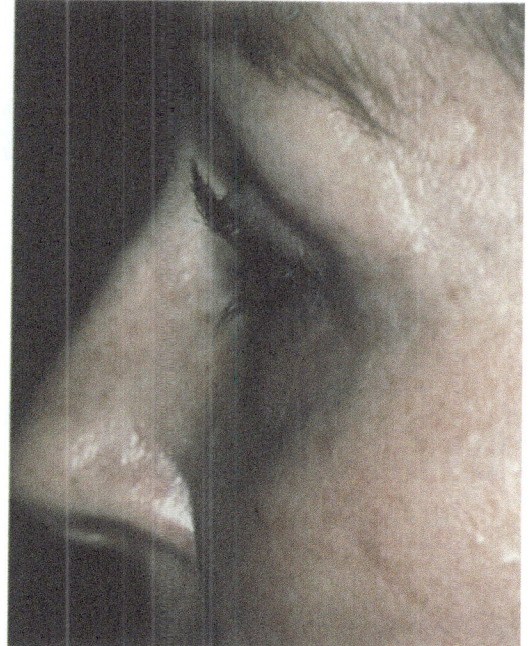

D

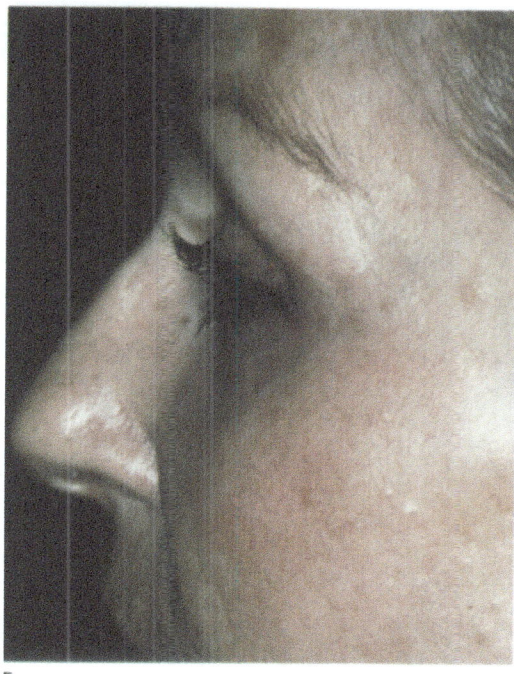

E

## Other Resurfacing Applications

While resurfacing skin surgically elevated in the subcutaneous plane is not recommended, excellent results are obtained when treating lax skin on the lower lid when performing a lower transconjunctival blepharoplasty (Figure 5-17 A–E). This procedure has become my standard treatment when the skin excess is not great and transposition of fat across the infraorbital rim is not necessary. Excellent results are also obtained when treating leukoplakia of the lip (Figure 5-18 A–B) and rhynophyma (Figure 5-19 A–B).

**Figure 5-18 A, B**
A) Patient has lower lip leukoplakia. B) Six months after resurfacing with two passes at 16 watts, 6 mm spot using the 200 mm handpiece.

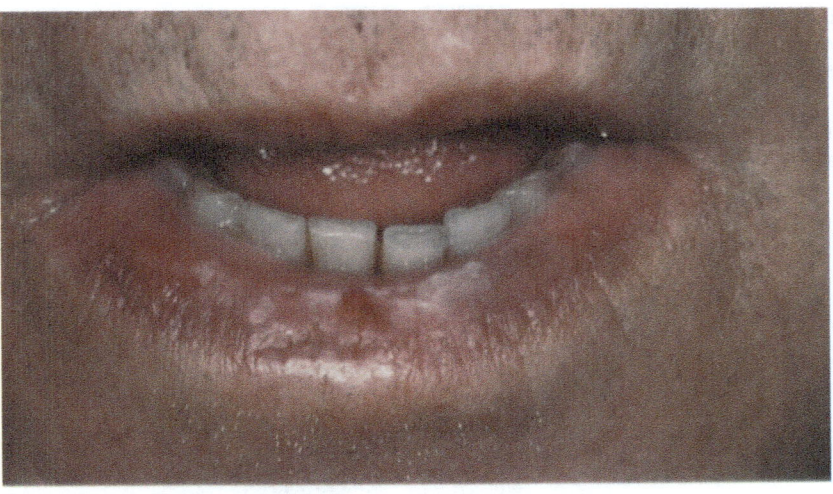

A

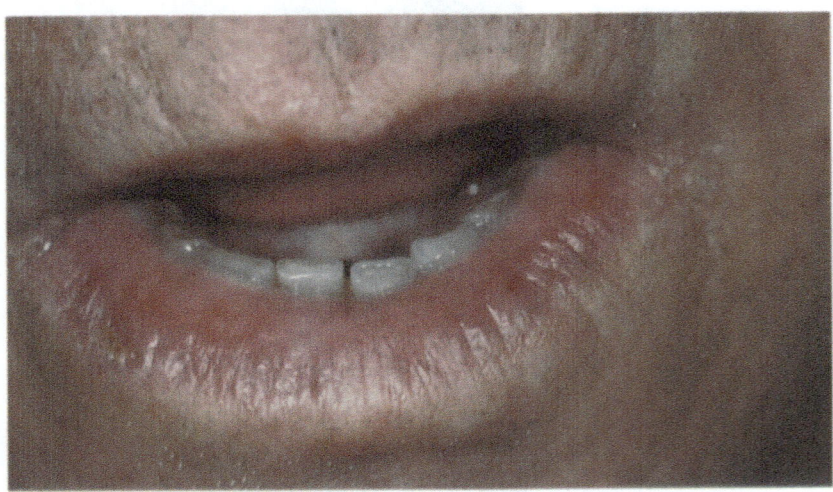

B

Chapter Five   **Laser Skin Resurfacing**

**Figure 5-19 A, B**
A) After two courses of Accutane, this man still had residual fullness of the nasal tip. B) Multiple passes were required to obtain the desired contour as shown three months after resurfacing.

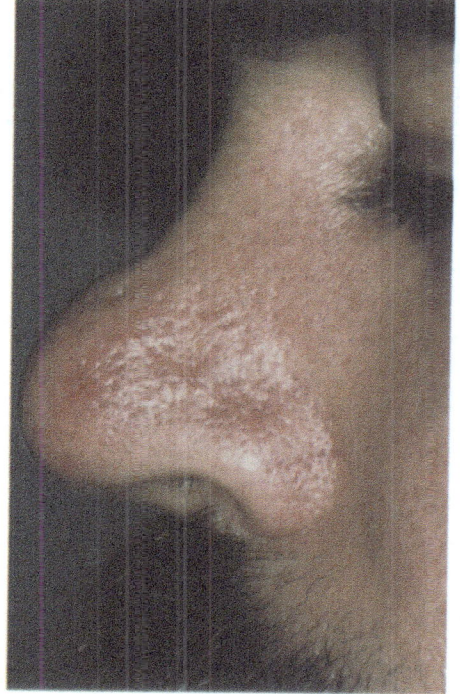

A

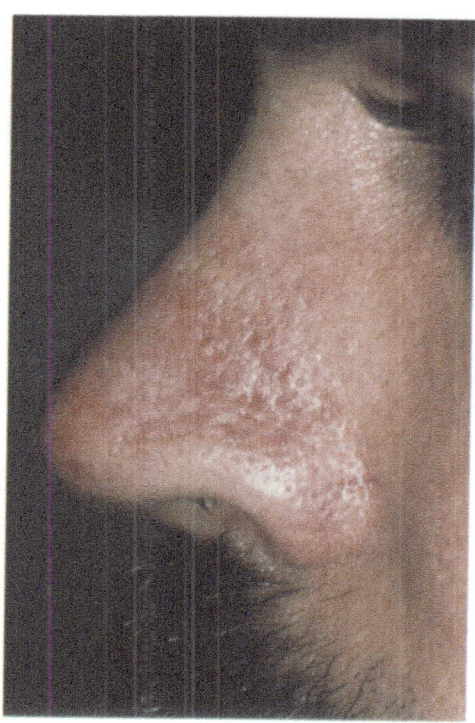

B

## Complications

Possible complications are similar to those that can occur following chemical peels. Obtained from personal communications and experience, the adverse effects observed in laser resurfacing include:

milia

skin burns/scarring

injury to dental structures

ocular injuries

hyper/hypopigmentation

infection (bacterial, fungal, or viral)/contact dermatitis

prolonged erythema

dermal sinus tract after treatment

increased scleral show along the lower eyelid

### Milia

Milia can be minimized by preparing the skin preoperatively and assessing the sebaceous gland activity. Patients with oily skin are prone to develop milia during the initial postoperative period. Unlike bacterial pustules which usually appear within the first two weeks, milia develop after the skin is healed. Postoperative treatments that encourage formation include topical application of steroids, Vaseline, or antibiotic ointments such as Bacitracin or Polysporin. Patients with oily skin have increased milia formation when occlusive dressings are used and not changed daily. Daily cleansing helps keep pores open during the initial recovery period.

### Skin Burns/Scarring

Full thickness skin burns are avoided by staying within the proper resurfacing guidelines. Testing the laser settings on a wet tongue blade prior to treating the skin should help avoid burns due to faulty settings. Turning the laser on stand-by during rest periods will avoid burns due to inadvertent laser firing. Patients must refrain from applying their "standard" skin care products following resurfacing since the skin is fragile (Figure 5-20 A–D).

Recognition of prolonged skin redness is important in avoiding the possibility of scarring. These red, raised areas represent deep dermal or significant thermal injury and can lead to hypopigmentation and, or hypertrophic scarring. I like to treat these areas early with Cordran tape for one to two weeks, examining the patient weekly. Instillation of a small amount Celestone or Aristicort is also an alternative but caution must be exercised to avoid overtreatment. There is some anecdotal recommendations to treat patients with raised red dermal areas with oral antihistamines to counter the activity of the mast cells in the inflamed tissue. The key is to follow your patients closely dur-

**Figure 5-20 A, B**
A) In the operating room, superficial depth was obtained in the cheek area (blue arrow, one pass, 200 mm handpiece, 9 mm spot, 18 watts) and the tan color evident in the area of additional passes over the rhytids near the mouth (red arrow). B) One week later, a light crust is noticed as she was treated with the open technique and topical application of Preparation H.

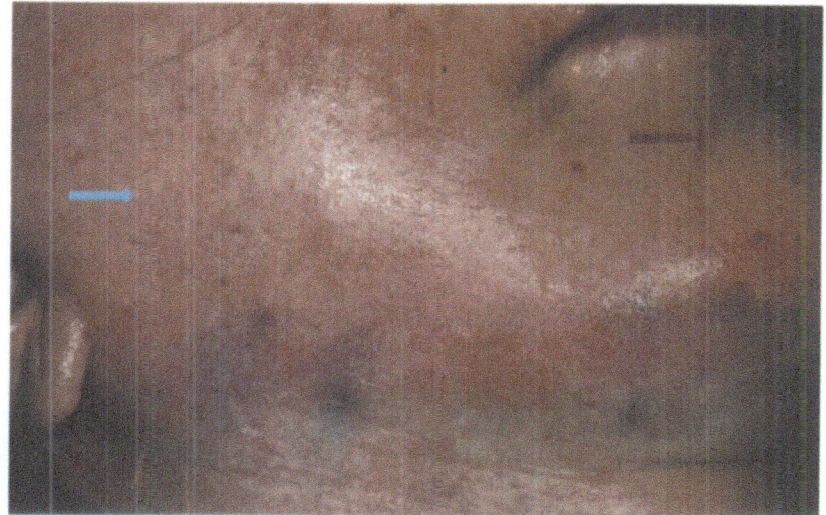

A

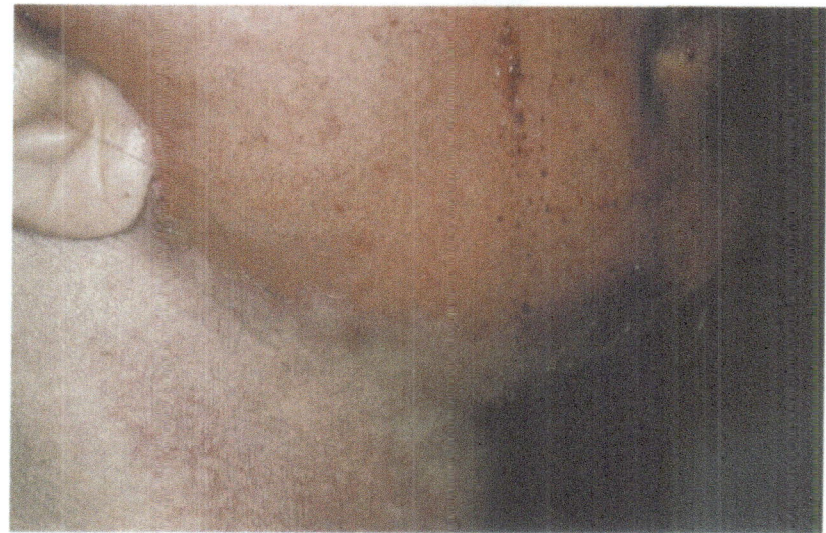

B

**Figure 5-20 C, D**

C) She returned one month post treatment with an ulcer. Questioning revealed that she decided to "clean" her face with her normal "green solution."
D) Shown at six months after resurfacing, the area went on to heal with local scar and alteration of pigmentation.

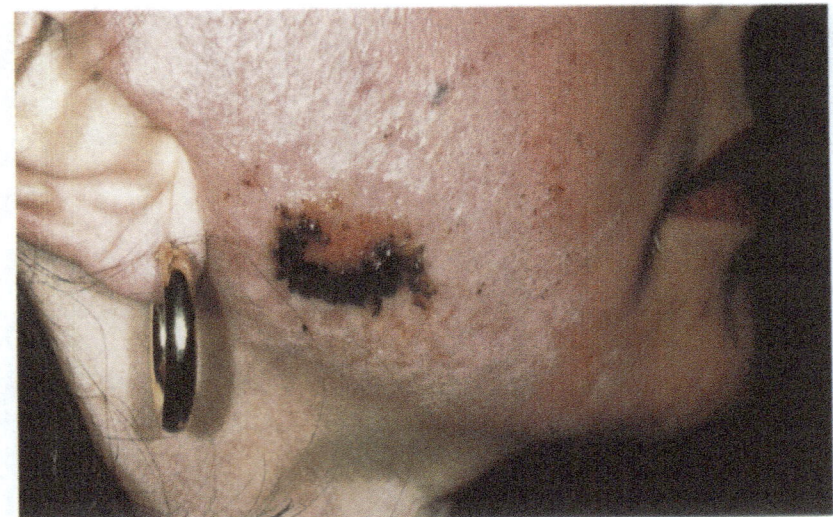

C

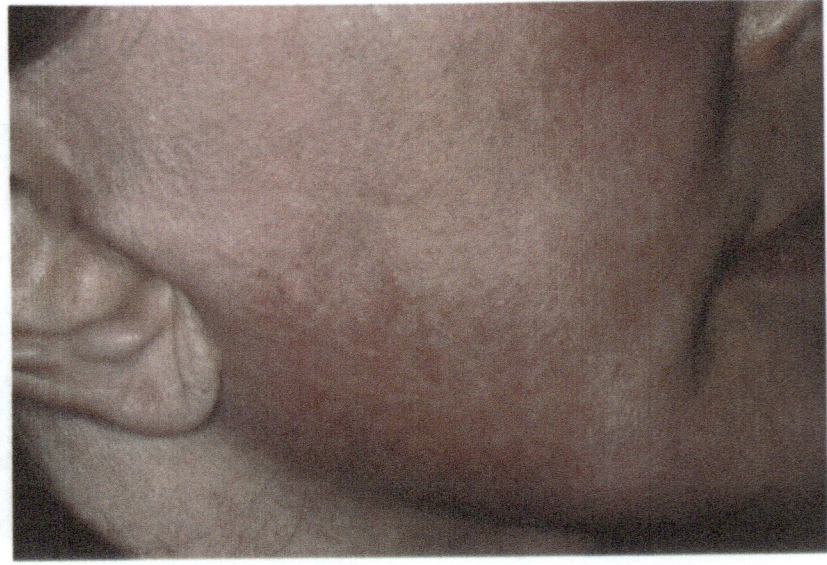

D

Chapter Five   **Laser Skin Resurfacing**

ing the immediate postoperative period and institute treatment as soon as possible to minimize the chance of a permanent problem.

## Dental Injuries

Dental injuries can be avoided by supporting the head and mandible during resurfacing of the peri-oral region. Another safety method is to place a moistened gauze in the patients labial sulcus covering the enamel dental surface.

## Ocular Injuries

Ocular injuries can be prevented by proper shielding prior to treatment. Secured moistened gauze covering the eyelid region is effective. However, I recommend a highly polished metal shield to cover the cornea and sclera with a matte outer surface. Prior to application, the shield's surface should be inspected to assure that there are no surface irregularities. Be aware of the possibility of the shields shifting during the case exposing the sclera to possible injury. To avoid the possibility of a hypersensitivity reaction, I do not use antibiotic ophthalmic ointments as a lubricant. Patients should be told of the possibility of transient postoperative lagophthalmus. When treating the peri-orbital region, patients should be given a prescription for artificial tears (i.e., Refresh drops during the day and Refresh PM prior to sleep) as skin shrinkage in the immediate post-treatment period may limit normal eyelid closure. Postoperative application should continue until normal eyelid function returns.

## Infection

Bacterial infection can be minimized with proper skin cleansing and prophylactic antibiotics, especially with the application of an occlusive dressing after resurfacing. Proper skin cleansing during the immediate postoperative period will keep debris on the skin to a minimum, reducing the nidus for bacterial proliferation. Clinically, the suspicion of a bacterial infection versus an exacerbation of rosacea or contact dermatitis is increased when patients complain of pain associated with a skin eruption. Viral eruptions are confirmed by a Tzanck stain and can occur following regional peri-oral or treatment of the entire face. The chance of herpetic breakout can be minimized by prophylactic treatment with acyclovir, 200 mg four times a day. Acyclovir is started the day before treatment and continued for the first week. This dose can be increased in patients with a propensity for breakouts or at the first sign of an eruption. Because of a relatively short half-life, 2.3 to 3.5 hours, a good alternative to Acyclovir is Famvir or Valtrex 500 mg bid. Fungal infections can occur and are differentiated from bacterial infections by culture (KOH prep). If present, they can be treated with topical Diflucan or Nysall cream. During the latter stages of healing, six to ten weeks after re-epithelialization, patients may develop a folliculitis or dermatitis lateral to the oral commissure. This is the area that often comes into contact with the telephone receiver. Gentle skin cleansing combined with disinfection of the phone mouth-piece or use of a headset has helped with this condition. Often after skin resurfacing, the skin is hypersensitive to topical agents. This may include creams and ointments the patient was able to apply prior to your treatment. This most likely represents a contact dermatitis which is transient vs. a true "allergic" reaction and may be due to the loss of the removal of the barrier function of the outer layers of the skin.

### Prolonged Redness

Some degree of redness after resurfacing is inevitable with current technology and treatment into the papillary dermis. The surgeon is creating a dermal injury with postinflammatory vascular changes. In addition, the epidermis and portions of the dermis which normally filter the color of the microvasculature are removed. The skin is very sensitive to topical agents after resurfacing, and creams normally tolerated prior to treatment can contribute to skin hyperemia.

There are ways to minimize the length of time the skin color is red/pink. Preoperatively, the sensitivity of the skin can be assessed by how the patient's skin reacts or responds to the tretinoin treatment. If the patient's skin becomes very red and desquamates rapidly with low concentrations (0.01 to 0.05%) beyond the initial seven to ten days of therapy, and continues to respond in this manner despite reducing the dosage and/or frequency, tretinoin treatment should be discontinued. In my experience, these patients and those that tolerate only once a day or every-other-day application tend to have prolonged redness after resurfacing unless the number of passes are reduced and/or the power settings are reduced by 1 to 2 watts from your standard maximum settings for a given handpiece, spot size, tissue type, and desired tissue effect. This results in a more superficial injury and retreatment may be more likely. However, patients may prefer this versus dealing with redness for four to six weeks or longer.

The number of passes and the power setting on the machine will also affect the length of postoperative redness. In general, the more passes over the same area or the higher the wattage settings, the more intense the redness will be and the longer it will last. A typical scenario for superficial rhytids in a patient with normal skin anatomy and preparation with tretinoins would be one to two weeks of redness on "crow's feet" wrinkles treated in the ST mode with one pass at 6 watts using the 125 mm handpiece, 3.7 mm spot, followed by one pass with the 200 mm handpiece, 6 mm spot size set at 17 watts. The redness is followed by a progressive fading, with resolution of the light pink color over the next six to eight weeks (Figure 5-21 A–C). Treatment of the deeper rhytids to a chamois color end point will result in redness that lasts two to four weeks following resurfacing. Leaving residual debris on the treatment site prior to an additional pass or application of the dressing also increases the length of time redness lasts.

**Figure 5-21 A, B, C**
A) Preoperative view of rhytids along the lower and lateral eyelid region in a 35-year-old female. B) Between weeks 2 and 3 the redness begins to fade, in this case with the use of 1% hydrocortisone. C) At the end of two months following a full face resurfacing, the pink color is essentially gone.

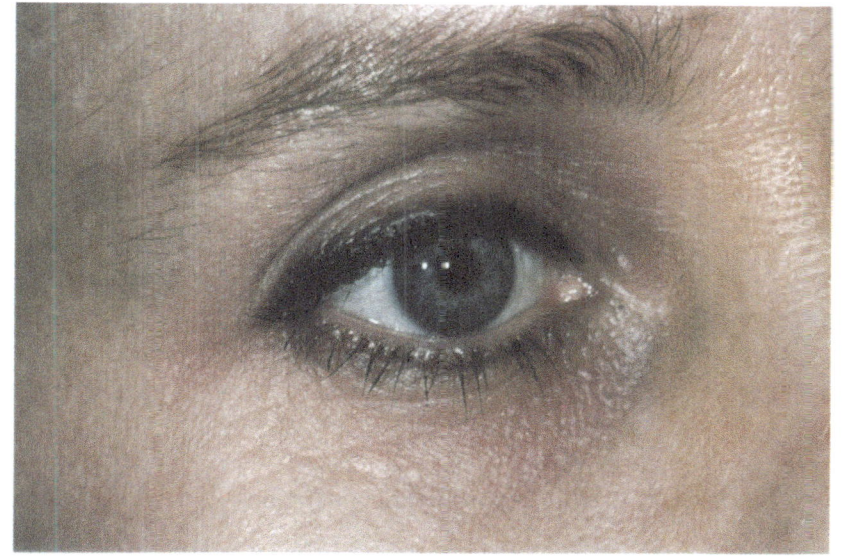

A

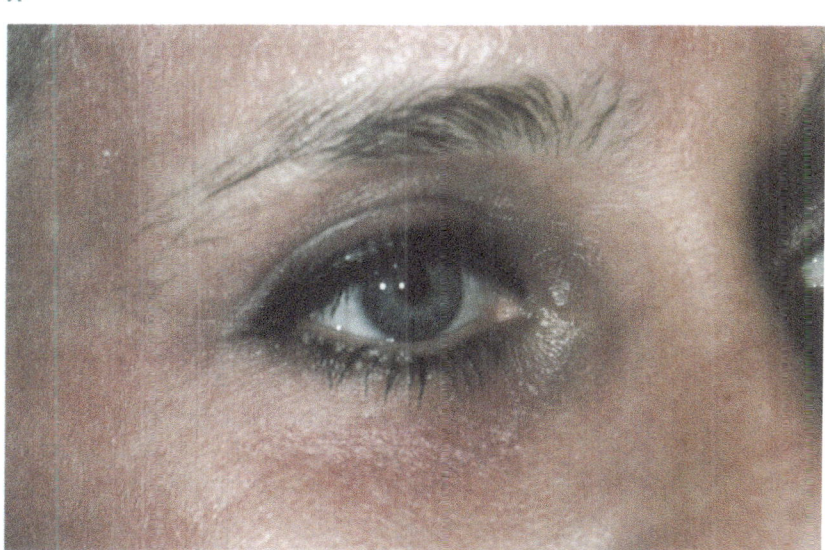

B

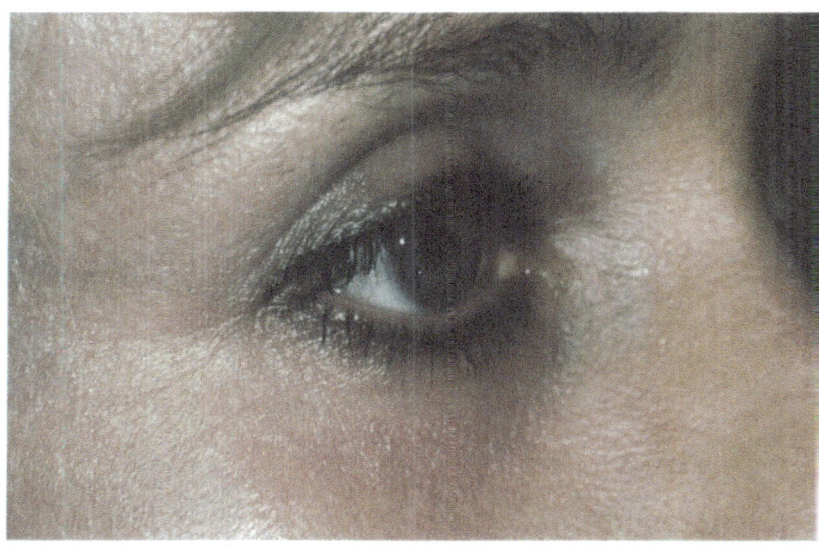

C

Postoperatively, redness can be minimized by avoiding possible irritants such as tretinoin, irritating soaps, and alcohol containing sun block in the immediate postoperative period. Nonperfumed, mild skin cleansers and sun block that do not contain alcohol or PABA are recommended. Topical steroids administered for a brief period of time are also beneficial. Once the skin has completely re-epithelialized, mild redness beyond ten days can be treated with 1% hydrocortisone cream applied twice a day. Redness usually fades to a light pink within one to two weeks. If the patient has significant redness, Temovate applied for seven days, twice a day, no treatment for one week, and then application for another seven days is very effective.

### Hyper/Hypopigmentation

The most common undesirable post-treatment sequela is hyperpigmentation, which is transient if treated properly. Melanogenesis is stimulated by hormones, ultraviolet light, increase in tyrosinase substrate, and repair of skin intracellular DNA damage [51]. Sun exposure increases the number of melanocytes, increases the amount of pigment within each cell, and increases the conversion of melanocytes to keritinocytes [52]. The melanogenic response is dependent on the spectral band of ultraviolet light. At suberythema doses, UVA increases melanogenesis more than UVB [53]. Therefore, a patient does not have to experience "redness" to experience ultraviolet effects on skin pigmentation. Within cells, the type of melanin also affects skin color and tissue injury due to radiation exposure. Eumelanin is found in greater proportion in patients with darker color and is photoprotective. Phaeomelanin is found in greater proportion in patients with red hair and fair skin and, when stimulated with ultraviolet light, produces free radicals which are damaging to the skin [54]. These patients tend to have a relatively prolonged post-resurfacing hyperemic phase.

Post-treatment inflammation plays an important role in the final skin color. Hyperpigmentation occurs following the production of arachidonic acid and its metabolites of the inflammatory cascade. The release of this component of the cell wall increases tyrosinase activity, which increases melanin formation [55]. Reduction of erythema with topical anti-inflammatory agents reduces postinflammatory hyperpigmentation [56]. Application of hydroquinone following steroid therapy is often necessary (Figure 5-22 A–E). Failure to wear sun block can also lead to hyperpigmentation. Patients return to work and return with what I describe as the "car sign," hyperpigmentaion on the side of the face corresponding to the side of the car the patient usually sits on. If recognized early, topical hydroquinone and sun block will resolve the hyperpigmentation. If three to four months transpire before hydroquinone is instituted, resolution may require retreatment or topical 20 to 30% TCA application.

**Figure 5-22 A, B**
A) Preoperative view of a hispanic female prior to skin care protocol. B) At the time of resurfacing, the skin is noticeably lighter following six weeks of preoperative skin treatment.

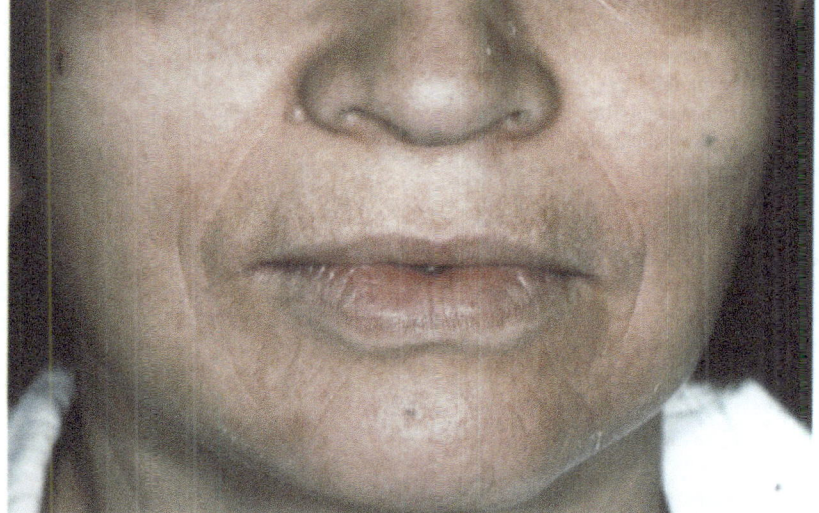

A

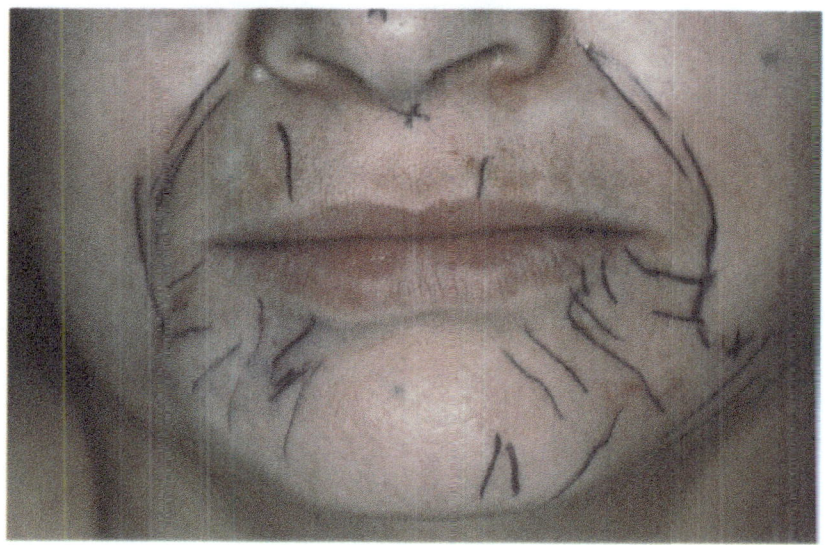

B

**Figure 5-22 C, D, E**
C) She failed to show for her scheduled follow-up visits and returned at one month post resurfacing with hyperpigmentation. D) Three weeks after initiating 4% hydroquinone application, the hyperpigmentation begins to resolve. E) Six months after resurfacing, and three months after stopping all skin treatments except sun block and moisturizers, the rhytids are reduced and the skin color is homogenous, approximating the color at the time of resurfacing (see B).

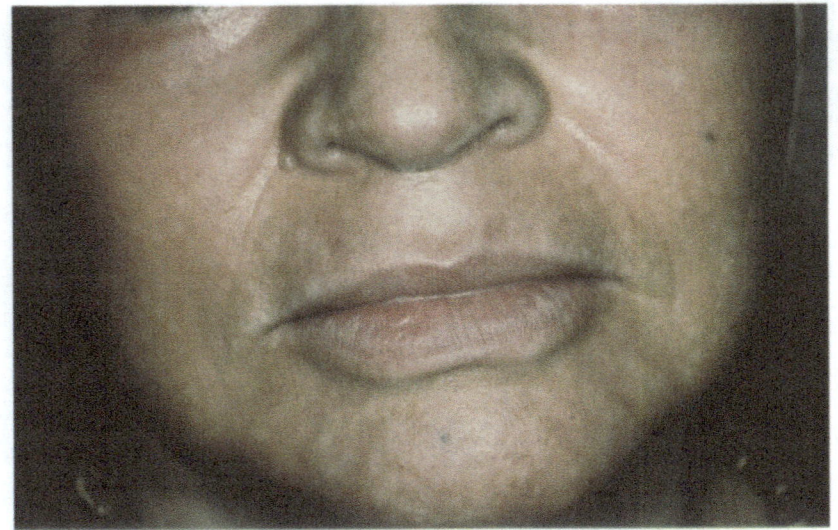

C

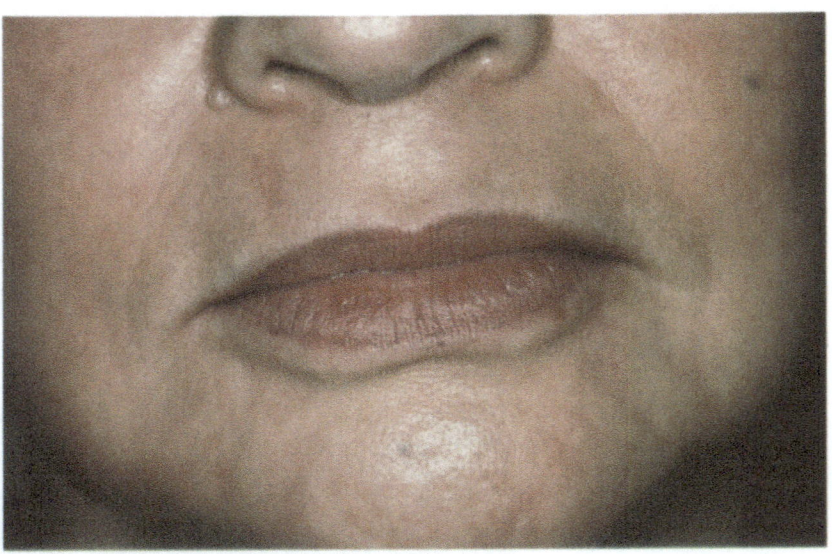

D

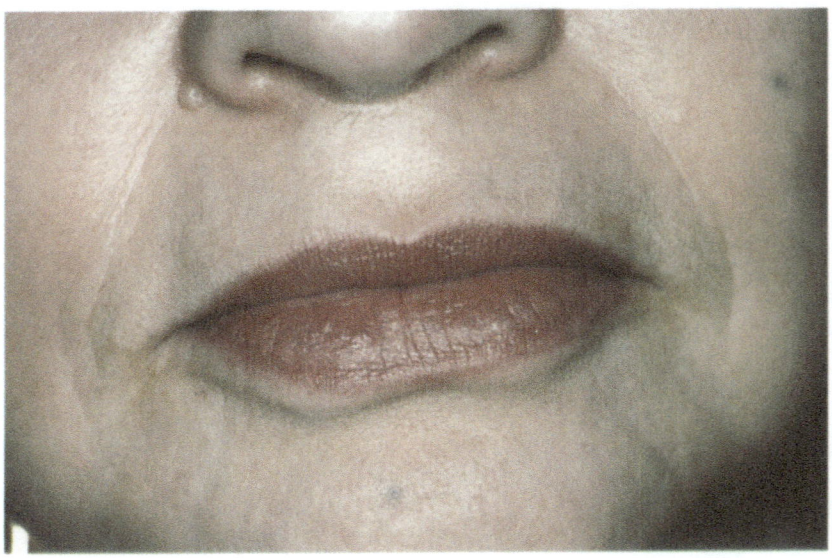

E

Chapter Five    **Laser Skin Resurfacing**

I have not obtained consistent, long term good results in treating melasma or chloasma with laser resurfacing. Be aware of the possibility of a patient having melasma which is camoufladged by simultaneous actinic skin damage. Initially, these patients obtain a good, confluent skin color. However with time, the blotchy hyperpigmentation skin color returns. Awareness of the possibility of chemically stimulated hyperpigmentation is important as many menopausal women on hormone supplements request laser resurfacing. In cases precipitated by hormone treatment, I have had some success when the precipitating medication has been reduced or eliminated.

Hypopigmentation can occur when the dermal injury penetrates too deep. This is observed through direct injury when laser energy settings are too high or when injury to the melanocytes occurs from incidental thermal injury or post-treatment complication, i.e., infection or prolonged inflammation. Thus, once re-epithelialization has occurred, it is helpful to limit the length of time erythema persists, whether caused by the laser treatment, post-treatment topical agents, or sun.

## Dermal Sinus Tract

A dermal sinus tract may develop after resurfacing when you have prolonged dermis–dermis contact immediately following resurfacing. The most common location is at the upper or lower eyelid region when there is a redundancy of skin prior to resurfacing i.e. the patient would optimally benefit from a blepharoplasty. Muscle activity during conversation, smiling, etc., may cause dermal–dermal contact during the time when there is no epithelial cover. Gentle separation of the skin and application of a topical nonirritating ointment (Vaseline, Preparation H, Crisco, etc.) is helpful. If recurrent, the redundant skin may have to be excised.

## Scleral Show

Temporary scleral show is a common finding following resurfacing of the lower eyelid (Figure 5-23 A–D). It is usually self-limiting unless skin scarring and contraction develops or muscle necrosis occurs following simultaneous transconjunctival blepharoplasty. Patients with a lax tarsal plate may have prolonged lid retraction following resurfacing and may require a subsequent suspension.

**Figure 5-23 A, B**
A) This 76-year-old patient did not want any surgical procedure for the brow and upper eyelid rhytids. She has significant lower lid scleral show following prior surgery and residual prominent lower eyelid fat. B) Four months following blepharoplasty with relocation of lower lid fat across the infraorbital rim and muscle suspension. She has also completed a four-week skin preparation protocol.

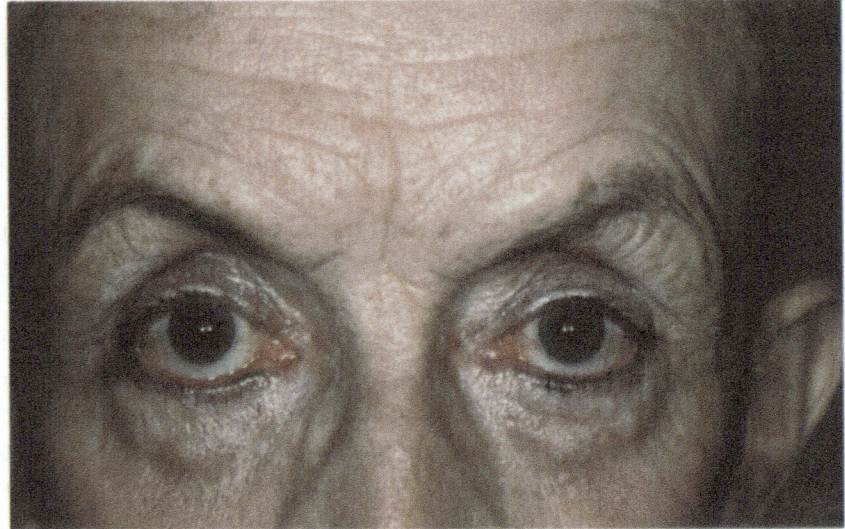

A

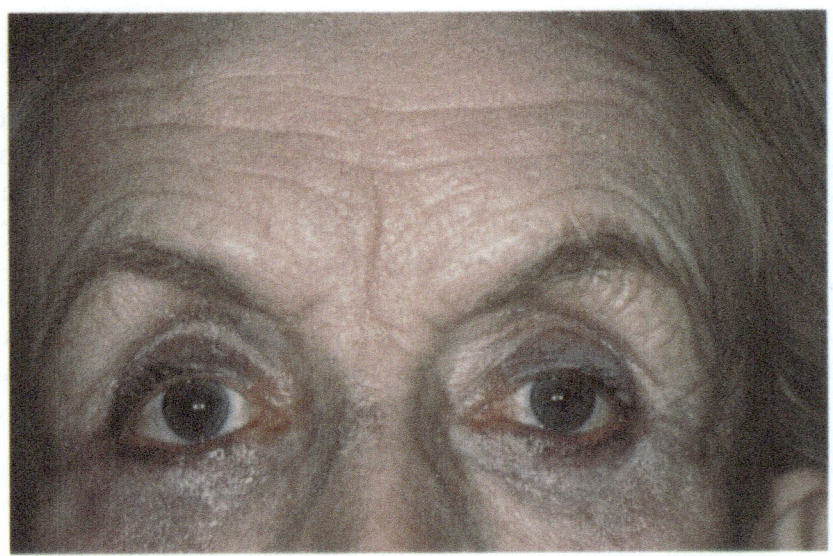

B

**Figure 5-23 C, D**
C) Two months after resurfacing, her skin is a light pink and she has increased lower eyelid scleral show. D) One year after resurfacing, significant rhytid reduction remains with a return of good lower eyelid position.

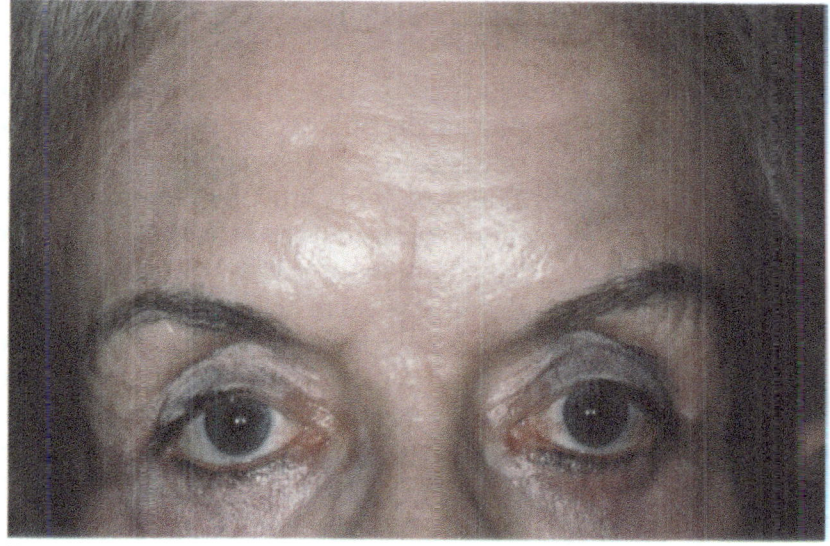

C

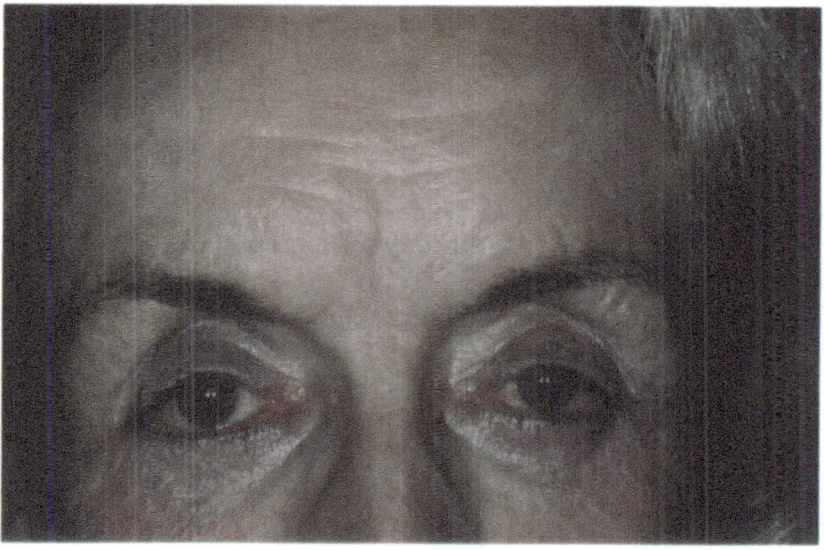

D

## Claustrophobia

Claustrophobia with the use of occlusive dressings is a phenomena that rarely occurs and is difficult to anticipate. In these situations, patients remove their dressings and call the office in a state of panic. These patients must be reassured that their final result should not be compromised as long as they follow your recommendations, although their length of recovery will be prolonged. Crusting on the skin can develop, similar to that found following a chemical peel. Resolution is facilitated with application of a washcloth soaked with a dilute white vinegar/water solution (1/50 concentration) three times a day for fifteen to twenty minutes. The treated area is kept as clean as possible and prophylactic antibiotics are continued until epithelialization is complete. A topical ointment is applied to the skin in between the above sessions. Patients are instructed not to pick off the scabs to avoid possible scarring and hypopigmentation.

In summary, I feel that laser resurfacing is an extremely effective method to treat rhytids and pigmentation disorders of the face. The intraoperative control and ability to treat areas selectively by varying the depth of dermal injury with an essentially bloodless field give this technology a distinct advantage over chemical peels and dermabrasion.

## Coherent Ultrapulse $CO_2$ Laser

### by Dr. David Apfelberg, M.D.

The Ultrapulse $CO_2$ laser (Coherent Medical, Palo Alto, CA) has been used in over 200 cases by me for resurfacing with resulting rejuvenation of the facial skin. Rhytids, photo-aging, and acne scarring can be markedly improved with the laser. In my practice, laser resurfacing has replaced chemical peel and dermabrasion as the procedure of choice. Initially starting with regional areas (peri-oral, peri-orbital), I now routinely perform full-face Ultrapulse $CO_2$ laser resurfacing. This is now routine for photo-aging, acne scars, and multiple fine rhytids. This procedure is ideal for those patients who are not candidates for facelift. A facelift is not an option for those who are too young or too old and/or have had repeated surgery resulting in the stretching of the skin.

### Description of the Coherent Ultrapulse Laser

This laser is able to remove 100 micron slices of skin in a bloodless manner. Since the ultra short pulse width ms is shorter than the TRT of tissue (695 ms), all heat is dissipated during vaporization, thus producing a truly "cold beam" with very little risk of thermal damage and subsequent burn scars. As each layer is precisely removed, the operator can observe the remaining tissue for high points and irregularities that can be selectively smoothed on subsequent passes until smooth upper dermal contour can be achieved. Depth through the epidermis and into the papillary or reticular dermis can be readily observed by color changes in the tissue as well as observations of shrinkage of collagen. Dual benefits of physical smoothing of the surface irregularities and heat shrinkage in Type 1 collagen secondary to heat production at 55 to 60° centigrade provide immediate and long lasting benefits.

The CPG (Computer Pattern Generator) is an automatic scanning device that allows for a rapid, repeatable, accurate geometric pattern of laser pulses (Figure 5-24). It produces up to 250 spots in a 4.8 cm$^2$ area. The time per spot is less than 1/1000th of a second, and the rate may be 300 spots per second. The CPG is integrated to the laser. The variables that can be utilized are for pattern, size, and density. Seven separate and distinct geometric patterns can be chosen, including triangles, squares, and wide or narrow lines in a variety of sizes, thus producing 100 selectable patterns (Figure 5-25). These patterns can be varied by size to accommodate small or large skin segments. The density or closeness of the spot can be set from widely spaced to slight (10%) overlap to more dense spacing at 60% overlap (Figure 5-26). The laser delivers approximately 7.5 joules/cm$^2$ of power at spot size 2.25 mm and 300 milli-joules. The critical vaporization fluence for char-free tissue ablation is 5 joules/cm$^2$ so that fluences produced are well above this threshold.

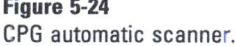

**Figure 5-24**
CPG automatic scanner.

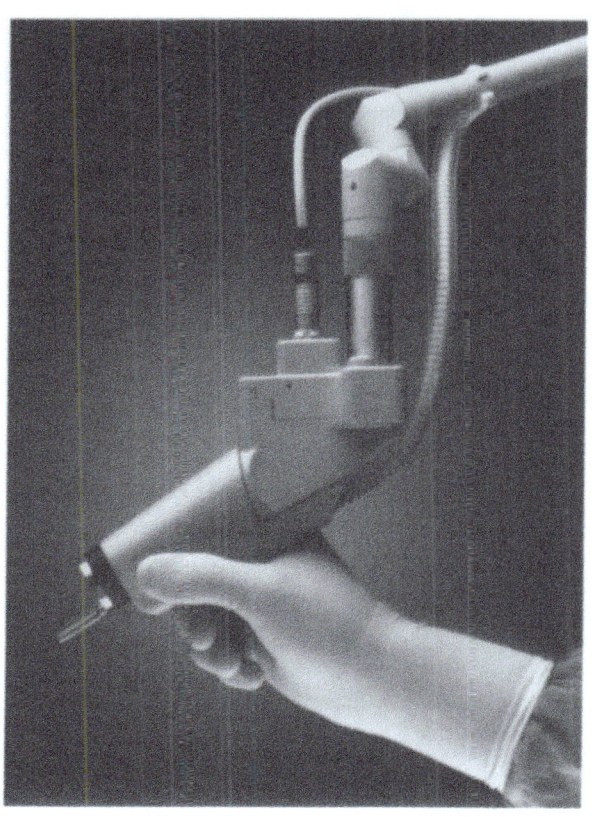

**Figure 5-25**
CPG patterns.

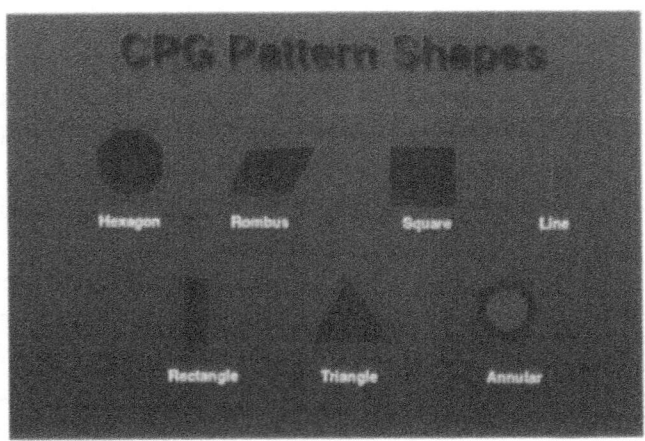

**Figure 5-26**
Density selections for overlap of spots.

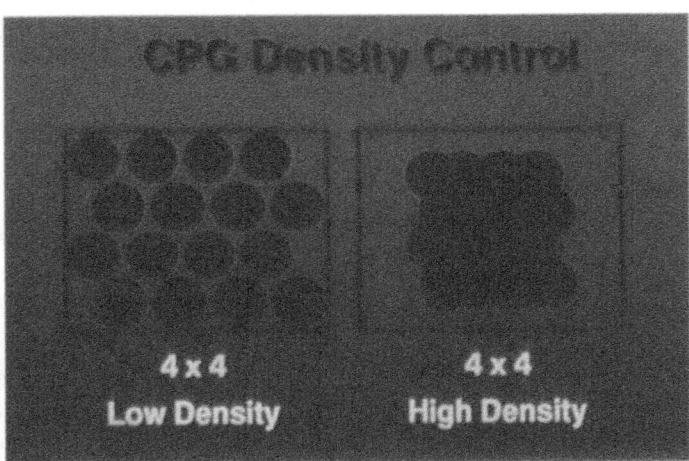

## Patient Selection

Patient selection for Ultrapulse laser abrasion is extremely important. Ideal patients have fine static rhytids, peri-oral or peri-orbital wrinkles, full face photo-aging, or acne scars. Patients with facial wrinkles who are not good candidates for surgical facelift because of medical contraindications or too many previous facelifts can also be helped. Patient selection is based on skin type and coloration. Individuals with thin fragile skin need to be treated very superficially or scarring is a risk. Darkly pigmented patients may need pre- and post-treatment skin preparation with bleaching agents to prevent postinflammatory hyperpigmentation. The zonal areas for resurfacing should be identified for skin type as well. A past history of keloid scarring should be sought, and patients with a positive history should be approached with caution or "test patched" first. A history of repeated oral herpes simplex infections indicates the need for anti-viral prophylaxis. Previous skin treatments such as chemical peel or dermabrasion may have already caused scarring or changes in texture or pigment which should be pointed out to the patient. Previous sun exposure with resultant photo-aging skin damage should be evaluated and the patient cautioned about limited sun exposure following the procedure. Any skin pathology such as scars, keratosis, rosacea, acne, or dyschromias should be diagnosed and treated prior to laser abrasion. Patients who have taken Accutane for up to twelve to eighteen months prior to surgery should not undergo laser abrasion as re-epithelialization is compromised and scarring is more prevalent. Finally, patients should have realistic expectations about the probable outcome of the procedure. In addition, they should understand the goals and also the limitations and possible side effects and complications.

## Preparation for Surgery

Preparation for surgery is another very important component of Ultrapulse laser care. Although some physicians do laser resurfacing without any preparation of the skin, my preference is for a two to three week regimen of good skin care prior to the procedure. A side benefit of this approach is the enlistment of the patient's cooperation and participation in the process, as well as an assessment of the patient's motivation and ability to follow instructions. My preference is for three weeks of twice a day use of "Kligman's solution" (Retin-A, 0.1% cream; hydroquinone, 4 to 5%; dexamethasone, 0.1% cream) [57]. Other surgeons use only hydroquinone or kojic acid for darkly pigmented patients, and some physicians add a glycolic acid regimen. Routine medication on the day of surgery includes a broad spectrum antibiotic, an anti-viral agent for herpes prophylaxis, and a mild analgesic. Systemic steroids to prevent swelling are not routine but may be considered in full-face laser abrasion.

## Description of Ultrapulse Procedure

The sequence and process of the Ultrapulse laser resurfacing as fairly standardized are accomplished as follows. Before regular or intravenous sedation anesthesia in the operating room, rhytids are first marked to identify them prior to distortion by the local anesthesia (Figure 5-27). A weak adrenaline solution (no stronger than a 1:200,000) is used so severe vasoconstriction will not obliterate the color indicators of depth. Complete superficial laser abrasion observing anatomical areas is done at 450 to 500 millijoules, 3 to 5 watts, 10% overlap (collimated handpiece) or pattern 3 (square) or pattern 4 (line), size 5 to 9, density 4 to 6 (CPG scanner) to remove the epidermis and reveal the underlying irregularities (Figure 5-28). The desiccated tissue is then wiped clean with a very moist saline gauze with complete removal (Figure 5-29). The surface is dried since excess water would absorb the laser energy. Two to four subsequent passes can be made at 350 millijoules, 3 to 5 watts with the collimated handpiece, or repeat CPG scanner parameters to remove the "shoulders" or high points of the rhytids, furrows, or scars (Figures 5-30 and 5-31). The thickness of the skin established in the preoperative evaluation must be respected, as well as observance of variation in zonal areas (i.e., fewer passes in the eyelid skin, more passes to thick photoaged cheeks). A reddish-pink color indicates removal of the epidermis. A uniform gray appearance signals achievement of the depth of the papillary dermis, and a chamois yellow appearance heralds tissue removal down to the deep papillary or upper reticular dermis (Figure 5-29). It is better to stop at this point and re-do the area in two to three months rather than risk scarring by too deep removal of tissue on the first treatment. Edges of the regular areas are feathered to prevent a sharp line of demarcation by either "paint brushing" a random pattern with gradual decreasing powers of the laser, random pattern with the same power, a combination of these two techniques, or by applying 35% TCA.

**Figure 5-27**
Rhytids are marked prior to injection/distortion with local anesthetic.

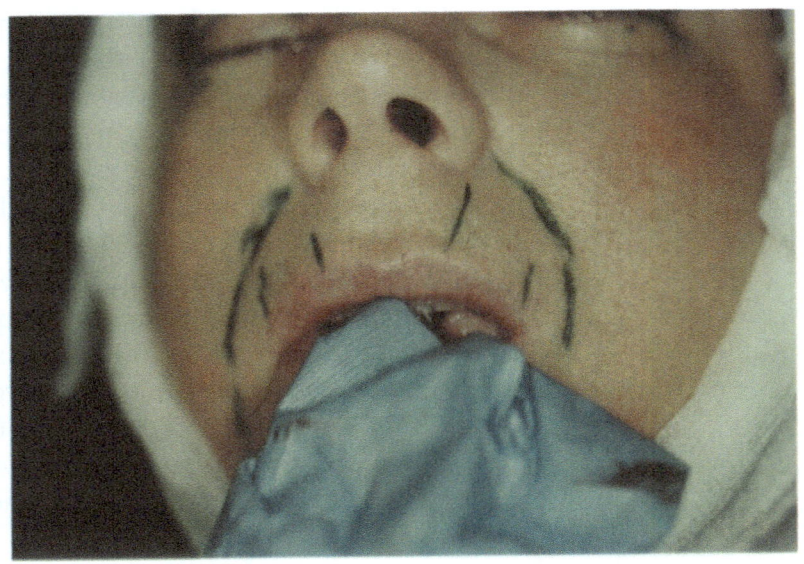

**Figure 5-28**
Complete superficial laser abrasion of the upper lip, first pass done with CPG or collimated handpiece.

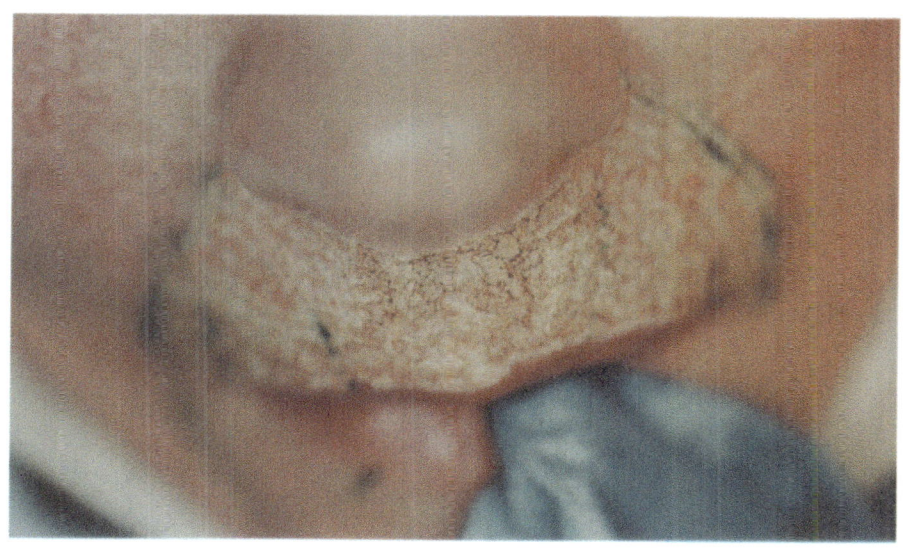

**Figure 5-29**
After moist saline gauze debridement of charred epidermis, several more passes are made to remove "shoulders" or high points of rhytids. Note color variations: pink—epidermis; gray—papillary dermis; yellow—reticular dermis.

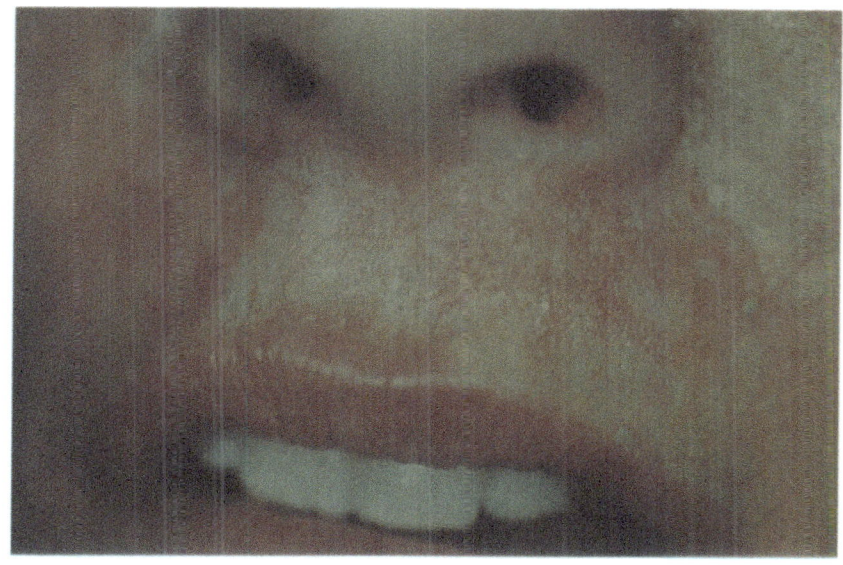

**Figure 5-30**
Schematic illustration of process of removing high points adjacent to rhytids to smooth out the area.

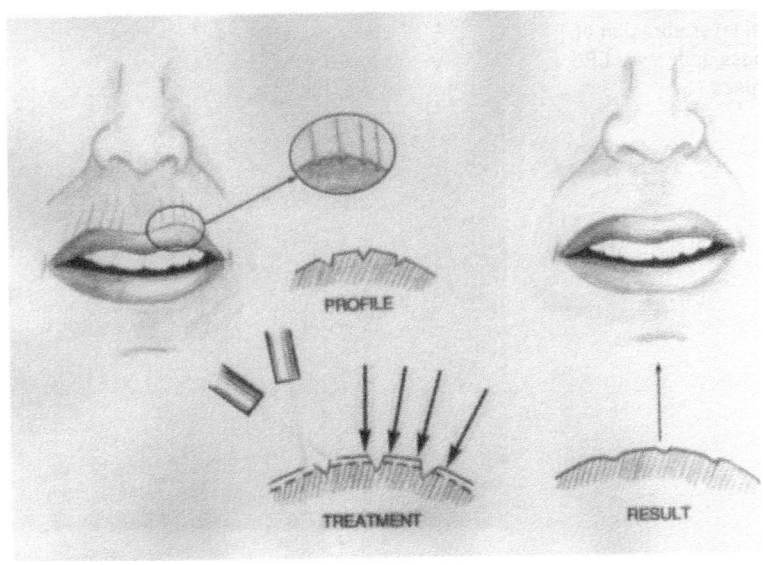

**Figure 5-31**
Schematic illustration of longitudinal or perpendicular removal of "shoulders" or high points next to rhytids but avoidance of depth.

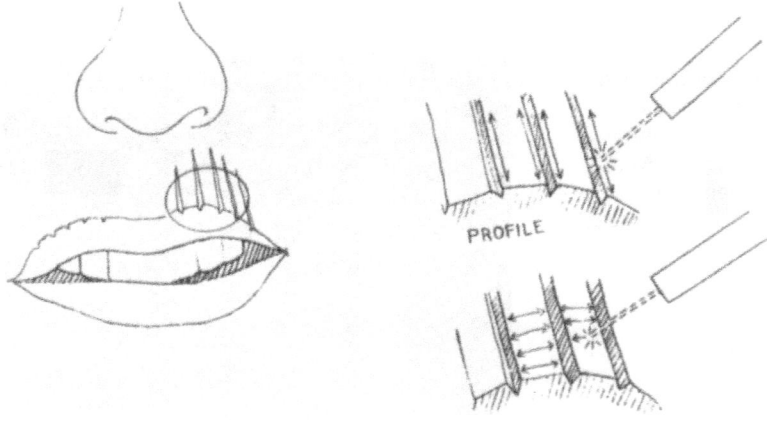

## Postoperative Care

Postoperative treatment consist of either open treatment with use of ice compresses and liberal topical ointments to keep the area moist (Bacitracin, Vaseline, Preparation H) or the application of an occlusive semi-permeable dressing (Omniderm, Vigilon, Flexzan, etc.). Antibiotics and anti-viral agents are routine, and analgesia is prescribed as needed. Some physicians prescribe a $\frac{1}{4}$ solution of acetic acid (1 tablespoon white vinegar in 8 to 12 ounces of water) as a compress four to six times a day to keep the area moist and clean and prevent scabs from forming. All agree that a moist environment under semi-permeable occlusive dressings or ointment aids in re-epithelialization. Drying, crusting, and scabbing are to be avoided.

Knowledge about and care of potential complications and side effects should be part of the learning process of any plastic surgeon doing Ultrapulse $CO_2$ laser resurfacing. Pain is usually mild to moderate, especially with occlusive dressings, but may require mild narcotics. Active herpes should be treated vigorously with oral agents (Zovirax and topical Zovirax ointment). Infections should be cultured and treated with appropriate antibiotics. Swelling often subsides after three to four days with application of ice only, but may require systemic steroids (Medrol Dosepak, Decadron) if persistent. Redness responds to topical mild steroids but normally persists in all patients for as long as eight to ten weeks (green make-up base is a good camouflage). Patients with Type III skin color (olive/dark) should routinely be treated with hydroquinone both prior to and immediately following re-epithelialization to prevent post-inflammatory hyperpigmentation. Physicians should be carefully pro-active in observance of any sign of hypertrophic or keloid scars. Areas with persistent erythema, texture change, firmness, or pain should be aggressively treated with intralesional steroids to prevent formation of keloids.

## Regional Treatment (Figures 5-32, 5-33, 5-34, and 5-35)

Regional treatment of limited anatomical segments is usually accomplished using the 3 mm collimated handpiece and 4 to 6 watts of continuous power. Alternately, the CPG scanner in a square (pattern #3) or linear (pattern #4) pattern, size 5 to 7, and density 4 to 6 (10 to 30% overlap) may be used. The regional anatomical unit is best treated and the edges feathered to prevent a sharp line of demarcation. The first pass at 350 to 450 millijoules with 10% overlap takes off the superficial epidermis down to the papillary dermis. Utilizing 4.5 X magnifying surgical loupes, the high points or "shoulders" of the rhytids are then taken down at 250 to 350 millijoules in several passes until either the area is smooth or a chamois yellow color is observed, indicating depth to the deep papillary or upper reticular dermis. This is the deepest endpoint. Random "paintbrush" for shrinkage is usually then done over the area. The edges can be feath-

**Figure 5-32**
Fine rhytids of upper lip and chin.

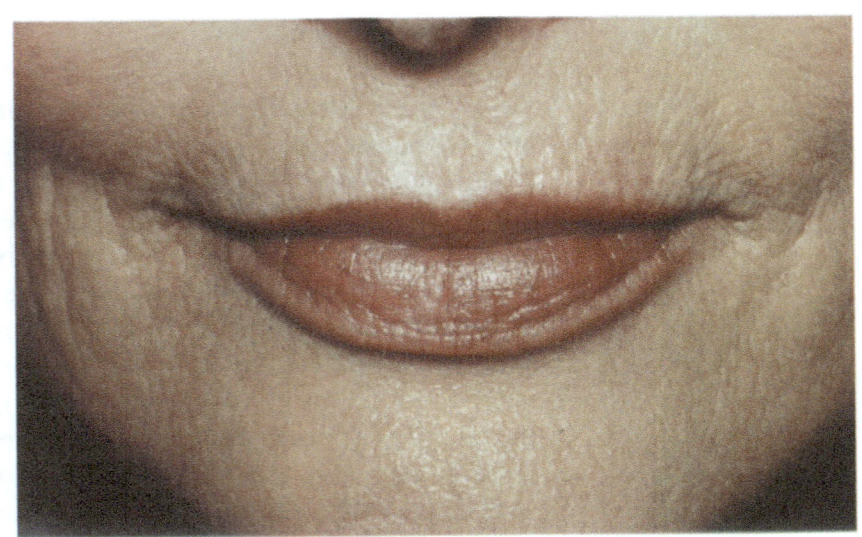

**Figure 5-33**
Marked improvement and smoothening
of peri-oral area without texture or
color change.

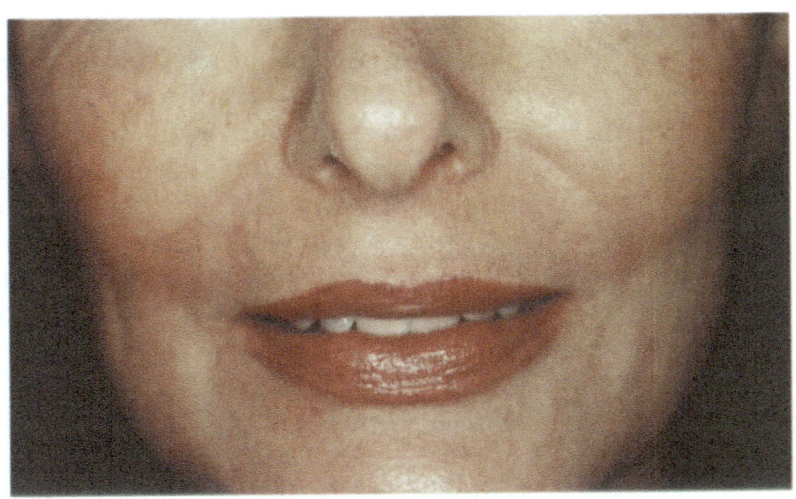

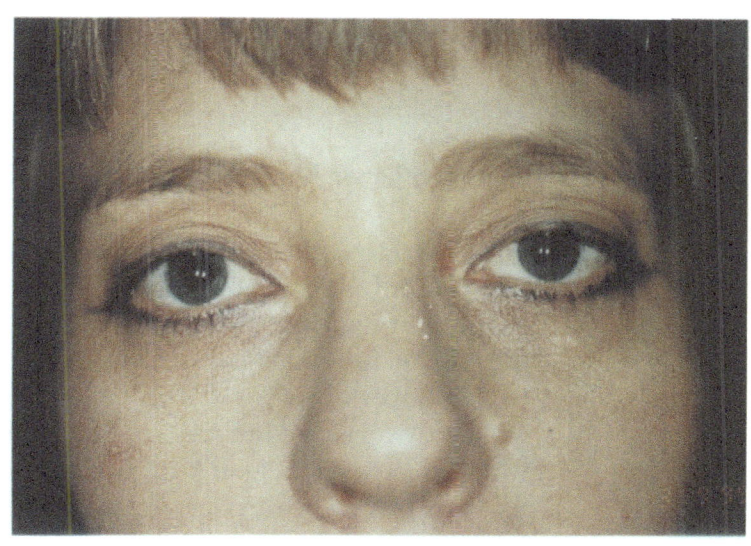

**Figure 5-34**
Upper eyelid hooding and fine wrinkles with mild fat herniations in lower eyelids. Note mild scleral show and position of lower lids.

**Figure 5-35**
Final result following UltraPulse $CO_2$ laser upper blepharoplasty and transconjunctival lower blepharoplasty with resurfacing. Lower lid position unchanged. (Note slight erythema present at six weeks.)

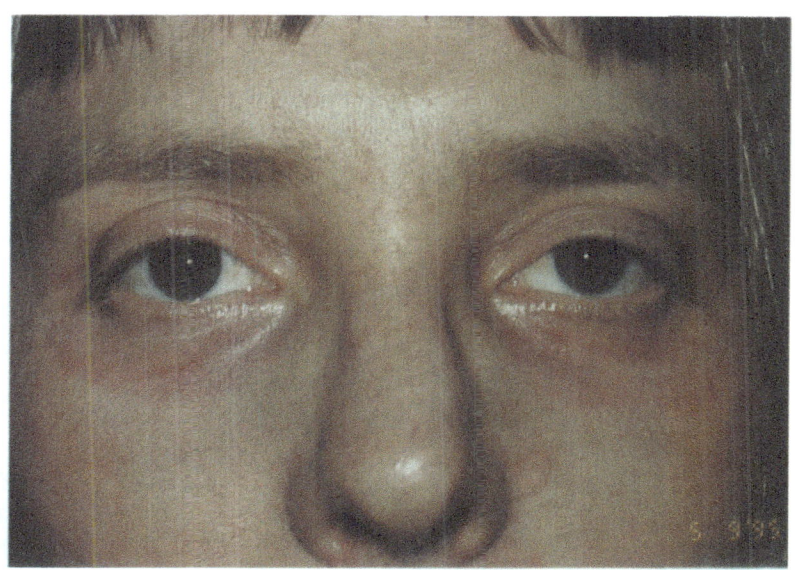

**Figure 5-35**
Final result following UltraPulse $CO_2$ laser upper blepharoplasty and transconjunctival lower blepharoplasty with resurfacing. Lower lid position unchanged. (Note slight erythema present at six weeks.)

ered by gradually decreasing power in millijoules of the laser or by random pattern.

### Full-Face Laser Abrasion (Figures 5-36, 5-37, 5-38, 5-39, 5-40, and 5-41)

Full-face laser abrasion is accomplished with the CPG scanner. The scanner is held perpendicular to the skin at the focal distance established by the guide and placed in a slow repeat mode. The usual laser setting for full-face laser abrasion is 3, 9, 5 to 6 (largest square with 10 to 20% overlap of spots). Each laser square is joined to the adjacent without overlap. After the entire area is vaporized, the vaporized epithelium is wiped clean with a very moist gauze. A smoke evacuator is used to remove the laser plume. A second pass is then made at similar settings, and one can observe shrinkage of the skin and collagen. Further passes are made in a more selective manner using a single spot or line to remove "shoulders" or high points on either sides of rhytids. It is not necessary or desirable to try to remove all wrinkles during the initial laser abrasion. Touch-up treatments can be done in three to six months. The appearance of the chamois yellow color marks the endpoint of the procedure. The face is then dressed with antibiotic ointment and Omniderm occlusive semi-permeable dressing, which is left in place for two to three days. The patient is then started on vinegar/water compresses and moisturizing creams.

**Figure 5-36**
Illustration of use of CPG scanner for full-face laser abrasion.

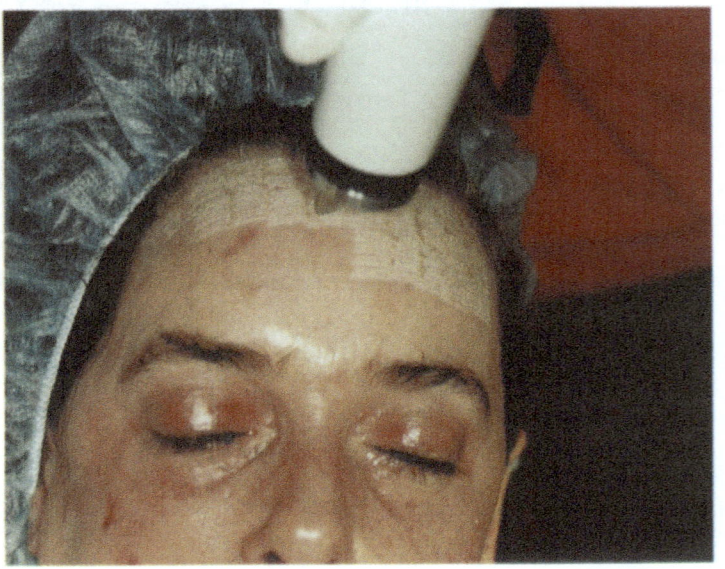

**Figure 5-37**
Full-face laser abrasion completed.
Note scleral eye shield protector (blue)
in eyes and careful approximation of
squares.

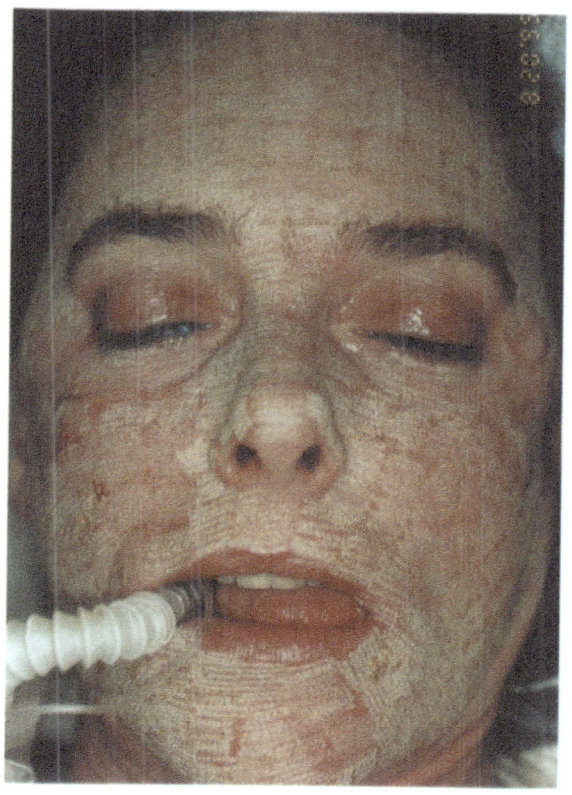

**Figure 5-38**
Appearance after three days with Om-
niderm/Bacitracin ointment dressing in
place.

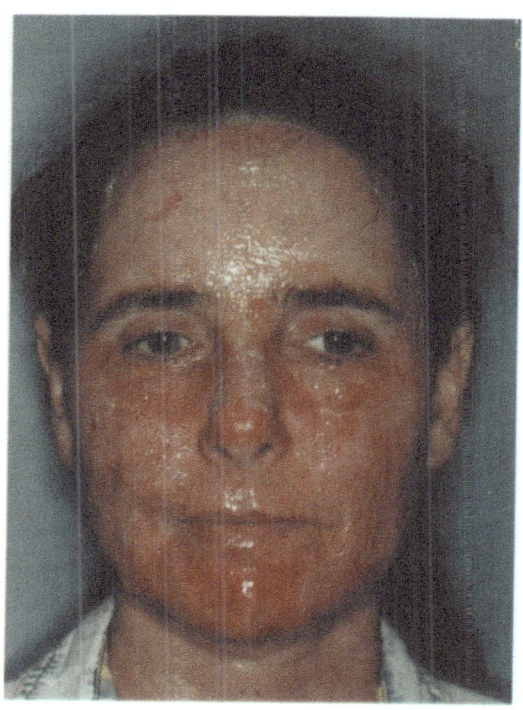

**Figure 5-39**
Re-epithelialization and healing by day 10.

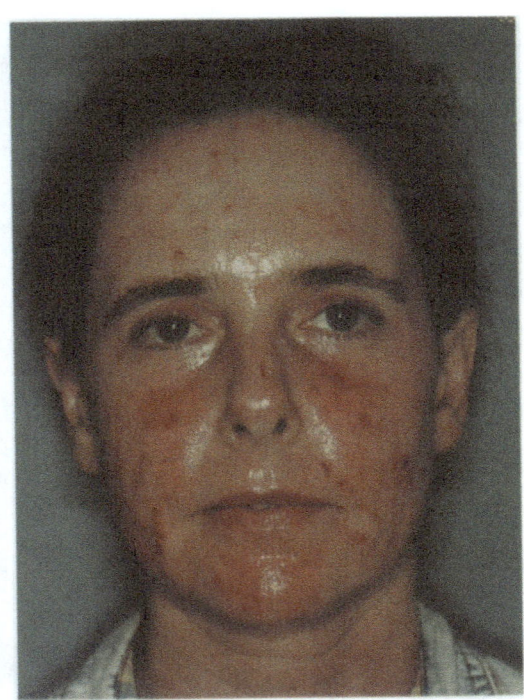

**Figure 5-40**
Elastosis and rhytids in preoperative patient.

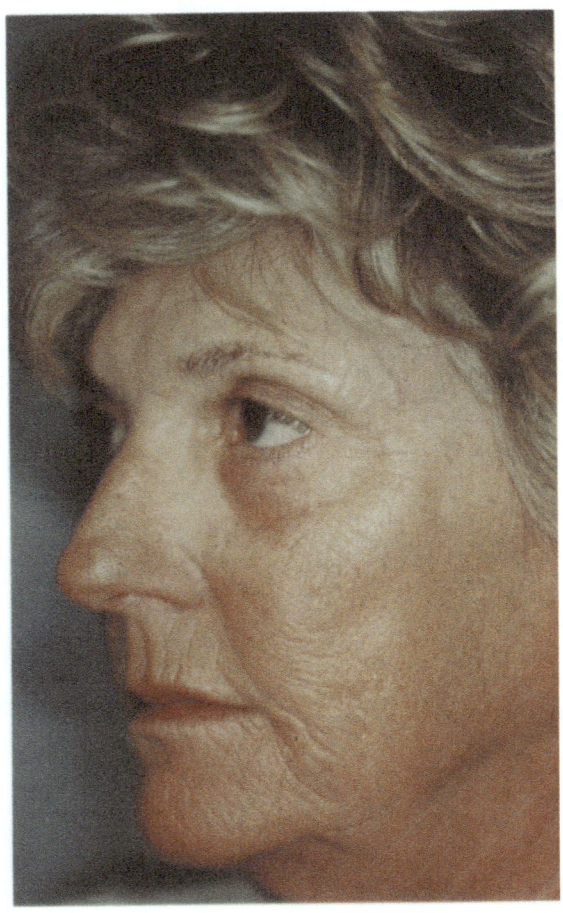

Chapter Five   **Laser Skin Resurfacing**

Figure 5-41
Elimination of most rhytids and skin
tightening after full-face UltraPulse
laser abrasion. (Cheek scar from separate cyst excision.)

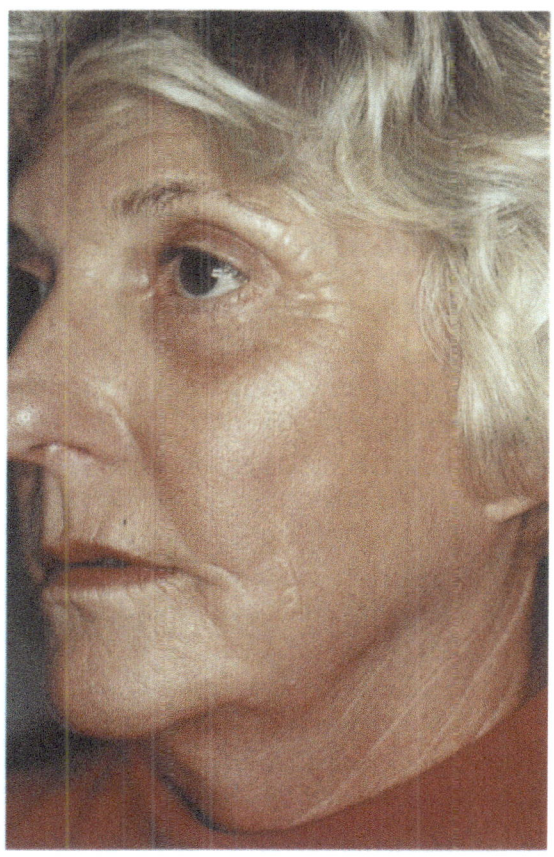

## References

1. Shapshay SM, Strong MS, Anastasi GW, et al. Removal of rhinophyma with the carbon dioxide laser. A preliminary report. *Arch Oto-
   laryngol* 1980;106:257–259.

2. Greenbaum SS, Krull EA, Watnick K. Comparison of $CO_2$ laser and
   electrosurgery in the treatment of rhinophyma. *J Am Acad Dermatol*
   1988;18:363–368.

3. Wheeland RG, Bailin PL, Ratz JL. Combined carbon dioxide laser
   excision and vaporization in the treatment of rhinophyma. *J Dermatol
   Surg Oncol* 1987;13:172–177.

4. David LM. Laser vermilion ablation for actinic cheilitis. *J Derm Surg
   Oncol* 1985;11:605–608.

5. Whitaker DC. Microscopically proven cure of actinic cheilitis by $CO_2$
   laser. *Laser Surg Med* 1987;7:520–523.

6. Dufresne RG Jr, Garrett AB, Bailin PL, Ratz JL. Carbon dioxide laser
   treatment of chronic actinic cheilitis. *J Am Acad Dermatol*
   1988;19:876–878.

7. Stanley RJ, Roenick RK. Actinic cheilitis—Treatment with the carbon
   dioxide laser. *Mayo Clin Proc* 1988;63:230–235.

8. David LM, Lask GP, Glassberg P, et al. Laser abrasion for cosmetic
   and medical treatment of facial actinic damage. *Cutis*
   1989;43:583–587.

9. Hobbs ER, Bailin PC, Wheeland RG, Ratz JL. Superpulsed lasers: Minimizing thermal damage with short duration, high irradiance pulses. *J Derm Surg Oncol* 1987;13:955–964.

10. Lanzafame RJ, Naim JO, Rogers DW, Hinshaw R. Comparison of continuous wave, shop-wave and superpulse laser wounds. *Laser Surg Med* 1988;8:119–124.

11. Fitzpatrick RE, Ruiz-Esparza J, Goldman MP. The depth of thermal necrosis using the $CO_2$ laser: A comparison of the superpulsed mode and conventional mode. *J Derm Surg Oncol* 1991;17:340–344.

12. Weinstein C. Ultrapulse carbon dioxide laser removal of periocular wrinkles in association with laser blepharoplasty. *J Clin Laser Med Surg* 1994;12:205–209.

13. Weinstein C, Alster TS. Skin resurfacing with high-energy, pulsed carbon dioxide lasers. In: Alster TS, Apfelberg DB, eds. *Cosmetic Laser Surgery*. New York: Wiley-Liss, 1995:9–24.

14. Fitzpatrick E, Goldman MP. $CO_2$ laser surgery. In: Goldman MP, Fitzpatrick RE, eds., *Cutaneous Laser Surgery*. St. Louis: Mosby, 1994: 198–258.

15. Schoenrock DL, Chernoff WG, Rubach BW. Cutaneous ultrapulse laser resurfacing of the eyelids. *Int J Aesth Restor Surg* 1995;3:31–36.

16. Apfelberg DB. Ultrapulse carbon dioxide laser resurfacing and facial cosmetic surgery. *Can J Plast Surg* 1995;3:1–4.

17. Apfelberg DB. Laser assisted meloplasty and blepharoplasty. In: Alster TS, Apfelberg DB, eds. *Cosmetic Laser Surgery*. New York: Wiley-Liss, 1995:29–41.

18. Apfelberg DB. The ultrapulse carbon dioxide laser for facial cosmetic surgery and resurfacing. *Ann Plast Surg* 1995 (in press).

19. Lask G, Keller G, Lowe N, et al. Laser skin resurfacing with the Silk-Touch flashscanner for facial rhytids. *Dermatol Surg* 1995;21:1021–1024.

20. Grevelink JM. Facial contouring using a flashscanner-enhanced carbon dioxide laser. *Facial Plast Surg Clin N Am* 1996;4:241–246.

21. Waldorf HA, Kauvar A, Geronemus RG. Skin resurfacing of fine to deep rhytides using a char-free carbon dioxide laser in 47 patients. *Dermatol Surg* 1995;21:940–946.

22. Ho C, Nguyen Q, Lowe NJ, et al. Laser resurfacing in pigmented skin. *Dermatol Surg* 1995;21:1035–1037.

23. Pathak MA, Fitzpatrick TB. Preventive treatment of sunburn, dermatoheliosis and skin cancer with sun-protective agents. In: Fitzpatrick TB, Eisen AZ, Wolff K, et al. eds. *Dermatology in General Medicine, 4th ed.* McGraw Hill, 1993;Vol. 1:1694.

24. Anderson RR, Parish JA. Selective photothermolysis: Precise microsurgery by selective absorption of pulsed radiation. *Science* 1983;220:524–527.

25. Walsh JT, Deutsch TF. Pulsed $CO_2$ laser tissue ablation: Measurement of the ablation rate. *Laser Surg Med* 1988;8:264–275.

26. Walsh JT, Flotte TJ, Anderson RR, et al. Plused $CO_2$ laser tissue abla-

tion: Effect of tissue type and pulse duration on thermal damage. *Laser Surg Med* 1988;8:108–118.

27. Kauvar AN, Waldorf HA, Geronemus RG. A histopathological comparison of "char-free" carbon dioxide lasers. *Dermatol Surg* 1996;22:343–348.

28. Jacques SL. "Water content and concentration profile in human stratum corneum." Ph.D. dissertation, University of California, Berkeley, 1984.

29. Warner RR, Morgan NE, Eby TA, et al. Water measurement in biological tissue. In: Romig AD, Chambers WF, eds. *Microbeam Analysis*, Vol. 21. San Francisco Press, Inc., 1986:238–240.

30. Sasaki G. Presentation at the California Society of Plastic Surgery, Palm Springs, CA, May 1996.

31. Kligman AM, Baker TJ, Gordon HL. Long-term histologic follow-up of phenol face peels. *Plast Recon Surg* 1985;75:652–659.

32. Klingman AM. Early destructive effects of sunlight on human skin. *JAMA* 1969;210:2377.

33. Zachariae H. Delayed wound healing and keloid formation following argon treatment or dermabrasion during isotretinoin treatment. *Br J Dermatol* 1988;118:703–706.

34. Roenigk H, et al. Acne, retinoids and dermabrasion. *J Derm Surg Oncol* 1985;11:396–398.

35. Wright M. Retinoic acid isomer shows no effect on wound healing rate. *Dermatol Times* 1988;9:35.

36. Griffiths WAD. Wound healing and the retinoids. *Retincias Today Tomorrow* 1986;4:26.

37. Katz BE, MacFarlane DF. Atypical facial scarring after isoretinoin therapy in a patient with previous dermabrasion. *J Am Acad Derm* 1994;30:852–853.

38. Rubenstein R, Roenigk H, et al. Atypical keloids after dermabrasion of patients taking isoretinoin. *J Am Acad Derm* 1986;15:280–285.

39. Rafal ES, Griffiths CE, Ditre CM, et al. Topical tretinoin (retinoic acid) treatment for liver spots associated with photodamage *N Engl J Med* 1992;326:368–374.

40. Noble S. Tretinoin. A review of its pharmacological properties and clinical efficacy in the topical treatment of photodamaged skin. *Drugs Aging* 1995;6:479–496.

41. Green LJ. Photoaging and the skin. The effects of tretinoin. *Dermatol Clin* 1993;11:97–105.

42. Kligman AM, Leyden JJ. Treatment of photoaged skin with topical tretinoin. *Skin Pharmacol* 1993;6:78–82.

43. Griffiths CE, Voorhees JJ. Topical retinoic acid for photoaging: Clinical response and underlying mechanisms. *Skin Pharmacol* 1993;6:70–77.

44. Fuchs E, Green H. Regulation of terminal differentiation of cultured human keratinocytes by vitamin A. *Cell* 1981;25:617.

45. Palumbo A, d'Ischia M. Mechanism of inhibition of melanogenesis by hydroquinone. *Biochim Biophys Acta* 1991;1073:85–90.

46. Smith CJ, O'Hare KB. Selective cytotoxicity of hydroquinone for melanocyte-derived cells is mediated by tyrosinase activity but independent of melanin content. *Pigment Cell Res* 1988;1:386–389.

47. Barber ED. The percutaneous absorption of hydroquinone through rat and human skin in vitro. *Toxicol Letters* 1995;80:17–72.

48. Cabanes J. Kojic acid, a cosmetic skin whitening agent, is a slow-binding inhibitor of catecholase activity of tyrosinase. *J Pharm Pharmacol* 1994;46:982–985.

49. Nakagawa M. Contact allergy to kojic acid in skin care products. *Contact Dermatitis* 1995;32:9–13.

50. Noble WC. Ecology and host resistance in relation to skin disease. In: Fitzpatrick TB, Eisen AZ, Wolff K, et al., eds. *Dermatology in General Medicine, 4th Ed.* 1993;Vol. 1:257.

51. Jimbow K. Regulatory factors of pheo- and eumelanogenesis in melanogenic compartments. *Pigment Cell Res* 1992;2:36–42.

52. Pawelek JM, Chakraborty AK. Molecular cascades in UV-induced melanogenesis: A central role for melanotropins? *Pigment Cell Res* 1992;5:348–356.

53. Bech-Thomsen N. A quantitative study of the melanogenic effect of multiple suberythemal doses of different ultraviolet radiation sources. *Photodermatol Photoimmunol Photomed* 1994;10:53–56.

54. Valverde P, Healy E, Jackson I. Variants of the melanocyte-stimulating hormone receptor gene are associated with red hair and fair skin in humans. *Nature Genetics* 1995;11:328–330.

55. Tomita Y, Maeda K. Melanocyte-stimulating properties of arachidonic acid metabolites: Possible role in postinflammatory pigmentation. *Pigment Cell Res* 1992;5:357–361.

56. Takiwaki H. The degrees of UVB-induced erythema and pigmentation correlate linearly and are reduced in parallel manner by topical anti-inflammatory agents. *J Investigative Dermatology* 1994;103:642–646.

57. Kligman AM, Willis I. A new formula for depigmenting human skin. *Arch Dermatol* 1975;III:40–48.

# Index

*Italic* page numbers indicate illustrations; page numbers with t indicate tables.

The manufacturer's authorised representative in the EU is Springer
Nature Customer Service Centre GmbH, Europaplatz 3, 69115 Heidelberg,
Germany. If you have any concerns regarding our products, please
contact ProductSafety@springernature.com

Printed and bound by CPI Group (UK) Ltd, Croydon, CR0 4YY

23/04/2026

02095658-0004